C000319853

VOLUNTARY AND INVOLUNTARY CHILDLESSNESS

VOLUNTARY AND INVOLUNTARY CHILDLESSNESS: THE JOYS OF OTHERHOOD?

EDITED BY

NATALIE SAPPLETON
Manchester Metropolitan University, UK

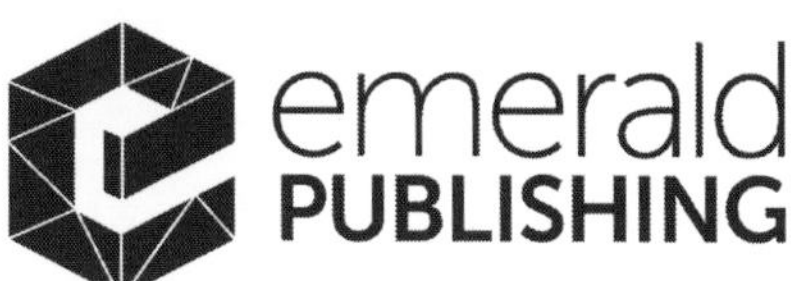

United Kingdom – North America – Japan – India – Malaysia – China

Emerald Publishing Limited
Howard House, Wagon Lane, Bingley BD16 1WA, UK

First edition 2018

Reprints and permissions service
Contact: permissions@emeraldinsight.com

British Library Cataloguing in Publication Data
A catalogue record for this book is available from the British Library

ISBN: 978-1-78754-362-1 (Print)
ISBN: 978-1-78754-361-4 (Online)
ISBN: 978-1-78754-363-8 (Epub)

Printed and bound by CPI Group (UK) Ltd, Croydon, CR0 4YY

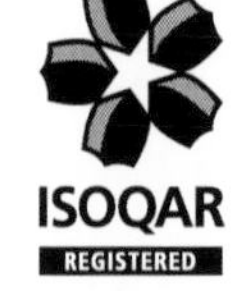

ISOQAR certified Management System, awarded to Emerald for adherence to Environmental standard ISO 14001:2004.

Certificate Number 1985
ISO 14001

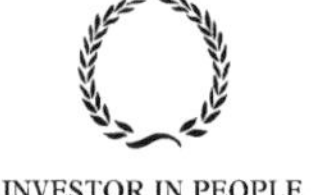

INVESTOR IN PEOPLE

Acknowledgements

The authors would like to thank the participants, both the parents and the childfree, for sharing their stories and experiences with us.

Contents

SECTION II: STRUCTURE, AGENCY AND CHILDLESSNESS

SECTION III: INTERSECTIONAL PERSPECTIVES ON CHILDLESSNESS

SECTION IV: LIVED EXPERIENCES OF CHILDLESSNESS

List of Figures

List of Tables

List of Contributors

Laura Carroll is an expert and leading voice on the intentionally childless choice. She is the author of *Families of Two: Interviews with Happily Married Couples without Children by Choice* (2000), which received international recognition. Since its publication, Laura (MS Psychology) has continued to conduct qualitative research on the intentionally childless, and is currently conducting a longitudinal study on intentionally childless women. Laura is also the author of *The Baby Matrix: Why Freeing Our Minds from Outmoded Thinking about Parenthood & Reproduction Will Create a Better World* (2012), which examines and challenges long-held social and cultural assumptions about parenthood and reproduction.

Megumi Fieldsend is a PhD student in Psychology at Birkbeck University of London, UK, working with Professor Jonathan A. Smith. She is currently conducting her research using Interpretative Phenomenological Analysis (IPA), exploring the experience of women living with involuntary childlessness. She is particularly interested in the dynamics of experiential adult development, meaning reconstruction, self and identity and the psychological impact on people living without the children they hoped for.

Anna Gotlib was born in the Soviet Union and immigrated to the United States with her family. She is currently an Assistant Professor of Philosophy at Brooklyn College, City University of New York, USA. Before joining the faculty at Brooklyn College, she was an Assistant Professor of Philosophy at Binghamton University (SUNY). Previous to her academic career, she was employed as an Attorney, specialising in International Law and Labor Law, working in the United States and abroad. Her recent research has appeared in the *International Journal for Feminist Approaches to Bioethics*, *Journal of Bioethical Inquiry*, *Humana Mente* and several volumes and collections. She is the Editor of *The Moral Psychology of Sadness* as well as *The Moral Psychology of Regret* (Rowman & Littlefield International, 2017, 2018).

Melissa Graham is an Associate Professor in the College of Science, Health and Engineering at LaTrobe University, Australia. She supervises honours, master's and PhD research students in the area of women's health. She is the Deputy Director, Centre for Health through Action on Social Exclusion (CHASE), a multi-disciplinary research centre which works collaboratively to promote social inclusion, in the School of Health and Social Development, Faculty of Health at Deakin University. Her research focuses on the exploration of the lives of women who do not have children, the role of policy on reproductive health, reproductive decision-making and the experiences of social in/exclusion. These research areas are interconnected and each consider and draw attention to the implications for health and well-being.

Nazli Kazanoglu is a third-year PhD student in the School of Social Policy at Ulster University, UK. Her current thesis is 'Europeanization Patterns of Gender Equality within Work and Family Life Reconciliation Policies in Germany and Turkey'. She received her bachelor's degree in Sociology from Middle East Technical University, her master's degree in Sociology of Mass Media and Communication Systems from Istanbul Bilgi University in Turkey and did her replacement in UC Berkeley, USA. Her research interests lie in the area of Europeanisation studies, comparative welfare regime analysis, new-institutionalism theory, gender equality, women's employment and reconciliation of work and family life.

Deborah Lowry is an Associate Professor of Sociology at the University of Montevallo, USA, where she teaches courses on social problems, ageing, environment, China and social change. Her research interests lie in rural sociology, East Asia, and the scholarship of teaching and learning. Lowry was an NIH (National Institutions of Health) Postdoctoral Fellow at the University of Michigan's Population Studies Center. She holds a BA degree from Grand Valley State University, an MA from Western Michigan University and a PhD from the Michigan State University.

Ingrid Lynch is a Senior Research Specialist at the Human Sciences Research Council (HSRC), in the Human and Social Development programme. She is also an Honorary Research Associate in the Critical Studies in Sexualities and Reproduction research programme at Rhodes University, South Africa. Her research interests include critical feminist approaches to genders and sexualities; queer family-making and social belonging; and sexual and reproductive justice. She is editor of the forthcoming book, *Queer Kinship: Perspectives on Sexualities, Families, and Reproduction in South Africa*, along with Tracy Morison and Vasu

Reddy, funded by the DST/NRF Centre of Excellence in Human Development.

Catriona Ida Macleod is a Professor of Psychology and SARChI Chair of the Critical Studies in Sexualities and Reproduction research programme at Rhodes University, South Africa. Her major scholastic contributions have been in two main areas: sexual and reproductive health, and feminist theory in psychology. She has written extensively in national and international journals in relation to teenage pregnancy, abortion, sexuality education, pregnancy support, feminist psychology and postcolonialist and poststructural theory. She is author of the multi award-winning book *'Adolescence', Pregnancy and Abortion: Constructing a Threat of Degeneration* (Routledge, 2011) and co-author (with Tracy Morison) of the book *Men's Pathways to Parenthood: Silence and Heterosexual Gendered Norms* (HSRC Press, 2015). She is Editor-in-Chief of the international journal *Feminism & Psychology*. She oversaw the formation of the Sexual Violence Task Team that was set up in response to the #RUReferenceList protests in South Africa. She is on the steering committee of the Sexual and Reproductive Justice Coalition and is an Executive Committee Member of the International Society of Critical Health Psychology and the International Society of Theoretical Psychology. She is the recipient of the VC's Distinguished Senior Research Award (2015) and the VC's Community Engagement Award (2015).

Hayley McKenzie is a Lecturer in the School of Health and Social Development, Faculty of Health at Deakin University, Australia. Dr McKenzie's research focuses on family and social policy, and exploring the inequities experienced by particular social groups who are reliant on social and institutional policies, including a specific focus on women's health and well-being. Dr McKenzie teaches at the undergraduate and postgraduate level and has supervised honours and master's students exploring social policy and the impacts on women's health and well-being.

Kate de Medeiros is an Associate Professor of Gerontology at Miami University, Ohio, USA. Her research includes narrative approaches to understanding later life; friendships among people with dementia; flourishing, suffering, precarity and frailty; and humanistic approaches to studying old age.

Jenny Mercer is a Principal Lecturer at Cardiff Metropolitan University, UK. She is a Social Psychologist, with a strong interest in qualitative research methods. Her work to date involves a range of qualitative approaches to understanding human experience in applied settings (e.g. thematic analysis, grounded theory, phenomenology and participatory designs). These have often been used to address unconventional areas such as coming to terms with death, the impact of having a traumatic childbirth experience and women who choose not to have children. It is hoped that such research is one way of raising awareness of topics which are not always widely discussed.

Magdalena Mijas is a psychologist specializing in the fields of Sexology and LGBTQ Psychology. She is currently pursuing her PhD in the field of health sciences from Jagiellonian University Medical College. Her research focuses on stigma and health disparities among LGBTQ populations. She is also involved in LGBTQ rights activism in Poland. She is the lead author of 'Language, Media, HIV: The Picture of Infection and Seropositive People in Newspaper Articles' (Mijas, Dora, Brodzikowska, & Żoładek, 2016) and co-author of 'Introduction to LGB Psychology' (Iniewicz, Mijas, & Grabski, 2012) and 'Human Sexuality: Selected Issues' (Iniewicz & Mijas, 2011).

Tracy Morison is a Social and Health Psychology Lecturer in the School of Psychology at Massey University, New Zealand, and an Honorary Research Associate in the Critical Studies in Sexualities and Reproduction research programme at Rhodes University, South Africa. Tracy's research focus falls within the broad area of sexual and reproductive health, with a particular interest in reproductive 'choice', stigma and marginalised identities. She works with critical feminist theories and qualitative methodologies. She is the co-author of *Men's Pathways to Parenthood: Silence and Heterosexual Gendered Norms* (Morison & Macleod, 2015, HSRC Press).

Alyssa Mullins is a PhD Graduate and Data Analyst at the University of Central Florida in Orlando, Florida, USA. Her research interests include relationships, family life, public health and policy initiatives and community programmes. Her current research focuses on experiences of voluntary childlessness in social arenas.

Rose O'Driscoll is a former Senior Lecturer in the School of Health Sciences at Cardiff Metropolitan University, UK. Her main areas of teaching were sociology, social care and mental health. She also worked as an Associate Lecturer with the Open University. Prior to this, she worked with people with learning disabilities, homeless women, older people and mental health service users in Ireland, England and Wales.

Her sociological research on why women choose not to have children was undertaken for her PhD. She continues to explore lesser-known areas of women's lives on a freelance basis.

Helen Peterson is Associate Professor in Sociology and Senior Lecturer in Work Science at the Department of Sociology and Work Science at the University of Gothenburg, Sweden. Her pioneering research on voluntary childlessness, funded by the Swedish Research Council for Health, Working Life and Welfare, was the first sociological study on the subject in Sweden. She co-authored the first anthology about voluntary childlessness in the Nordic countries, published in 2010 (written in Swedish). Since its publication, her research has earned international recognition and has been published in several distinguished journals, such as *Journal of Family and Economic Issues*, *Women's Studies International Forum*, the *European Journal of Women's Studies*, and *Feminist Media Studies*.

Robert L. Rubinstein is a Professor of Anthropology at the University of Maryland Baltimore County (UMBC), USA. He has carried out research on Alzheimer's disease and dementia, assisted living and many other topics related to ageing and old age.

Natalie Sappleton is a Senior Lecturer at Manchester Metropolitan University, UK. Her research interests are in the intersections between social networks, gender segregation and gender stereotyping in the context of entrepreneurship. Her research programmes have included Women Audio Visual Engineers (WAVE), Women in North West Engineering and numerous investigations into sex discrimination at the Equality and Human Rights Commission. Natalie received her MA (Hons.) in Economics and Politics at the University of Glasgow and her master's in Research from Manchester Metropolitan University. Her PhD thesis investigates the role of gender role (in)congruency on the ability to acquire resources among New York City entrepreneurs.

Simi Seemanthini (PhD) is a Consultant Clinical Psychologist (Registered with the RCI & NZPB). Prior to this she taught in the Department of Psychiatry at Kasturba Medical College, India. She completed her PhD in 2014 at Mangalore University, India.

Ivett Szalma holds a PhD in Sociology from the Corvinus University of Budapest. She is Researcher at the Institute of Sociology, Centre for Social Sciences, Hungarian Academy of Sciences (http://www.tk.mta.

hu/kutato/szalma-ivett). Previously, she worked at the Swiss Centre of Expertise in the Social Sciences (FORS) as Postdoctoral Researcher. Her research topics include childlessness, work-life conflicts, the measurement of homophobia, adoption by same-sex couples and fatherhood practices. She is the Head of the Family Sociology Section of the Hungarian Sociological Association. Her most recent publications have featured in *Values and identities in Europe. Evidence from the European Social Survey* (2017, Routledge) and *Archives of Sexual Behavior*, *45*(7), (2016).

Judit Takács is a Research Chair at the Institute of Sociology, Centre for Social Sciences, Hungarian Academy of Sciences, and is responsible for leading research teams and conducting independent research on family practices, work-life balance issues and childlessness as well as the social history of homosexuality, social exclusion/inclusion of LGBTQ+ people and HIV/AIDS prevention. Her most recent publications include 'Trans Citizenship in Post-Socialist Societies' (in *Critical Social Policy*; with R. Kuhar and S. Monro, 2018), 'Social Attitudes toward Adoption by Same-Sex Couples in Europe' (in the *Archives of Sexual Behavior*; with I. Szalma and T. Bartus, 2016) and 'Disciplining Gender and (Homo)Sexuality in State Socialist Hungary in the 1970s' (published in the *European Review of History*, 2014). Currently, she works as a seconded National Expert at the ECDC in Stockholm.

Ann Taket is the Director of Centre for Health through Action on Social Exclusion (CHASE), School of Health and Social Development, Faculty of Health at Deakin University, Australia. Professor Taket has over 30 years' experience in public health-related research. Her research has included studies of a wide variety of issues in health policy, service planning and service evaluation, and health-related education in the UK, Australia and other countries. These studies have involved a wide range of different methodologies, both qualitative and quantitative. She has particular interests in research directed at understanding the complex interactions between social exclusion and health, prevention and intervention in violence and abuse and the value of human rights-based approaches in policy and practice.

Kimiko Tanaka is an Associate Professor of Sociology at the James Madison University, USA. Her research focuses on issues related to family, gender and health in Japan's past and present. She has authored papers in the area of demography, family and public health. Dr Tanaka was NIA (National Institute on Aging) Postdoctoral Research Fellow at the University of Wisconsin-Madison. Previously, she has taught at the Rochester Institute of Technology. She holds a BA degree from International Christian University and an MA and PhD in Sociology from the Michigan State University, East Lansing.

Ryan du Toit is a PhD Candidate at Rhodes University, South Africa. His research explores how pre-termination of pregnancy counselling is conducted in the South African context, specifically in the Eastern Cape. Ryan is also registered as an Intern Research Psychologist with the Health Professions Council of South Africa (HPCSA) and is an Editorial Assistant for Feminism and Psychology. He conducts post-graduate quantitative research seminars and is a Facilitator for the gender and sex project. Ryan's research interests include pre-termination of pregnancy, discursive psychology, conversation analysis, pornography and media representation of sexuality and the psychology of the internet.

Beth Turnbull is a PhD Candidate in the School of Health and Social Development, Faculty of Health, Deakin University, Australia. Her research takes quantitative and qualitative approaches to understand the social connection and exclusion in different areas of life of women and men with no children. Beth's PhD seeks to explore the extent and quality of women's and men's resources and participation in employment based on whether they have children.

Introduction: Childlessness through a Feminist Lens

Natalie Sappleton

Childlessness and Feminism

The issue of childlessness is now firmly on the academic agenda and is receiving equally intense scrutiny in media commentary. Doubtless, this unprecedented level of focus is being driven by the remarkable upsurge in childlessness, and especially voluntary childlessness, that has been witnessed virtually across the globe since around the 1980s (Kreyenfeld & Konietzka, 2017). In the United States, there has been an increase in childlessness among women aged between 40 and 44 from 10.2% in 1976 to 15.1% in 2012 (Monte & Mykyta, 2016). In Spain, Austria and the United Kingdom, more than one-fifth of women aged between 40 and 44 are childless (OECD, 2015). In India, the proportion of women between the ages of 35 and 39 that are not mothers doubled from 3.86% in 1981 to 7.28% in 2011 (Sarkar, 2016). It has been predicted that the next Russian census, due to be undertaken in 2020, will reveal that the proportion of women passing reproductive age without bearing children will reach 10% for the first time (Fakhrislamova, 2016). In fact, one analysis of childlessness trends in 35 OECD countries between the mid-1990s and 2010 revealed that only four countries – Slovenia, Turkey, Chile and Luxembourg – had witnessed a fall in childlessness rates over that time period (OECD, 2015).

Yet childlessness is far from a new phenomenon. For instance, Sobotka's (2017) European-wide cohort analysis reveals that childlessness levels have been as high as 25% among French women born around the turn of the twentieth century, Belgian woman born around 1910 and Irish women born during the inter-war period. May reports that childfree lifestyles were more common in the 1930s in North America than they are today (May, 1997). Fakhrislamova's (2016) historical analysis of patterns of childlessness in Russia reveal that in spite of the enforcement of the steep *nalog na bezdetnost* ('childlessness tax') in the Soviet Era, many women of childbearing age still opted to remain childfree. The media and scholarly attention that childlessness is currently attracting can therefore not entirely be attributable to the escalation in the numbers and proportions of the childfree, but perhaps to their increased visibility (Furstenberg, 2014).

Feminism and its adherents have undoubtedly played a key role in illuminating the childfree from the societal shadows. Second wave (largely white, colonial) feminists, whose campaigns intensified in the 1960s and 1970s, placed reproductive rights and sexual freedom at the heart of their crusade, and associated with the subjugation of women with domestic roles and normative heterosexuality carved out within a patriarchal order. Consciousness-raising and grassroots-level campaign groups were established to theorise their ideologies, promote and solicit support for their ideas, and to defend individual rights. For example, the National Organization for Non-Parents (NON), America's first childfree activist group was established in 1972 (Healey, 2016). From the 1990s onwards, third-wave feminists (even those that reject the label), informed by post-modern ideologies, sought to subvert sexist cultures and to destabilise constructs of heteronormativity and universal womanhood and to transverse and celebrate differences across multiple lines of identity – class, sexual orientation and ethnicity, as well as gender. In this, the decision (or not) to remain childless should be seen as a form of empowerment and a means for women to reify themselves as active subjects.

It is perhaps unsurprising then, that a recent cacophony of calls to address growing levels of childlessness, lays the blame for the phenomenon squarely on the shoulders of those that promote and adhere to the feminist project. In the American conservative news portal, *The Daily Wire*, and under the headline, 'Feminism Is Leaving a Wake of Unhappy, Unmarried, and Childless Women in Its Path', for instance, Amanda Prestigiacomo writes that modern, childless women are 'unhappy and alone' and in 'sadness and isolation', and suggests that feminism 'is to blame for this onslaught of college-educated yet terribly empty women'. Such viewpoints are not restricted to the right-wing press, however. Several recent tomes and critics have propagated this blame narrative, attributing the alleged growing unhappiness of women, the fertility crisis and the denigration of motherhood on feminists who told young women that they could 'have it all' (see e.g. Dux & Simic, 2008; Szalai, 2015). Wood and Newton (2006, p. 347), for instance, contend that 'of perhaps most import is the failure of feminist approaches to really challenge motherhood, and in fact their tendency to valorize women's procreative potential and mothering practices'. As Campo

(2005) has argued, this narrative has become so dominant in public and scientific discourse to the extent that alternative explanations have been overlooked.

Also sidelined is the theoretical and empirical work being undertaken by researchers of different stripes who are using feminist epistemology, feminist theories and feminist frameworks to explain, account for, and understand the consequences of childlessness. Researchers from a wide range of scholarly disciplines, including, but not limited to, psychology, sociology, gender studies, social work and social policy have concerned themselves with a range of issues relevant to childlessness, such as the impact it has on lives and emotional states, the implications for personal and relational networks and occupational mobility, and the way in which it is represented and depicted in popular culture. This volume brings together these myriad perspectives under the unifying umbrella of a feminist perspective. By providing an in-depth and interdisciplinary overview of the state-of-the-art of the field, the tome hopes to illuminate how feminism as a method of scientific enquiry, rather than a mere political movement, is contributing to knowledge production in the area of childlessness.

This Volume

Fifteen original chapters make up this volume. The collection is structured around five key principles of feminist enquiry: the pursuit of the theoretical; consideration to the intertwining of processes of structure and agency; intersectionality; a concern for understanding lived experiences and efforts to 'unsilence' the marginalised.

Section 1: Theoretical Perspectives on Voluntary and Involuntary Childlessness

The three chapters in the opening section of the book serve as an introduction to key theories and concepts within the broader topic of childlessness. In Chapter 1, Ingrid Lynch and colleagues trace developments in research in the field of voluntary childlessness from 1920 to 2013. The chapter highlights the transdisciplinary nature of research enquiry, as well as methodological diversity, but points out the dominance of the Global North as a site of enquiry. In Chapter 2, Megumi Fieldsend offers a similar analysis of the field of knowledge production, but this time pertaining to involuntary childlessness and focusing on the psychological and psychosocial perspectives. Aspects examined include the competing psychological emotions of desire and regret, as well as the impact that involuntary childlessness has on self and identity and personal relationships. Drawing on a philosophical feminist value theory, Anna Gotlib philosophises on the concept of free will in Chapter 3, exploring the way in which voluntarily childless women grapple with internal narratives of desiring their choices to remain childfree.

Section 2: Structure, Agency and Childlessness

A tension exists in the feminist literature between those that highlight the importance of social structures in constraining and shaping action, opportunity and choice and those that emphasise the importance of individual agency in the struggle against dominant societal forces (Clegg, 2006). It is, of course, beyond the scope of this collection to seek to resolve that debate. Rather, the chapters that are presented in Section 2 are designed to reflect the complex overlappings of structure and agency in determining outcomes of motherhood and 'otherhood'. First, taking a Bourdeuisian approach, in Chapter 4, Alyssa Mullins constructs pronatalism as a field in which the habitus of childbearing is driven by consideration to Bourdieu's four forms of capitalism. Continuing the theme of pronatalism, and focusing on one particular type of capital – social capital – in Chapter 5, Melissa Graham and colleagues examine how childfree women experience social networks, social connectedness and support. Chapter 6, also by Alyssa Mullins, emphasises the contradictions that women face in pronatalist societies.

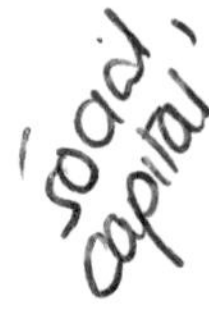

Section 3: Intersectional Perspectives on Childlessness

Gender is not the only source of individuals' social identities. Intersectionalist feminist scholars are united by their rejection of the feminist metonymic fallacy; their belief that the category 'woman' does not adequately describe a common experience of oppression, and the need to include multiple axes of identity and experience in order to develop a fuller understanding of women's lived experiences (McCall, 2005). The two chapters in this section represent a response to that call, by examining how gender and age intersect in the production of narratives and outcomes relating to childlessness. In Chapter 7, Rose

O'Driscoll and Jenny Mercer report on the perceptions and insights of women in Britain, over the age of 45, who have made the decision not to have children. In Chapter 8, Kate de Medeiros and Robert L. Rubinstein adopt a similar focus, exploring narratives of ageing among American women and including race and ethnicity as a specific intersection.

Section 4: Lived Experiences of Childlessness

Lived realities and everyday experiences play a crucial role in shaping individuals' multiplex, complex and layered personal and social identities. Therefore, investigating and accounting for individuals' lived experiences is critical for feminist research. This is reflected in Stanley and Wise's (1993, p. 146) argument that knowledge can be progressed by developing a language of experience, and 'this must come from our exploration of the personal, and the everyday, and what we experience – women's lived experiences'. In that spirit, the four chapters in Section 4 present accounts of the experiences of the childfree within structural and institutional frameworks such as marriage, employment and entrepreneurship. In Chapter 9, Laura Carroll reflects on agency and decision-making processes within the context of the voluntary childless marriage. The chapter exposes how voluntarily childless heterosexual couples arrive at the decision to not have children, and the response that they receive from society. Chapter 10, authored by Helen Peterson, and referring to the Swedish context, looks at a hitherto under-investigated decision-making process – the way in which women who would prefer to remain childfree seek out partners for love, companionship and marriage. The employment arena is the focus of the next two chapters. In Chapter 11, Beth Turnbull and colleagues explore how women who have no children navigate employment and occupational arenas. In Chapter 12, the focus of attention turns to entrepreneurship. Natalie Sappleton explores how remaining childfree is a way for gender-role violating women entrepreneurs to gain access to the resources that they need for business survival and success.

Section 5: National Perspectives on Childlessness

Feminists espousing an intersectionalist epistemology emphasise the importance of privileging the voice of the 'subaltern' (Spivak, 1988). It is important to adopt the discourse and experiences of the marginalised 'other', especially those beyond the current dominant geopolitical structures of knowledge production. Therefore, the final section of the book presents three chapters that examine childlessness within specific national contexts. In Chapter 13, Ivett Szalma and Judit Takács examine childlessness in the context of Hungary, which has a curiously low fertility rate. Drawing on both quantitative and qualitative sources of data, and with specific reference to men and women, the authors explore the extent to which there is a voluntary dimension to childlessness in that geographical context, and what the drivers of that choice might be. A different approach is adopted by Kimiko Tanaka and Deborah Lowry in Chapter 14. This chapter presents a theoretical and historical chronicle of childlessness in Japan, beginning in the Tokugawa period, and concluding with a discussion of the contemporary period. Although the stigma that often accompanies childlessness is found in Japan as in many other regions of the world, this chapter demonstrates historical flux and development in terms of social expectations placed upon the Japanese woman. In Chapter 15, Nazli Kazanoglu explores developments in childcare welfare policy in Germany, examining the link between public policy and Germany's high rate of childlessness. This chapter explores how ideology-driven policy produces and reinforces processes of de-familialisation as well as familialisation.

This book represents the start of a transdisciplinary conversation on an issue that has wide implications and ramifications for individual lives, societies and economies. Since it is only possible to touch upon just a small subset of the research questions childlessness creates, we end this book with a call to action for feminist researcher and scholars.

References

Campo, N. (2005). 'Having it all', or had enough? Rethinking feminism: A review essay. *Lilith: A Feminist History Journal*, *14*, 105–113.

Clegg, S. (2006). The problem of agency in feminism: A critical realist approach. *Gender and Education*, *18*(3), 309–324.

Dux, M., & Simic, Z. (2008). *The great feminist denial*. Melbourne: Melbourne University Publishing.

Fakhrislamova, R. T. (2016). The phenomenon of childlessness in Russia: Historical and social background. *Sociological Research*, *55*(6), 430–449.

Furstenberg, F. F. (2014). Fifty years of family change: From consensus to complexity. *The Annals of the American Academy of Political and Social Science*, *654*(1), 12–30.

Healey, J. (2016). Rejecting reproduction: The national organization for non-parents and childfree activism in 1970s America. *Journal of Women's History*, *28*(1), 131–156.

Kreyenfeld, M., & Konietzka, D. (2017). *Childlessness in Europe*. Cham: Springer.

May, E. T. (1997). *Barren in the promised land: Childless Americans and the pursuit of happiness*. Cambridge, MA: Harvard University Press.

McCall, L. (2005). The complexity of intersectionality. *Signs: Journal of Women in Culture and Society*, *30*(3), 1771–1800.

Monte, L. M., & Mykyta, L. (2016). The occupational attainment of mid-career childless women, 1980-2012. Paper presented at the Work and Family Researchers Network (WFRN) Conference, June 23, Washington, DC.

OECD. (2015). *OECD family database*. Retrieved from http://www.oecd.org/els/family/database.htm#structure

Sarkar, K. (2016). Fertility transition in India. Emerging significance of infertility and childlessness. In A. R. B. K. Singh (Ed.), *India 2016: Population transition* (pp. 87–102). Bhopal: MLC Foundation.

Sobotka, T. (2017). Childlessness in Europe: Reconstructing long-term trends among women born in 1900–1972. *Childlessness in Europe: Contexts, causes, and consequences* (pp. 17–53). Berlin: Springer.

Spivak, G. C. (1988). Can the subaltern speak? In: L. Grossberg & C. Nelson (Eds.), *Marxism and the interpretation of culture* (pp. 271–313). Urbana: University of Illinois Press.

Stanley, L., & Wise, S. (1993). *Breaking out again*. London: Routledge.

Szalai, J. (2015). The complicated origins of 'having it all'. *The New York Times*, p. 2.

Wood, G. J., & Newton, J. (2006). Childlessness and women managers: 'Choice', context and discourses. *Gender, Work & Organization*, *13*(4), 338–358.

SECTION I
THEORETICAL PERSPECTIVES ON VOLUNTARY AND INVOLUNTARY CHILDLESSNESS

Chapter 1

From Deviant Choice to Feminist Issue: An Historical Analysis of Scholarship on Voluntary Childlessness (1920–2013)

Ingrid Lynch, Tracy Morison, Catriona Ida Macleod, Magdalena Mijas, Ryan du Toit and Simi Seemanthini

Abstract

Existing reviews of research on voluntary childlessness generally take the form of narrative summaries, focusing on main topics investigated over time. In this chapter, the authors extend previous literature reviews to conduct a systematic review and content analysis of socio-historical and geopolitical aspects of knowledge production about voluntary childlessness. The dataset comprised 195 peer-reviewed articles that were coded and analysed to explore, inter alia: the main topic under investigation; country location of authors; sample characteristics; theoretical framework and methodology. The findings are discussed in relation to the socio-historical contexts of knowledge production, drawing on theoretical insights concerned with the politics of location, representation and research practice. The shifts in the topics of research from the 1970s, when substantial research first emerged, uphold the view of voluntary childlessness as non-normative. With some regional variation, knowledge is dominated by quantitative, hard science methodologies and mostly generated about privileged, married women living in the global North. The implications of this for future research concerned with reproductive freedom are outlined.

Keywords: Childfree; voluntary childlessness; feminist theory; pronatalism; knowledge production; literature review; content analysis

Introduction

Exploring the history of public thinking about voluntary childlessness can provide important insights for the feminist project of reproductive freedom (Moore & Geist-Martin, 2013). To date, several scholars have explored representations of voluntary childlessness in a range of contexts, such as media representations (Moore & Geist-Martin, 2013), textbooks (Chancey & Dumais, 2009), student perceptions (Koropeckyj-Cox, Çopur, Romano, & Cody-Rydzewski, 2015) and other public talk (Morison, Macleod, Lynch, Mijas, & Shivakumar, 2015). In this chapter, we address scholarly constructions of voluntary childlessness as a form of public representation by turning our attention to research conducted on the topic spanning a period of 93 years (1920–2013).

Our work is guided by the post-structural feminist view of knowledge production as a socio-political project. From this perspective, research is seen as 'intricately interwoven with the socio-historical and socio-economic power relations of modern society' (Macleod, 2004, p. 615). This theoretical lens treats research as simultaneously reflecting and producing particular power relations (in this case with regard to gender, sexuality and reproduction), rather than as value-neutral or objective.

The rise of research on voluntary childlessness is documented in several reviews of the literature, most conducted fairly recently and using a narrative approach to reflect on this growing body of work. These include reviews aimed at identifying research trends (Agrillo & Nelini, 2008; Blackstone & Stewart, 2012; Macklin, 1980), synthesising findings across studies (Bloom & Pebley, 1982), critically analysing key debates in scholarship (Shapiro, 2014) and identifying different discursive constructions of voluntarily childless women over time in both the popular and academic press (Moore & Geist-Martin, 2013). In this chapter, we extend past narrative reviews by means of a systematic review and content analysis of literature going back to the earliest article we could locate (in the 1920s). Our analysis allows us to attend to socio-historical and geopolitical aspects shaping research about voluntary childlessness in relation to the politics of knowledge production, treating the published work as data, thus troubling 'the epistemic privilege of academic discourse' (Macleod, Bhatia, & Kessi, 2017, p. 309).

Voluntary Childlessness as a Topic of Enquiry

Researchers have noted that scholarship reflects the ideological preoccupations of the places and historical moments within which it has been produced (Macleod & Howell, 2013). At a particular time, researchers' assumptions appear as common sense and so go unquestioned. These taken-for-granted assumptions shape the kinds of knowledge that are produced, as well as future research trajectories and how research is taken up beyond the academy.

Within reproductive research, questions have been shaped by a pronatalist bent, which is steeped in taken-for-granted (gendered, class- and race-based) assumptions about who should and should not reproduce and, accordingly, whose fertility should be curbed or encouraged (see e.g. Lowe, 2016; Macleod, 2011; Morison, 2013). Consequently, researchers have explored the reproductive decision-making of those conventionally deemed 'unfit' parents – such as those who are young, disabled, of colour, economically disadvantaged or other than heterosexual. Little to no research has explicitly considered white, heterosexual, middle-class, married women's/couple's motivations to have children and their associated decision-making (Morison, 2013). Women from this socially privileged group of potentially 'fit' parents 'are seldom asked to explain their choice to have children, in contradistinction to those who cannot *or do not want to* have children' (Sevón, 2005, p. 463, our emphasis).

Childlessness – both voluntary or not – has therefore generally been treated as a problem or social issue primarily in relation to white, heterosexual, middle-class and married women/couples (Shapiro, 2014). For instance, only a very small number of studies have focused on lesbian women and gay and heterosexual men who are voluntarily childless (Shapiro, 2014), with research tending to focus initially on heterosexual women and later (in the 1980s) expanding to include studies with heterosexual couples (Blackstone & Stewart, 2012).

Reviews have shown how research on voluntary childlessness in the 1970s was framed within an assumption of deviance and made curious the decision of fertile, childbearing-age women to deliberately forego parenthood (Blackstone & Stewart, 2012; Moore & Geist-Martin, 2013; Shapiro, 2014). More recent scholarship has, however, seen a shift from this 'deviance' view to more positive depictions of childfree women (Moore & Geist-Martin, 2013). Blackstone and Stewart (2012) further note that new research topics emerged by the 2000s, including: a focus on the well-being of an aging population of voluntarily childless adults; research exploring the gendered nature of voluntary childlessness and the impact of family-oriented workplace policies on the childfree. Moore and Geist-Martin (2013) maintain that these changing patterns demonstrate some accommodation of shifts in sexual and reproductive health and rights. In this chapter, we argue that there is extensive work to be done before these kinds of claims can be made.

The common themes addressed in the body of scholarship include: the demographic incidence and correlates of voluntary childlessness (Bloom & Pebley, 1982); different pathways to becoming voluntarily childless; motivations and reasons for being childfree; the physical and mental health consequences of being childfree and stigmatisation of childfree individuals and their responses to such stigma (Agrillo & Nelini, 2008; Blackstone & Stewart, 2012; Kelly, 2009; Macklin, 1980; Shapiro, 2014). Many of these common topics point to pronatalism in the corpus of work, particularly so in studies seeking correlates of voluntary childlessness, the motivations and reasons for being childfree and the physical and mental health consequences of being childfree (Shapiro, 2014). Interest in these issues indicates a need to 'explain' the phenomenon of voluntary childlessness, and the assumption that it would probably have negative consequences. These are questions seldom posed regarding parenthood.

The extant reviews highlight the main themes explored in childfree scholarship over time and provide some insight into the dynamic manner in which such scholarship is constructed in relation to public concerns, as well as mapping some opportunities for further study. However, these reviews do not clearly explicate the process of selecting texts for analysis or include a rigorous analysis of methodological or theoretical characteristics of available scholarship. Building on the insight of prior reviews, our study responds to these gaps through a systematic review and content analysis of research about voluntary childlessness, with the aim of illuminating how this body of knowledge, as a socio-political and socio-historical project, informs contemporary understandings of voluntary childlessness.

Methodology

In this chapter, as indicated above, we investigate scholarship on voluntary childlessness as a socio-political and socio-historical project. Accordingly, the broad questions that we sought to answer were:

- How is this work shaped by the politics of knowledge production?
- How does this knowledge inform contemporary understandings of voluntary childlessness and ultimately speak to feminist understandings of the issue?

Following Macleod et al. (2017), we seek to illuminate the politics surrounding the production of knowledge on this topic in terms of location, representation and practice. Though we discuss each of these separately below, it must be noted that they are inextricably interlinked with one another. As Borsa (1990, p. 36) asserts:

> Where we live, how we live, our relation to the social systems and structures that surround us are deeply embedded parts of everything we do and remain integral both to our identity or sense of self and to our position or status within a larger cultural and representational field.

First, in analysing of the politics of location, the aim is to establish the ways that location (understood broadly) may work in the interest of privilege and power. Analysis of the politics of location includes the interrogation of the researcher's situation in relation to power, and how this might shape the interpretation of data, as well as the community of people being studied. To this end, we question how socio-structural, historical and economic differences set the parameters of inquiry and ultimately favour particular readings while undermining or silencing others (Macleod et al., 2017). This means rendering visible the power relations and dominant cultural codes implicated when knowledge producers are located in different sites (be they geographic or particular cultural, political or textual) and through such a critical awareness, developing frameworks that may function as productive sites of resistance (Borsa, 1990; Giroux, 1992).

Second, the analysis of the politics of representation rests on the premise that the act of representation – in the sense of presenting something/somebody in language, discourse, texts, images and so on – is a re/production rather than a reflection of reality (Danielsen, Jegerstedt, Muriaas, & Ytre-Arne, 2016). Consequently, such an analysis involves interrogating the type of world that is constructed through the process of knowledge production, including the particular identities made available to subjects (Denzin & Lincoln, 2011). In post-colonial contexts, representational practices are largely shaped by socially constructed categories of race/ethnicity, class, gender, sexuality and dis/ability (among others). For instance, much of social science research has historically framed reproduction and parenthood in heteronormative ways, positioning those outside of normative notions of 'family', such as teenage mothers, single-parent fathers or queer-identified parents, as unnatural, shameful, abnormal or pathological (Landau, 2009; Macleod, 2011; Silverstein, 1996). Attending to the politics of representation means interrogating such positionings and the power relations underpinning them.

Third and finally, the analysis of the politics of research practices implies thinking through the methodologies that enable particular kinds of representations. Most simply this involves illuminating how research is done as an epistemic practice. To do so 'we have to pay close attention to the politics of data, methods, subjects, theories, and epistemological visions' (Petrina, 1998, p. 51). Such an analysis attends to how and why certain knowledges continue to be produced in particular ways through particular practices and processes in order to collude with (or possibly trouble) hegemonic knowledges (Winkler, 2017, p. 3).

Drawing on the framework outlined above, we treated the literature as data and made use of both integrative and interpretive analytical approaches (Dixon-Woods, Agarwal, Jones, Young, & Sutton, 2005). Our dataset comprised 195 peer-reviewed journal articles about voluntary childlessness published between 1920 (when the earliest article we could locate was published) and 2013 (the analysis was conducted in 2014) within a range of disciplines and primarily in the global North. The dataset includes articles reporting on empirical work – qualitative and quantitative studies with participants as well as document or media analyses – and non-empirical contributions – that is theoretical, conceptual or methodological articles, meta-analyses or literature reviews. (A list of these articles appears in Appendix.)

The exclusion of other formats (e.g. books, chapters), 'grey' literature and peer-reviewed articles not published in English could be seen as limiting. We argue, however, that focusing on published academic journal articles does provide a reasonable indication of the state of research on the subject. English-language journals tend to carry higher impact factors and to dominate in terms of knowledge production (Gupta, 2007). It is also likely that published academic journal articles are generally more widely accessible to academic communities.

The data were located through systematic searches of social science and humanities databases. In order to include publications that would contain research on 'childlessness' as a social phenomenon our search covered fields such as psychology, social work, sociology, gender studies, reproductive health and sexuality studies, but excluded medical articles, which dealt largely with infertility.

Our literature search was not restricted to any time period or geographical location, since we were interested in ascertaining the extent of the research produced over time and across regions. The key words 'childfree', 'voluntary childlessness' and 'voluntarily childless' yielded a corpus of 307 texts from which we eliminated a further 112 texts that were irrelevant or (e.g. covering topics such as infertility/involuntary childlessness, fertility trends) or not peer-reviewed (e.g. book reviews, editorials and letters to the editor). We attempted to locate full-text versions of articles as far as possible, in some cases directly from the author. In cases where full-texts were unavailable (mostly for older/out-of-print journals), we used abstracts to identify certain variables (e.g. country in which research is produced) where possible. In cases where information was missing, this is indicated in coding and the presentation of results.

We took a deductive, but iterative, approach to coding, developing a set of a priori codes and refining these to ensure they captured evolving complexity and unanticipated nuances. The coding process was designed to promote reliability, using coding pairs and multiple rounds of coding.[1] Throughout the process, discrepancies between coders were dealt with in close consultation with the codebook and the research questions to determine whether the original code was perhaps ambiguous or inadequate. When codes were refined during coding, all cases using the code were verified against the new code. (The main variables used for the codebook appear in Table 1.)

Using these codes, we captured descriptive information about each article in order to identify general trends and patterns in the dataset related to authorship, theoretical framing and methods. We also captured information about sampling in empirical studies, but coded this as 'not applicable' for non-empirical articles. Each variable was disaggregated and assigned a numerical code. For example, the gender of the first author was distinguished as female = 1, male = 2 and indiscernible = 3.

[1]The coding process began with each author independently coding articles and then discussing these in pairs, with the aim of reaching consensus in relation to any discrepancies between them. Cases were recorded when agreement could not be reached and attended to by a separate coder in a further round of coding. Any discrepancies remaining after this additional round of coding were discussed as a team.

Table 1. Summary of Main Coding Categories.

Variable Type	Variable	Variable Descriptions
The politics of location	Date	Year of publication
	First author's country	Institutional affiliation of the first author
	Sample country	Geographic location of the researched sample
The politics of research practices, including sample for empirical studies with human participants	Article type	Empirical or non-empirical nature of the article
	Method	Method of data collection and analysis
	Theoretical framework	Theoretical framework informing the study
	Sample size	The size of the researched sample
	Sample race	Race of participants as described in the article
	Socio-economic status (SES)	The SES of the participants as described in the article
	Sample age	The age of the participants in the study
	Sample sexuality	Sexual 'orientation' of the participants in the study
	Sample gender	Gender of the participants in the study
	Sample relationship status	Relationship status of the participants in the study (e.g. cohabiting, married and single)
	Sample reproductive status	Reproductive status of the participants in the study (e.g. voluntarily childless, parents and child-anticipating)
The politics of representation	Topic	Main focus of the articles

When authors did not provide specific information (in the full-text article or abstract) the codes 'not stated' or 'inferred' were applied. For instance, when participant sexuality was not described, sometimes inferences could be made in relation to references to 'husbands' and 'wives' (or similar) and the code 'heterosexual – inferred' was applied (as opposed to the other possibilities of 'unstated' or 'heterosexual–stated'). Including such codes ('unstated', 'inferred') allowed us to attend to the ways that particular normative social categories, such as whiteness or heterosexuality, were either made explicit or taken for granted. The coded texts were analysed descriptively according to the variables listed above (Table 1). Cross-tabulations were conducted to explore relationships between variables of interest.

The Politics of Location: When, and by Whom Was Research Produced?

The first study to treat voluntary childlessness as a topic in its own right appeared in 1920, but the subject appears to have received virtually no substantial academic attention until the 1970s. Only six articles (3% of the entire dataset) where published in the 49-year period from 1920 to 1969. The remaining 44 years of the period under study (1970–2013) saw the bulk of the research produced, as illustrated in Figure 1 below. During this time, the number rose from 11.3% in the 1970s and peaked in the 1980s at 39%. It tapered off in the 1990s (9.2%), and then began gradually increasing again in the early 2000s (28.7%). During the period 2010–2013, we located 17 published articles (8.7%).

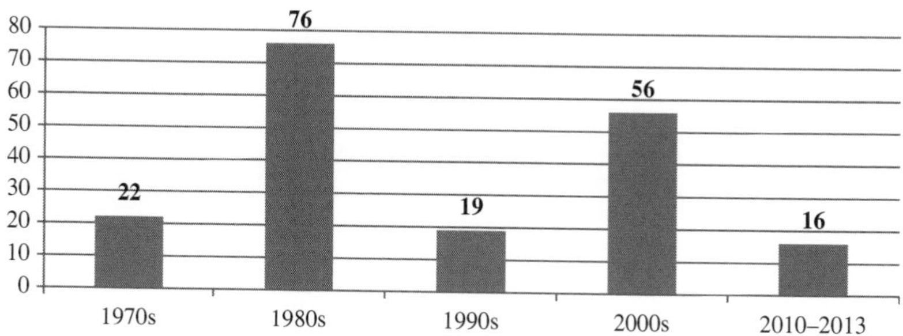

Figure 1. Number of Articles Published per Decade from the 1970s Onwards.

The rise of interest in the 1970s corresponds with what has been called the Second Demographic Transition that took place in 'Western' countries, emerging in the 1950s, but gaining momentum in the late 1960s and 1970s: 'sustained sub-replacement fertility, a multitude of living arrangements other than marriage, the disconnection between marriage and procreation, and no stationary population' (Lesthaeghe, 2010, p. 211). The emergence of voluntary childlessness in research from the 1970s onwards, therefore, occurs in the context of national and regional concerns around threats to the 'traditional' nuclear family as well as anxiety over women's reproductive rights and shifting gender roles. The increased interest in the 1980s could have to do with the global trend of concentrating on reproductive issues (as opposed to population control) that led up to the International Convention on Population and Development held in Cairo in 1994 (Shalev, 2000).

Information about who produces knowledge about voluntary childlessness was inferred from the first (or sole) author's affiliation.[2] In a small percentage of cases, it was not possible to discern the primary author's affiliation (1.5%). The analysis demonstrates the dominance of North American knowledge production (in English-language journals at least): almost two-thirds (64.6%) of authors have United States or Canadian affiliations, followed by Australian and New Zealand (12.8%), continental Europe (10.8%) and the United Kingdom (10.3%).

Most articles (145) rely on empirical data generated with participants. When considering the location of the participants from whom data were collected in these articles, these correspond largely with author affiliation. Accordingly, there is a dominance of samples from North America (57.9%), followed by Australia and New Zealand (13.1%), continental Europe (12.4%) and the UK (6.9%). There is only one article with African (Ethiopian) participants, representing the entirety of research conducted in poorer resourced settings (the global South). This means that the overwhelming majority of the participants were from well-resourced, industrialised countries (the global North).

What knowledge is ultimately produced is related to the kinds of questions that hold sway in particular spaces at particular historical moments, in this case the global North from the 1970s onwards. It is

[2]While there is obviously overlap between sample and author locations, these are not necessarily always the same. For instance, the sole African study is written by an author located outside Africa.

also intimately connected to resources to publish and who is in the position to publish (Macleod, 2004). The notable absence of global South voices as authors and participants can be considered in relation to regional concerns and global funding imperatives. While lowering of fertility rates has historically been a priority in wealthier, industrialised countries (Marshall, 2015), sexual and reproductive health researchers in poor-resourced countries have concentrated on the adverse consequences of rapid population growth (Ezeh, Bongaarts, & Mberu, 2012) and HIV prevention, which tend to receive more funding (Griffin, 2006). This means that there is far less research across a range of contexts that provides insight into nuances of reproductive decision-making.

The Politics of Research Practices: Type, Method, Theory and Sample

The majority of the articles are unsurprisingly empirical (77.5%), with a much smaller proportion tackling theoretical or conceptual issues or consolidating knowledge through meta-analyses or reviews (22.6%). The theoretical categorisations that were applied during the coding process appear in Table 2 (see also method section).

The preponderance of quantitatively oriented research is clear from the frequency with which 'hard science' theories are drawn on. This is highlighted when the theoretical framing is viewed in relation to the methodologies that are drawn on in the articles. These are outlined in Table 3.

When viewed in relation to one another the data in Tables 2 and 3 show that knowledge production around voluntary childlessness is dominated by quantitative, positivist research. In contrast, only about a fifth of the work is comprised of qualitative research and the critical and social theories typically employed within this paradigm, such as feminist, post-modern and systems theories.

We noted some other interesting trends when cross-tabulating the articles' theoretical framing with their decade of publication. The share of articles using a hard science framework remains relatively consistent over the decades from the 1970s. Individual-focused theories spike in the 1980s, being used by 34.2% of articles in that decade. Systems-oriented theories debut in the 1990s, while classic and post-modern/critical theories first appear in the 2000s.

Table 2. Theoretical Frameworks Used.

Theoretical Frameworks Used	**Description**	**Frequency**	**Percentage**
'Hard science' frameworks	Positivist, psychometric, psychiatric and evolutionary psychology	85	43.6
Individual-focused theory	Attitudes and perceptions, identity, personality, wellness, developmental, risk/resilience and motivations	38	19.5
Ambiguous/unstated	Difficult to infer the theoretical framework	26	13.3
Unavailable	Full - text not available and information not in the abstract	17	8.7
Feminist	Various feminist theories (including explicitly feminist studies making use of post-modern or critical frameworks)	9	4.6
Social theories	Symbolic interactionism and social identity theory	6	3.1
Post-modern/critical frameworks	Social constructionism, post-structuralism, post-colonialism, masculinities studies and general gender studies (but not explicitly feminist)	5	2.6
Systems-orientated theory	Socio-ecological, cultural, community, health systems and organisational	3	1.5
Classic theories	Existentialism, phenomenology, psychodynamic, hermeneutic and cognitive-behavioural	3	1.5
Communication studies	Communication theories, communication privacy management theories and media study theories	3	1.5
Total		*195*	*100*

Table 3. Methodologies Used.

Methodology Used	Frequency	Percentage
Quantitative	110	56.4
Not applicable	36	18.5
Not available	22	11.3
Qualitative	22	11.3
Mixed methods	5	2.6
Total	*195*	*100*

The use of feminist theories is remarkably low, given the topic. These are applied in only a small fraction of articles in the 1970s (9.1%); 1990s (5.3%) and 2000s (10.7%), meaning that in the 1980s, the decade with the most number of articles, no feminist theories were used. The use of feminist approaches seems to coincide with particular socio-political changes: the 1970s 'sexual revolution' and increased availability of hormonal contraception in the global North; some resurgence in the 2000s in restrictions of women's sexual and reproductive health and rights (e.g. access to contraception and abortion); and lowered fertility rates coupled with the revitalisation of appeals to the preservation of the traditional heterosexual nuclear family across regions (Pollitt, 2014).

In terms of methodologies, the changes in those employed (when using human participants) over time are shown in Table 4. This cross-tabulation shows that quantitative methods have remained popular over the decades. The use of qualitative methods, however, steadily rises as they are used initially in mixed-method designs, but increasingly in their own right (likely due to their growing credibility and popularity in social research more broadly).

In terms of methodologies, a cross-tabulation of methodology and author location (Table 5) shows that the mixed-method studies are exclusively conducted by authors located in North America, although these are still a small proportion of the total (4.3%). An exclusively qualitative approach was most common in the United Kingdom, where one-third (33.3%) of British studies is qualitative.

There is also regional variation in the theoretical frameworks used, as shown in Table 6. Authors from North America and continental Europe concentrate on 'hard science' frameworks. Researchers in Australia, New Zealand and the United Kingdom tend to use individual-focused theories.

Table 4. Cross-tabulation of Decade and Method (for Empirical Articles Relying on Participant Data).

Decade	Qualitative (%)	Quantitative (%)	Mixed Method (%)	Not Available (%)	Total No. of Empirical Articles
<1970s	0	2	0	2	4
1970s	13.3	66.7	13.3	6.7	15
1980s	3.1	75.4	1.6	23.4	64
1990s	14.3	71.4	7.1	7.1	14
2000s	30	67.5	2.5	0	40
>2010s	21.4	78.6	0	0	14

Table 5. Cross-tabulation of Methodology of Empirical Articles by Author Location.

Author Location	Qualitative (%)	Quantitative (%)	Mixed Method (%)	Not Available (%)	Total No. of Empirical Articles in Author Location
Australia/New Zealand	9.1	59.1	0	31.8	22
North America	10.6	77.7	4.3	7.5	94
United Kingdom	33.3	25.0	0	41.7	12
Europe Continental	6.7	93.3	0	0	15
Not stated	50.0	50.0	0	0	2

Table 6. Cross-tabulation of Author Location and Theoretical Framework, Indicating the Most and the Least Used.

Region	Most Used Theoretical Framework	% of Articles	Least Used Theoretical Framework	% of Articles
North America	Hard science framework	49.2	Post-modern/critical theory	0.8
Australia/ New Zealand	Individual-focused theory	52	Social theories, systems-orientated theory, classic theories, feminist theory and communication studies	0
Continental Europe	Hard science framework	61.9	Individual-focused theory, classic theories, post-modern/critical theory, feminist theory and communication studies	0
United Kingdom	Individual-focused theory	20	Social theories	0

Authors in North America and the United Kingdom use a larger range of theories than authors in Australia, New Zealand and continental Europe, with a spread of theories most even in the United Kingdom (e.g. postmodern/critical theory and feminist frameworks accounted for 15% of articles each and 'hard science' frameworks for 10% of articles).

Given that the focus of the research is on voluntary childlessness, it is to be expected that the majority of articles (84.8%) would discuss participants' reproductive status. Just under half (40%) of all the empirical articles with human participants have mixed samples comprising of childfree people and one other category, such as involuntary childless people and parents. A much smaller proportion of the empirical studies (18.6%) focuses exclusively on childfree participants, while only 8.3% has general population samples (these studies explore, for example, attitudes to, or acceptance of, voluntary childlessness). The remainder of empirical articles includes combinations of childless and child-anticipating participants, as well as parents (17.9%).

Participants' gender is nearly always reported (95.2% of articles), and authors also usually explicitly report on or allude to relationship status (i.e. widowed, single, divorced, partnered/cohabiting and married), age and socio-economic status. Since the majority of the studies concern fertility trends, most report diverse samples and more than half of the studies (51%) included both female and male participants. As we discuss later, when articles that make use of mixed samples – that is studies relying on survey or population-based data – are excluded, the numbers of the groups that are focused on become more significant. In the remainder of the studies, the number of female-only samples (59% or 40.7%) far outweighs male-only samples (5% or 3.4%). Almost a third (31.7%) of these had married-only participants. This research mainly includes people in early adulthood (9.7%) or middle adulthood (6.9%) and then late adulthood (2.8%). Some studies (21.4% of articles) also include participants from middle to upper socio-economic status, with 7.6% not reporting on the socio-economic status of their participants.

In contrast to the categories mentioned above, there were two variables that authors were less likely to report on or to mention explicitly, namely, participants' race and/or sexuality. Around a third of articles (32.4%) do not state the race of the participants and when it is mentioned this refers to mixed race/population sampling (36.5%). Only one article specifically focuses on an exclusively Black sample – interestingly, this is also the sole study conducted in an African country, and is focused on family size preferences – while 10.3% has exclusively White participants.

Just over three quarters (75.9%) of the articles do not refer to the participants' sexuality at all. Only a small proportion of articles (2.8%) directly state that participants are heterosexual, but this could be inferred in well over a further 37.9% of the full-text articles. A small proportion of articles (6.2%) reports on mixed samples (participants who are heterosexual along with lesbians, those 'in a same-gendered relationship', or lesbians and bisexual persons).

Our analysis, thus, shows that the studies tend to narrowly focus on specific groups (when participant characteristics are reported on). Other scholars have also noted this trend (Blackstone & Stewart, 2012; Shapiro, 2014). While some attempts have been made to widen the focus and include heterosexual couples, lesbians and gay and heterosexual men, our (and others') findings show that these studies remain in the minority. Moreover, because of the frequent reliance on data from population surveys the extent of the lack of diversity is often obscured. When we exclude studies drawing on these data, however, it becomes clear that women, middle- to upper-class participants, those who are young adults through to middle adulthood, and married individuals or couples remain the focus of research.

The fact that many authors do not specify participants' sexuality or racial identifications is also telling. We can speculate that most participants are White and (assumed to be) heterosexual, but that these characteristics go unmentioned because of their privileged normative status. The assumption of heterosexuality may inadvertently obscure diverse sexualities within samples. The focus on married, heterosexual, middle-class women can also be understood in relation to the aforementioned concerns about declining fertility rates and preserving 'traditional' families with their conventional gendered roles.

The Politics of Representation: What Topics Have Been of Interest?

In Table 7, we outline the main focus of articles. Other than studies of general fertility patterns that include voluntary childlessness, researchers have largely focused on: (1) explaining voluntary childlessness; (2) explicating the outcomes or consequences of deliberately not having children and (3) decision-making around, and the pathways to, voluntary childlessness.

In contrast to the work attempting to explain or account for voluntary childlessness, there appears to be less research that considers

Table 7. The Main Focus of Articles.

Main Focus of Article	Code for Articles that…	Count	%
Explaining voluntary childlessness	Explain voluntary childlessness or voluntarily childless people and including comparative studies (e.g. voluntarily childless with involuntarily childless, child-anticipating and parents)	36	18.5
'Outcomes' of being voluntarily childless	Highlight the 'outcomes' or consequences of being voluntarily childless including psychological and social concerns, well-being, quality of life, life satisfaction, relationships and adjustment; including comparative studies with involuntarily childless, child-anticipating, parents, etc.	27	13.8
Fertility trends or prevalence studies, with reference to voluntary childlessness	Explain general fertility or reproductive intentions, decisions and outcomes; and these studies all include reference to voluntary childlessness – at micro (personal) or macro (societal) level	27	13.8
Explaining general fertility, with reference to voluntary childlessness	Refer to trends or prevalence in fertility, population or demographics related to childlessness (including voluntary childlessness); macro level statistical, sociological, psychological and population or historical analyses within or across countries	21	10.8

Decision-making, pathways	Refer to decision-making: choice (including type or timing of choice) and pathways towards childlessness (including postponing, delaying and ambivalence and voluntary sterilisation)	20	10.3
Attitudes, perceptions towards, acceptance of, voluntary childlessness	Concerned with attitudes towards or perceptions and acceptance of voluntarily childless people	17	8.7
Voluntary childlessness as phenomenon	Generally discuss the phenomenon of being voluntarily childless and including literature reviews	13	6.7
Gender/'sex roles'	Foreground gender or 'sex roles', or gendered ideology in relation to voluntary childlessness	10	5.1
Race	Foreground race by exploring connections between voluntary childlessness and racial or ethnic identity	5	2.6
Social representations and discourses	Speak to social representations, discourses and constructions of voluntarily childless people (e.g. in the media)	4	2.1
Other foci	Fewer than five articles each: age, life-course issues, stigma, subjective experiences, laws and policies and family forms	15	7.6
Total		*195*	*100*

personal experiences or social meanings of voluntary childlessness and the potential implications of these for childfree people. The minority of articles focus specifically on contextual issues, dealing with voluntarily childless people's subjective experiences and personal narratives; social stigma, stigma management and disclosure (communication) of voluntary childlessness; legal aspects (e.g. workplace policies); childless couples as 'alternative' families and changing family forms; age, life-course or developmental issues; and childlessness in later years. These trends confirm observations in the recent literature reviews referred to earlier.

The focus on possible negative outcomes, and therefore the need to 'explain' voluntary childlessness, can be understood in relation to the dominance of research from the global North, where 'since the 1970s, expressions of state concern over low fertility have greatly increased' (Marshall, 2015, p. 1541). Western Europe and North America saw significant transformations in family formation and childbearing after World War II. After a brief post-war marriage rush and 'baby-boom' in the 1950s, subsequent decades

> brought a reversal of those trends in the form of later marriage, a great increase in nonmarital cohabitation, a large rise in divorce, and a sharp fall in fertility to below the replacement level. (Cherlin & Furstenberg, 1988, p. 291)

Regional variation in research interests can be seen when cross-tabulating empirical articles' most commonly researched topics with the sample location. North American and British research has mostly tried to explain voluntary childlessness (26.5% and 30% of studies, respectively) or considered it in relation to other fertility trends (15.7% and 20%, respectively). Most attention in continental Europe and Australasia has been captured by decision-making or pathways to voluntary childlessness (25% and 26.3%, respectively) or investigating fertility patterns with reference to voluntary childlessness (31.2% and 21%, respectively).

The main topics under investigation have also shifted over time, as revealed by a cross-tabulation (main topic by decade of publication, shown in Table 8) which identifies the most and least researched topics related to voluntary childlessness from the 1970s onwards. When research interest first takes hold in the 1970s, most of the focus is on establishing the prevalence of this phenomenon as a fertility trend in relation to other shifts in fertility at the population level (18.2% of articles). Interest then shifts to explanations of voluntary childlessness in

Table 8. Cross-tabulation of Main Focus and Decade: Indicating the Most and the Least Researched Topics.

Decade	Most Researched per Decade	Articles per Decade (%)	Least Researched per Decade	Articles per Decade (%)
1970s	• Fertility prevalence	18.2	• Age/life-course • Race • Stigma • Social representations • Subjective experience	0
1980s	• Explaining voluntary childlessness	22.4	• Family forms • Stigma • Subjective experience • Laws/policies	0
1990s	• Explaining voluntary childlessness	36.8	• Explaining fertility • Family forms • Age/life-course • Race • Gender • Social representations • Subjective experience • Laws/policies	0

Table 8. (*Continued*)

Decade	Most Researched per Decade	Articles per Decade (%)	Least Researched per Decade	Articles per Decade (%)
2000s	• Explaining fertility • Consequences of voluntary childlessness	12.5	• Family forms • Age/life-course • Race	1.8
>2010	• Consequences of voluntary childlessness	25	[a]	

Note: [a]As this is not a full decade, the number of categories with no research is relatively high, so we do not report on them here.

the 1980s (22.4% of articles), peaking in the 1990s (38.6% of articles). Thereafter, attention turns to the outcomes or consequences of remaining childfree in the 2000s (12.5% of articles), continuing into the 2010s (25% of articles). These findings confirm the recent reviews of research referred to above, which describe a shifting research focus that aligns with global changes in thinking about sexuality and reproduction. The research trajectory follows a developmental logic of first 'discovering' the phenomenon, then attempting to account for or explain its occurrence, and finally considering its (generally negative) consequences.

It is only in later decades, with the rise of qualitative methodologies, that interest in some of the under-researched areas of investigation emerges. An interest in stigma first appears only in the 1990s and childfree people's experiences only in the 2000s. While these kinds of topics add nuance and allow for the explication of power relations concerning reproduction, they have still to make a significant impact on the major knowledge production concerning voluntary childlessness.

Prior to the 1970s, a few early studies highlight mostly negative concerns: the preservation of heterosexual marriage as ideal context for childbearing, with voluntary childlessness within a marriage seen as denigrating that ideal (1920s); voluntary childlessness and low birth rates as threatening Western civilisation (1930s); voluntary childlessness as motivated by individualism, infantile and neurotic attitudes and materialism (1930s and 1940s); and the foregrounding of race (1960s).

Conclusion

Our findings identify a trajectory of topical interest from the 'discovery' of the phenomenon (1970s), to explaining voluntary childlessness (1980s, 1990s and 2000s), to concerns with (mostly negative) consequences (2000s onwards). Quantitative, 'hard science' articles dominate the production of knowledge, with a short supply of feminist and qualitative research. Participants tend to be women, privileged, married and assumed to be White and heterosexual. In contrast, not only are poorer, Black, queer people and/or men relatively absent from the articles that formed our dataset, voluntarily childless people in the global South have virtually no representation either. Other than the smoothing over of difference and complexity that this implies, there is the danger of extending conclusions to groups outside of this relatively small group of people.

Given the topics of interest and the politics of fertility in the global North where the vast majority of research was conducted, the concentration on these participants is perhaps not entirely opportunistic. We argue, therefore, that the focus on these persons – and the concomitant lack of attention on others – points to pronatalist and heteronormative assumptions that shape the knowledge produced about voluntary childlessness. Together these sets of norms create the assumption of procreation and biological parenthood as an expected part of heterosexual adulthood. What is problematic, and thereby 'research-worthy', alongside topics such as infertility or use of reproductive technologies, is wilful non-reproduction among those ordinarily entitled and encouraged to do so: married, White, middle-class, able-bodied, heterosexual women/couples (Morison, 2013). Most of the research on voluntary childlessness can therefore be considered as largely coming from a 'problem perspective', not only in relation to concerns about fertility rates, but also the implied deviance of particular childfree individuals who form the main research focus. As alluded to in the background discussion at the beginning of this article, pronatalist assumptions – which are interwoven with hetero-gendered, class- and race-based ideas about who is fit to reproduce – inform the ways that voluntary childlessness is approached by researchers. In contrast, non-reproduction is less problematic among those deemed less 'fit to reproduce', whom we also alluded to in the opening discussion, and they received far less attention in the literature on voluntary childlessness.

While the current research concentrates on those most likely to experience stigma and negative sanction for non-reproduction (Morison et al., 2015), at the same time it inadvertently repeats and reinforces the very assumptions that create such responses. We have argued elsewhere that '[r]esearchers working in the areas of families and reproduction should critically assess the implicit assumptions upon which their work is based to ensure that they do not inadvertently reiterate pronatalist norms' (Morison et al., 2015, p. 13). To this end, in researching voluntary childlessness, it would be valuable to increase the use of critical social theory and feminist frameworks, currently under-utilised in existing scholarship. Research framed by feminist theories can assist with exploring the hetero-gendered norms that often underpin research, as well as family formation and reproductive politics more broadly. Feminist investigations can thus provide valuable insights for the fields of family studies and reproductive health (Ferree, 1990; Riessman, 2000).

Along the same lines, the growth in studies employing qualitative methodologies to explore voluntary childlessness is to be welcomed and further encouraged. Qualitative methodologies allow for depth and complexity in investigations (Gough & Lyons, 2016). Research exploring the subjective experiences and meaning-making in narratives and autobiographies of voluntary childless people can contribute to depth of understanding of an issue that involves the complex interweaving of social dynamics.

Finally, research is also needed within a range of settings with participants from various social locations, including the global South. Riessman's (2000) work on childlessness in South India suggests that these voluntarily childless individuals' experiences may be markedly different to those in Westernised, industrialised contexts, but that there may also be similarities. There is also a need for comparisons across contrasting geopolitical settings which would allow researchers interested in social justice to illuminate (rather than conceal) 'the ways that pronatalist discourses impact on people in different ways, and [...] to spotlight common causes and injustices' (Morison et al., 2015, p. 12) located in a range of structural, gendered, class- and race-based inequities that impinge upon reproductive freedom.

Acknowledgements

The authors gratefully acknowledge funding support from the Department of Science and Technology (DST) and National Research Foundation (NRF) of South Africa, obtained through the South African Research Chairs Initiative and the Centre of Excellence in Human Development.

References

Agrillo, C., & Nelini, C. (2008). Childfree by choice: A review. *Journal of Cultural Geography*, *25*(3), 347–363. doi:10.1080/08873630802476292

Blackstone, A., & Stewart, M. D. (2012). Choosing to be childfree: Research on the decision not to parent. *Sociology Compass*, *6*(9), 718–727.

Bloom, D. E., & Pebley, A. R. (1982). Voluntary childlessness: A review of the evidence and implications. *Population Research and Policy Review*, *1(3)*, 203–224.

Borsa, J. (1990). .Towards a politics of location: Rethinking marginality. *Canadian Woman Studies*, *11*(1), 36–39.

Chancey, L., & Dumais, S. A. (2009). Voluntary childlessness in marriage and family textbooks, 1950–2000. *Journal of Family History*, *34*(2), 206–223.

Cherlin, A., & Furstenberg, F. F. (1988). The changing European family: Lessons for the American reader. *Journal of Family Issues*, *9*(3), 291–297.

Danielsen, H., Jegerstedt, H., Muriaas, R. L., & Ytre-Arne, B. (2016). Gendered citizenship: The politics of representation. In H. Danielsen, K. Jegerstedt, R. L. Muriaas, & B. Ytre-Arne (Eds.), *Gendered citizenship and the politics of representation* (pp. 1–13). New York: Springer.

Denzin, N. K., & Lincoln, Y. S. (2011). *The Sage handbook of qualitative research*. London: Sage.

Dixon-Woods, M., Agarwal, S., Jones, D. R., Young, B., & Sutton, A. J. (2005). Synthesising qualitative and quantitative evidence: A review of methods. *Journal of Health Services Research and Policy*, *10*, 45–53.

Ezeh, A. C., Bongaarts, J., & Mberu, B. (2012). Global population trends and policy options. *Lancet*, *380*, 142–148.

Ferree, M. M. (1990). Beyond separate spheres: Feminism and family research. *Journal of Marriage and the Family*, *52*, 866–884.

Giroux, H. A. (1992). Paulo Freire and the politics of postcolonialism. *Journal of Advanced Composition*, *12*(1), 15–26.

Gough, B., & Lyons, A. (2016). The future of qualitative research in psychology: Accentuating the positive. *Integrative Psychological and Behavioral Science*, *50*(2), 234–243. doi:10.1007/s12124-015-9320-8

Griffin, S. (2006). *Literature review on sexual and reproductive health rights: Universal access to services, focusing on East and Southern Africa and South Asia*. London: Department for International Development.

Gupta, N. (2007). The poser: Universalising and indigenising social knowledge: Breaking the western hegemony. *Sociological Bulletin*, *56*(3), 426–430.

Kelly, M. (2009). Women's voluntary childlessness: A radical rejection of motherhood? *Women's Studies Quarterly*, *37*(3/4), 157–172.

Koropeckyj-Cox, T., Çopur, Z., Romano, V., & Cody-Rydzewski, S. (2015). University students' perceptions of parents and childless or childfree couples. *Journal of Family Issues*. Advance online. doi:10.1177/0192513X15618993

Landau, J. (2009). Straightening out (the politics of) same-sex parenting: Representing gay families in US print news stories and photographs. *Critical Studies in Media Communication*, *26*(1), 80–100.

Lesthaeghe, R. (2010). The unfolding story of the second demographic transition. *Population and Development Review*, *36*, 211–251.

Lowe, P. (2016). *Reproductive health and maternal sacrifice: Women, choice and responsibility*. London: Palgrave Macmillan.

Macklin, E. D. (1980). Nontraditional family forms: A decade of research. *Journal of Marriage and the Family*, *42*(4), 905–922.

Macleod, C. (2004). South African psychology and 'relevance': Continuing challenges. *South African Journal of Psychology*, *34*(4), 613–629.

Macleod, C. (2011). *'Adolescence', pregnancy and abortion: Constructing a threat of degeneration*. London: Routledge.

Macleod, C., Bhatia, S., & Kessi, S. (2017). Postcolonialism and psychology: Growing interest and promising potential. In C. Willig & W. Stainton-Rogers (Eds.), *The Sage handbook of qualitative research in psychology* (pp. 306–317). London: Sage.

Macleod, C., & Howell, S. (2013). Reflecting on South African psychology: Published research, 'relevance', and social issues. *South African Journal of Psychology*, *43*(2), 222–237. doi:10.1177/0081246313482630

Marshall, E. A. (2015). When do states respond to low fertility? Contexts of state concern in wealthier countries, 1976–2011. *Social Forces*, *93*(4), 1541–1566. doi:10.1093/sf/sov060

Moore, J., & Geist-Martin, P. (2013). Mediated representations of voluntary childlessness, 1900–2012. In D. Castañeda (Ed.), *The essential handbook of women's sexuality* (pp. 233–251). Santa Barbara, CA: Praeger.

Morison, T. (2013). Heterosexual men and parenthood decision making in South Africa: Attending to the invisible norm. *Journal of Family Issues*, *34*(8), 1125–1144.

Morison, T., Macleod, C., Lynch, I., Mijas, M., & Shivakumar, S. (2015). Stigma resistance in online childfree communities: The limitations of choice rhetoric. *Psychology of Women Quarterly*, *40*(2), 184–198. doi:10.1177/0361684315603657

Petrina, S. (1998). The politics of research in technology education: A critical content and discourse analysis of the *Journal of Technology Education*, volumes 1–8. *Journal of Technology Education*, *10*(1), 27–57.

Pollitt, K. (2014). Reclaiming abortion rights. *Dissent*, *62*(4), 15–44.

Riessman, C. K. (2000). Stigma and everyday resistance practices: Childless women in South India. *Gender & Society*, *14*(1), 111–135.

Sevón, E. (2005). Timing motherhood: Experiencing and narrating the choice to become a mother. *Feminism & Psychology*, *15*(4), 461–482.

Shalev, C. (2000). Rights to sexual and reproductive health: The ICPD and the convention on the elimination of all forms of discrimination against women. *Health and Human rights*, *4*(2), 38–66.

Shapiro, G. (2014). Voluntary childlessness: A critical review of the literature. *Studies in the Maternal*, *6*(1), 1–15.

Silverstein, L. B. (1996). Fathering is a feminist issue. *Psychology of Women Quarterly*, *20*, 3–37.

Winkler, T. (2017). Black texts on white paper: Learning to see resistant texts as an approach towards decolonising planning. *Planning Theory*, https://doi.org/10.1177/1473095217739335.

Appendix: Articles Analysed for Systematic Literature Review

Abbott, D. A., & Brody, G. H. (1985). The relation of child age, gender, and number of children to the marital adjustment of wives. *Journal of Marriage and the Family*, *47*(1), 77–84.

Abma, J. C., & Martinez, G. M. (2006). Childlessness among older women in the United States: Trends and profiles. *Journal of Marriage and Family*, *68*, 1045–1056.

Agrillo, C., & Nelini, C. (2008). Childfree by choice: A review. *Journal of Cultural Geography*, *25*(3), 347–363.

Bachrach, C. A. (1980). Childlessness and social isolation among the elderly. *Journal of Marriage and the Family*, *42*(3), 627–637.

Barnett, L. D., & Macdonald, R. H. (1986). Value structure of social movement members: A new perspective on the voluntary childless. *Social Behavior and Personality*, *14*(2), 149–159.

Baum, F. (1982a). Voluntarily childless marriages. *International Journal of Sociology and Social Policy*, *2*(3), 40–54.

Baum, F., & Cope, D. R. (1980). Some characteristics of intentionally childless wives in Britain. *Journal of Biosocial Science*, *12*(03), 287–300.

Baum, F. E. (1982). Voluntary childlessness and contraception: Problems and practices. *Journal of Biosocial Science*, *14*(01), 17–23.

Baum, F. E. (1983a). Orientations towards voluntary childlessness. *Journal of Biosocial Science*, *15*(02), 153–164.

Baum, F. E. (1983b). The future of voluntary childlessness in Australia. *Australian Journal of Sex, Marriage and Family*, *4*(1), 23–32.

Bernardi, L. (2003). Channels of social influence on reproduction. *Population Research and Policy Review*, *22*(5–6), 427–555.

Blackstone, A., & Stewart, M. D. (2012). Choosing to be childfree: Research on the decision not to parent. *Sociology Compass*, *6*(9), 718–727.

Blake, J. (1979). Is zero preferred? American attitudes toward childlessness in the 1970s. *Journal of Marriage and Family*, *41*(2), 245–257.

Bloom, D. E. (1982). What's happening to the age at first birth in the United States? A study of recent cohorts. *Demography*, *19*(3), 351–370.

Bloom, D. E., & Pebley, A. R. (1982). Voluntary childlessness: A review of the evidence and implications. *Population Research and Policy Review*, *1*(3), 203–224.

Bloom, D. E., & Trussell, J. (1984). What are the determinants of delayed childbearing and permanent childlessness in the United States? *Demography*, *21*(4), 591–611.

Boddington, B., & Didham, R. (2009). Increases in childlessness in New Zealand. *Journal of Population Research*, *26*(2), 131–151.

Boyd, R. L. (1989a). Racial differences in childlessness: A centennial review. *Sociological Perspectives*, *32*(2), 183–199.

Boyd, R. L. (1989b). Childlessness and social mobility during the baby boom. *Sociological Spectrum*, *9*, 425–438.

Boyd, R. L. (1989c). Minority status and childlessness. *Sociological Inquiry*, *59*(3), 331–342.

Bram, S. (1984). Voluntarily childless women: Traditional or non-traditional? *Sex Roles*, *10*(3–4), 195–206.

Bram, S. (1985). Childlessness revisited: A longitudinal study of voluntarily childless couples, delayed parents, and parents. *Lifestyles*, *8*(1), 46–66. doi:10.1007/BF01435914

Calhoun, L. G., & Selby, J. W. (1980). Voluntary childlessness, involuntary childlessness, and having children: A study of social perceptions. *Family Relations*, *29*(2), 181–183.

Callan, V. J. (1982). How do Australians value children? A review and research update using the perceptions of parents and voluntarily childless adults. *Journal of Sociology*, *18*(3), 384–398.

Callan, V. J. (1983a). Childlessness and partner selection. *Journal of Marriage and Family*, *45*(1), 181–186.

Callan, V. J. (1983b). Perceptions of parenthood and childlessness: A comparison of mothers and voluntarily childless wives. *Population and Environment*, *6*(3), 179–189. doi:10.1007/BF01258959

Callan, V. J. (1983c). Factors affecting early and late deciders of voluntary childlessness. *The Journal of Social Psychology*, *119*(2), 261–268. doi:10.1080/00224545.1983.9922830

Callan, V. J. (1983d). The voluntarily childless and their perceptions of parenthood and childlessness. *Journal of Comparative Family Studies*, *XIV*(1), 87–96.

Callan, V. J. (1984a). Childlessness and marital adjustment. *Australian Journal of Sex, Marriage and Family*, *5*(4), 210–214.

Callan, V. J. (1984b). Voluntary childlessness: Early articulator and postponing couples. *Journal of Biosocial Science*, *16*(4), 501–509.

Callan, V. J. (1985). Perceptions of parents, the voluntarily and involuntarily childless: A multidimensional scaling analysis. *Journal of Marriage and the Family*, *47*(4), 1045–1050. doi:10.2307/352349

Callan, V. J. (1986a). Pregnancy as seen by mothers wanting one or two children, voluntarily childless wives and single women. *Australian Journal of Sex, Marriage and Family*, *7*(2), 83–89.

Callan, V. J. (1986b). Single women, voluntary childlessness and perceptions about life and marriage. *Journal of Biosocial Science*, *18*(04), 479–487.

Callan, V. J. (1986c). The impact of the first birth: Married and single women preferring childlessness, one child, or two children. *Journal of Marriage and the Family*, *48*(2), 261–269.

Callan, V. J. (1987). The personal and marital adjustment of mothers and of voluntarily and involuntarily childless wives. *Journal of Marriage and Family*, *49*(4), 847–856.

Callan, V. J., & Hennessey, J. F. (1989). Psychological adjustment to infertility: A unique comparison of two groups of infertile women, mothers and women childless by choice. *Journal of Reproductive and Infant Psychology*, *7*(2), 105–112.

Callan, V. J., & Que Hee, R. W. (1984). The choice of sterilization: Voluntarily childless couples, mothers of one child by choice, and males seeking reversal of vasectomy. *Journal of Biosocial Science*, *16*(2), 241–248.

Campbell, E. (1983). Becoming voluntarily childless: An exploratory study in a Scottish city. *Social Biology*, *30*(3), 307–317.

Carlisle, E. (1982). Fertility control and the voluntarily childless: An exploratory study. *Journal of Biosocial Science*, *14*(02), 203–212.

Carmichael, G. A., & Whittaker, A. (2007). Choice and circumstance: Qualitative insights into contemporary childlessness in Australia. *European Journal of Population*, *23*(2), 111–143.

Casper, W. J., Weltman, D., & Kwesiga, E. (2007). Beyond family-friendly: The construct and measurement of singles-friendly work culture. *Journal of Vocational Behavior*, *70*(3), 478–501. doi:10.1016/j.jvb.2007.01.001

Chancey, L., & Dumais, S. A. (2009). Voluntary childlessness in marriage and family textbooks, 1950–2000. *Journal of Family History*, *34*(2), 206–223.

Connidis, I. A., & McMullin, J. A. (1999). Permanent childlessness: Perceived advantages and disadvantages among older persons. *Canadian Journal on Aging*, *18*(04), 447–465.

Daniluk, J. C., & Herman, A. L. (1984). Parenthood decision-making. *Family Relations*, *33*(4), 607–612.

De Jong, G. F., & Sell, R. R. (1977). Changes in childlessness in the United States: A demographic path analysis. *Population Studies*, *31*(1), 129–141.

DeLyser, G. (2011). At midlife, intentionally childfree women and their experiences of regret. *Clinical Social Work Journal*, *40*(1), 66–74. doi:10.1007/s10615-011-0337-2

De Rose, A., & Racioppi, F. (2001). Explaining voluntary low fertility in Europe: A multilevel approach. *Genus*, *57*(1), 13–32.

DeVellis, B. M. E., Wallston, B. S., & Acker, D. (1984). Childfree by choice: Attitudes and adjustment of sterilized women. *Population & Environment*, *7*(3), 152–162.

Dietz, T. (1984). Normative and microeconomic models of voluntary childlessness. *Sociological Spectrum*, *4*(2–3), 209–228. doi:10.1080/02732173.1984.9981719

Durham, W., & Braithwaite, D. (2009). Communication privacy management within the family planning trajectories of voluntarily child-free couples. *Journal of Family Communication*, *9*(1), 43–65. doi:10.1080/15267430802561600

Durham, W. T. (2008). The rules-based process of revealing/concealing the family planning decisions of voluntarily child-free couples: A communication privacy management perspective. *Communication Studies*, *59*(2), 132–147.

Dykstra, P. A., & Hagestad, G. O. (2007). Childlessness and parenthood in two centuries different roads—Different maps? *Journal of Family Issues*, *28*(11), 1518–1532.

Englund, C. L. (1983). Parenting and parentage: Distinct aspects of children's importance. *Family Relations*, *32*(1), 21–28.

Feldman, H. (1981). A comparison of intentional parents and intentionally childless couples. *Journal of Marriage and Family*, *43*(3), 593–600.

Fost, D. (1996). Child-free with an attitude. *American Demographics*, *18*(4) 15–17.

Gee, E. M. (1986). The life course of Canadian women: An historical and demographic analysis. *Social Indicators Research*, *18*(3), 263–283.

Geiss, L. S., McSeveney, D. R., & Floyd, H. H. (1983). Parenthood and marital happiness. *International Journal of Sociology of the Family*, *13*(1), 159–176.

Gillespie, R. (1999). Voluntary childlessness in the United Kingdom. *Reproductive Health Matters*, *7*(13), 43–53.

Gillespie, R. (2000). When no means no: Disbelief, disregard and deviance as discourses of voluntary childlessness. *Women's Studies International Forum*, *23*(2), 223–234.

Gillespie, R. (2001). Contextualizing voluntary childlessness within a postmodern model of reproduction: Implications for health and social needs. *Critical Social Policy*, *21*(2), 139–159.

Gillespie, R. (2003). Childfree and feminine: Understanding the gender identity of voluntarily childless women. *Gender & Society*, *17*(1), 122–136. doi:10.1177/0891243202238982

Gold, J. M., & Wilson, J. S. (2002). Legitimizing the child-free family: The role of the family counselor. *The Family Journal*, *10*(1), 70–74.

Goodbody, S. T. (1977). The psychosocial implications of voluntary childlessness. *Social Casework*, *58*(7), 426–434.

Greenglass, E. R., & Borovilos, R. (1985). Psychological correlates of fertility plans in unmarried women. *Canadian Journal of Behavioural Science*, *17*(2), 130–139.

Griffith, J. D., Koo, H. P., & Suchindran, C. M. (1984). Childlessness and marital stability in remarriages. *Journal of Marriage and the Family*, *46*(3), 577–585.

Hagewen, K. J., & Morgan, S. P. (2005). Intended and ideal family size in the United States, 1970–2002. *Population and Development Review*, *31*(3), 507–527. doi:10.1111/j.1728-4457.2005.00081.x

Harper, S. (2003). Changing families as European societies age. *European Journal of Sociology*, *44*(2), 155–184. doi:10.1017/S0003975603001231

Heaton, T. B., Jacobson, C. K., & Fu, X. N. (1992). Religiosity of married couples and childlessness. *Review of Religious Research*, *33*(2), 244–255.

Heaton, T. B., Jacobson, C. K., & Holland, K. (1999). Persistence and change in decisions to remain childless. *Journal of Marriage and the Family*, *61*(2), 531–539.

Heller, P. L., Tsai, Y. M., & Chalfant, H. P. (1986). Voluntary and non-voluntary childlessness: Personality vs. structural implications. *International Journal of Sociology of the Family*, *16*(1), 95–110.

Hird, M. J. (2003). Vacant wombs: Feminist challenges to psychoanalytic theories of childless women. *Feminist Review*, *75*(1), 5–19.

Hird, M. J., & Abshoff, K. (2003). Women without children: A contradiction in terms? *Journal of Comparative Family Studies*, *31*(3), 347–366.

Hoffman, S. R., & Levant, R. F. (1985). A comparison of childfree and child-anticipated married couples. *Family Relations*, *34*(2), 197–203.

Holahan, C. E. (1983). The relationship between information search in the childbearing decision and life satisfaction for parents and nonparents. *Family Relations*, *32*(4), 527–535.

Holton, S., Fisher, J., & Rowe, H. (2011). To have or not to have? Australian women's childbearing desires, expectations and outcomes. *Journal of Population Research*, *28*(4), 353–379.

Houseknecht, S. K. (1977). Reference group support for voluntary childlessness: Evidence for conformity. *Journal of Marriage and Family*, *39*(2), 285–292.

Houseknecht, S. K. (1979). Childlessness and marital adjustment. *Journal of Marriage and the Family*, *41*(2), 259–265.

Houseknecht, S. K. (1982a). Voluntary childlessness in the 1980s: A significant increase? *Marriage & Family Review*, *5*(2), 51–69.

Houseknecht, S. K. (1982b). Voluntary childlessness: Toward a theoretical integration. *Journal of Family Issues*, *3*(4), 459–471.

Jacobson, C. K., & Heaton, T. B. (1991). Voluntary childlessness among American men and women in the late 1980's. *Social Biology*, *38*(1–2), 79–93.

Jacobson, C. K., Heaton, T. B., & Taylor, K. M. (1988). Childlessness among American women. *Social Biology*, *35*(3–4), 186–197.

Jamison, P. H., Franzini, L. R., & Kaplan, R. M. (1979). Some assumed characteristics of voluntarily childfree women and men. *Psychoanalytic Inquiry*, *4*(2), 266–272.

Jeffries, S., & Konnert, C. (2002). Regret and psychological well-being among voluntarily and involuntarily childless women and mothers. *The International Journal of Aging and Human Development*, *54*(2), 89–106.

Johnson, G., Roberts, D., Brown, R., Cox, E., Evershed, Z., Goutam, P., & Swan, K. (1987). 'Infertile or childless by choice?', A multipractice survey of women aged 35 and 50. *British Medical Journal*, *294*(6575), 804–806.

Juhasz, A. M. (1980). Adolescent attitudes toward childbearing and family size. *Family Relations*, *29*(1), 29–34.

Kamalamani, E. P. (2009). Choosing to be childfree. *Therapy Today*, *20*(6), 30–33.

Kearney, H. R., & Annandale, V. (1979). Feminist challenges to social structure and sex roles. *Psychology of Women Quarterly*, *4*(1), 16–30.

Keith, P. M. (1983). A comparison of the resources of parents and childless men and women in very old age. *Family Relations*, *32*(3), 403–409.

Keizer, R., Dykstra, P. A., & Jansen, M. D. (2008). Pathways into childlessness: Evidence of gendered life course dynamics. *Journal of Biosocial Science*, *40*(6), 863–878. doi:10.1017/S0021932007002660

Keizer, R., Dykstra, P. A., & Poortman, A.-R. (2009). Life outcomes of childless men and fathers. *European Sociological Review*, *26*(1), 1–15. doi:10.1093/esr/jcn080

Keizer, R., Dykstra, P., & Poortman, A. R. (2011). Childlessness and norms of familial responsibilities in the Netherlands. *Journal of Comparative Family Studies*, *42*(4), 421–438.

Kelly, M. (2009). Women's voluntary childlessness: A radical rejection of motherhood? *Women's Studies Quarterly*, *37*(2), 157–172.

Kemkes, A. (2008). Is perceived childlessness a cue for stereotyping? Evolutionary aspects of a social phenomenon. *Biodemography and Social Biology*, *54*(1), 33–46.

Kemkes-Grottenthaler, A. (2003). Postponing or rejecting parenthood? Results of a survey among female academic professionals. *Journal of Biosocial Science*, *35*(2), 213–226. doi:10.1017/S002193200300213X

Kenkel, W. F. (1985). The desire for voluntary childlessness among low income youth. *Journal of Marriage and Family*, *47*(2), 509–512. doi:10.2307/352151

Kiernan, K. E. (1989). Who remains childless? *Journal of Biosocial Science*, *21*(4), 387–398.

Kingsley, K. D. (1938). Parents go on strike. *The North American Review*, *245*(2), 221–239.

Kiser, C. V. (1939). Voluntary and involuntary aspects of childlessness. *The Milbank Memorial Fund Quarterly*, *80*(4), 50–68.

Knodel, J., & Wilson, C. (1981). The secular increase in fecundity in German village populations: An analysis of reproductive histories of couples married 1750–1899. *Population Studies*, *35*(1), 53–84.

Knox, D. (1980). Trends in marriage and the family: The 1980's. *Family Relations*, *29*(2), 145–150.

Koepke, L., Hare, J., & Moran, P. B. (1992). Relationship quality in a sample of lesbian couples with children and child-free lesbian couples. *Family Relations*, *41*(2), 224–229.

Kohli, M., & Albertini, M. (2009). Childlessness and intergenerational transfers: What is at stake? *Ageing and Society*, *29*(8), 1171–1183. doi:10.1017/S0144686X09990341

Koropeckyj-Cox, T. (2012). Beyond parental status: Psychological well-being in middle and old age. *Journal of Marriage and Family*, *64*(4), 957–971.

Koropeckyj-Cox, T., & Pendell, G. (2007). The gender gap in attitudes about childlessness in the United States. *Journal of Marriage and Family*, *69*(4), 899–915.

Koropeckyj-Cox, T., Romano, V., & Moras, A. (2007). Through the lenses of gender, race, and class: Students' perceptions of childless/childfree individuals and couples. *Sex Roles*, *56*(7–8), 415–428. doi:10.1007/s11199-006-9172-2

Krishnan, V. (1993). Religious homogamy and voluntary childlessness in Canada. *Sociological Perspectives*, *36*(1), 83–93.

Kunz, P. R., & Brinkerhoff, M. B. (1969). Differential childlessness by color: The destruction of a cultural belief. *Journal of Marriage and Family*, *31*(4), 713–719.

Lampman, C., & Dowling-Guyer, S. (1995). Attitudes toward voluntary and involuntary childlessness. *Basic and Applied Social Psychology*, *17*(1–2), 213–222.

Lawrence, E., Rothman, A. D., Cobb, R. J., Rothman, M. T., & Bradbury, T. N. (2008). Marital satisfaction across the transition to parenthood. *Journal of Family Psychology*, *22*(1), 41–50. doi:10.1037/0893-3200.22.1.41

Letherby, G. (1999). Other than mother and mothers as others: The experience of motherhood and non-motherhood in relation to 'infertility' and 'involuntary childlessness'. *Women's Studies International Forum*, *22*(3), 359–372.

Letherby, G. (2000). Images and representation of non-motherhood. *Reproductive Health Matters*, *8*(13), 143.

Letherby, G. (2002). Childless and bereft? Stereotypes and realities in relation to 'voluntary' and 'involuntary' childlessness and womanhood. *Sociological Inquiry*, *72*(1), 7–20. doi:10.1111/1475-682X.00003

Lundquist, J. H., Budig, M. J., & Curtis, A. (2009). Race and childlessness in America, 1988–2002. *Journal of Marriage and Family*, *71*(3), 741–755.

Macklin, E. D. (1980). Non-traditional family forms: A decade of research. *Journal of Marriage and Family*, *42*(4), 905–922.

Magarick, R. H., & Brown, R. A. (1981). Social and emotional aspects of voluntary childlessness in vasectomized childless men. *Journal of Biosocial Science*, *13*(2), 157–167.

Majumdar, D. (2004). Choosing childlessness: Intentions of voluntary childlessness in the United States. *Michigan Sociological Review*, *18*, 108–135.

Marciano, T. D. (1975). Variant family forms in a world perspective. *Family Coordinator*, *24*(4), 407–420.

Marciano, T. D. (1979). Male influences on fertility: Needs for research. *Family Coordinator*, *28*(4), 561–568.

May, E. T. (1997). The politics of reproduction. *Irish Journal of American Studies*, *6*, 1–37.

McQuillan, J., & Greil, A. L. (2012). Does the reason matter? Variations in childlessness concerns among US women. *Journal of Marriage*, *74*, 1166–1181. doi:10.1111/j.1741-3737.2012.01015.x

McQuillan, J., Greil, A. L., Shreffler, K. M., & Tichenor, V. (2008). The importance of motherhood among women in the contemporary United States. *Gender & Society*, *22*(4), 477–496.

Mencarini, L., & Tanturri, M. L. (2006). High fertility or childlessness: Micro-level determinants of reproductive behaviour in Italy. *Population*, *61*(4), 389–415.

Merz, E.-M., & Liefbroer, A. C. (2012). The attitude toward voluntary childlessness in Europe: Cultural and institutional explanations. *Journal of Marriage and Family*, *74*(3), 587–600. doi:10.1111/j.1741-3737.2012.00972.x

Meyers, D. T. (2001). The rush to motherhood: Pronatalist discourse and women's autonomy. *Signs*, *26*(3), 735–773.

Mezey, N. J. (2005). Conducting multiracial feminist family research: Challenges and rewards of recruiting a diverse sample. *Michigan Family Review*, *10*, 45–65.

Mezey, N. J. (2008). The privilege of coming out: Race, class, and lesbians' mothering decisions. *International Journal of Sociology of the Family*, *34*(2), 257–276.

Miettinen, A. (2010). Voluntary or involuntary childlessness? Socio-demographic factors and childlessness intentions among childless Finnish men and women aged 25–44. *Finnish Yearbook of Population Research*, *46*, 5–24.

Mollen, D. (2006). Voluntarily childfree women: Experiences and counseling considerations. *Journal of Mental Health Counseling*, *28*(3), 269–283.

Mosher, W. D., & Bachrach, C. A. (1982). Childlessness in the United States estimates from the national survey of family growth. *Journal of Family Issues*, *3*(4), 517–543.

Movius, M. (1976). Voluntary childlessness: The ultimate liberation. *Family Coordinator*, *2*(1), 57–63.

Mueller, K. A., & Yoder, J. D. (1997). Gendered norms for family size, employment, and occupation: Are there personal costs for violating them? *Sex Roles*, *36*(3–4), 207–220.

Noordhuizen, S., de Graaf, P., & Sieben, I. (2010). The public acceptance of voluntary childlessness in the Netherlands: From 20 to 90 per cent in 30 years. *Social Indicators Research*, *99*(1), 163–181. doi:10.1007/s11205-010-9574-y

Oakley, D. (1986). Low-fertility childbearing decision-making. *Social Biology*, *33*(3–4), 249–258.

Ory, M. G. (1978). The decision to parent or not: Normative and structural components. *Journal of Marriage and Family*, *40*(3), 531–539.

Park, K. (2002). Stigma management among the voluntarily childless. *Sociological Perspectives*, *45*(1), 21–45.

Park, K. (2005). Choosing childlessness: Weber's typology of action and motives of the voluntarily childless. *Sociological Inquiry*, *75*(3), 372–402.

Parr, N. (2010). Childlessness among men in Australia. *Population Research and Policy Review*, *29*(3), 319–338.

Patterson, L. A., & Defrain, J. (1981). Pronatalism in high school family studies texts. *Family Relations*, *30*(2), 211–217.

Pearce, L. D. (2002). The influence of early life course religious exposure on young adults' dispositions toward childbearing. *Journal for the Scientific Study of Religion*, *41*(2), 325–340. doi:10.1111/1468-5906.00120

Pelton, S. L., & Hertlein, K. M. (2011). A proposed life cycle for voluntary childfree couples. *Journal of Feminist Family Therapy*, *23*(1), 39–53. doi:10.1080/08952833.2011.548703

Peterson, B. D., Pirritano, M., Tucker, L., & Lampic, C. (2012). Fertility awareness and parenting attitudes among American male and female undergraduate university students. *Human Reproduction*, *27*(5), 1375–1382. doi:10.1093/humrep/des011

Philipov, D., Spéder, Z., & Billari, F. C. (2006). Soon, later, or ever? The impact of anomie and social capital on fertility intentions in Bulgaria (2002) and Hungary (2001). *Population Studies*, *60*(3), 289–308. doi:10.1080/00324720600896080

Philliber, S. G., & Philliber, W. W. (1985). Social and psychological perspectives: A review on voluntary sterilization. *Studies in Family Planning*, *16*(1), 1–29.

Polit, D. F. (1978). Stereotypes relating to family-size status. *Journal of Marriage and the Family*, *40*(1), 105–114.

Polonko, K. A., Scanzoni, J., & Teachman, J. D. (1982). Childlessness and marital satisfaction: A further assessment. *Journal of Family Issues*, *3*(4), 545–573.

Popenoe, P. (1936). Motivation of childless marriages. *Journal of Heredity*, *27*(12), 469–472.

Popenoe, P. (1943). Childlessness: Voluntary or involuntary? *Journal of Heredity*, *34*(3), 83–85.

Poston, D. L. (1974). Income and childlessness in the United States: Is the relationship always inverse? *Social Biology*, *21*(3), 296–307.

Poston, D. L., & Gotard, E. (1977). Trends in childlessness in the United States, 1910–1975. *Social Biology*, *24*(3), 212–224.

Poston, D. L., & Kramer, K. B. (1983). Voluntary and involuntary childlessness in the United States, 1955–1973. *Social Biology*, *30*(3), 290–306.

Poston, D. L., & Szakczai, A. (1986). Patterns of marital childlessness in Hungary, 1930 to 1980. *Genus*, *35*(3–4), 267–284.

Poston, D. L., & Trent, K. (1982). International variability in childlessness: A descriptive and analytical study. *Journal of Family Issues*, *3*(4), 473–491.

Ramu, G. N. (1984). Family background and perceived marital happiness: A comparison of voluntary childless couples and parents. *Canadian Journal of Sociology*, *9*(1), 47–67.

Ramu, G. N. (1985). Voluntarily childless and parental couples: A comparison of their lifestyle characteristics. *Lifestyles*, *7*(3), 130–145. doi:10.1007/BF00986582

Ramu, G. N., & Tavuchis, N. (1986). The valuation of children and parenthood among the voluntarily childless and parental couples in Canada. *Journal of Comparative Family Studies*, *XVII*(1), 99–116.

Read, D. M. Y., Crockett, J., & Mason, R. (2012). 'It was a horrible shock': The experience of motherhood and women's family size preferences. *Women's Studies International Forum*, *35*(1), 12–21. doi:10.1016/j.wsif.2011.10.001

Reading, J., & Amatea, E. S. (1986). Role deviance or role diversification: Reassessing the psychosocial factors affecting the parenthood choice of career-oriented women. *Journal of Marriage and Family*, *48*(2), 255–260.

Ritchey, P. N., & Stokes, C. S. (1974). Correlates of childlessness and expectations to remain childless: U.S. 1967. *Social Forces*, *52*(3), 349–356.

Robb, J. E. (1920). Having right and being right. *International Journal of Ethics*, *30*(2), 196–212.

Ross, C. E., & Van Willigen, M. (1997). Education and the subjective quality of life. *Journal of Health and Social Behavior*, *38*(3), 275–297.

Ross, J., & Kahan, J. P. (1983). Children by choice or by chance: The perceived effects of parity. *Sex Roles*, *9*(1), 69–77. doi:10.1007/BF00303111

Rostad, B., Schei, B., & Sundby, J. (2006). Fertility in Norwegian women: Results from a population-based health survey. *Scandinavian Journal of Public Health*, *34*(1), 5–10. doi:10.1080/14034940510032383

Rovi, S. L. (1994). Taking 'no' for an answer: Using negative reproductive intentions to study the childless/childfree. *Population Research and Policy Review*, *13*(4), 343–365.

Rowland, D. T. (2007). Historical trends in childlessness. *Journal of Family Issues*, *28*(10), 1311–1337.

Rowland, R. (1982a). An exploratory study of the childfree lifestyle. *Journal of Sociology*, *18*(1), 17–30.

Rowland, R. (1982b). The childfree experience in the aging context: An investigation of the pronatalist bias of life-span developmental literature. *Australian Psychologist*, *17*(2), 141–150.

Rowlands, I., & Lee, C. (2006). Choosing to have children or choosing to be childfree: Australian students' attitudes towards the decisions of heterosexual and lesbian women. *Australian Psychologist*, *41*(1), 55–59. doi:10.1080/000500605 00391860

Russell, M. G., Hey, R. N., Thoen, G. A., & Walz, T. (1978). The choice of childlessness: A workshop model. *Family Coordinator*, *27*(2), 179–183.

Russo, N. F. (1979). Overview: Sex roles, fertility and the motherhood mandate. *Psychology of Women Quarterly*, *4*(1), 7–15.

Sahleyesus, D. T., Beaujot, R. P., & Zakus, D. (2006). Attitudes toward family size preferences in urban Ethiopia. *PSC Discussion Papers Series*, *19*(10), 5–10.

Schapiro, B. (1980). Predicting the course of voluntary childlessness in the 21st century. *Journal of Clinical Child & Adolescent Psychology*, *9*(2), 155–157.

Seccombe, K. (1991). Assessing the costs and benefits of children: Gender comparisons among childfree husbands and wives. *Journal of Marriage and Family*, *53*(1), 191–202.

Shaw, R. L. (2011). Women's experiential journey toward voluntary childlessness: An interpretative phenomenological analysis. *Journal of Community & Applied Social Psychology*, *21*(2), 151–163. doi:10.1002/casp

Shea, G. A. (1983). Voluntary childlessness and the women's liberation movement. *Population & Environment*, *6*(1), 17–26.
Shields, S. A., & Cooper, P. E. (1983). Stereotypes of traditional and nontraditional childbearing roles. *Sex Roles*, *9*(3), 363–376. doi:10.1007/BF00289671
Silka, L., & Kiesler, S. (1977). Couples who choose to remain childless. *Family Planning Perspectives*, *9*(1), 16–25.
Somers, M. D. (1993). A comparison of voluntarily childfree adults and parents. *Journal of Marriage and the Family*, *55*(3), 643–650.
Stobert, S., & Kemeny, A. (2003). Childfree by choice. *Canadian Social Trends*, (69), 7–11.
Tan, T. C., Tan, S. Q., & Wei, X. (2011). Cross-sectional pregnancy survey on fertility trends and pregnancy knowledge in Singapore. *The Journal of Obstetrics and Gynaecology Research*, *37*(8), 992–996. doi:10.1111/j.1447-0756.2010.01471.x
Tanturri, M. L., De Santis, G., & Seghieri, C. (2008). Economic well-being in old age in Italy: Does having children make a difference? *Genus*, *64* (1/2), 75–99.
Tanturri, M. L., & Mencarini, L. (2008). Childless or childfree? Paths to voluntary childlessness in Italy. *Population and Development Review*, *34*(1), 51–77.
Taylor, E. N. (2003). Throwing the baby out with the bathwater: Childfree advocates and the rhetoric of choice. *Women & Politics*, *24*(4), 49–76.
Terry, G., & Braun, V. (2011). Sticking my finger up at evolution: Unconventionality, selfishness, and choice in the talk of men who have had 'preemptive' vasectomies. *Men and Masculinities*, *15*(3), 207–229. doi:10.1177/1097184X11430126
Testa, M. R., & Grilli, L. (2006). The influence of childbearing regional contexts on ideal family size in Europe. *Population*, *61*(1/2), 109–137.
Testa, M. R., & Toulemon, L. (2006). Family formation in France: Individual preferences and subsequent outcomes. *Vienna Yearbook of Population Research*, *4*, 41–75.
Thompson, R., & Lee, C. (2011). Fertile imaginations: Young men's reproductive attitudes and preferences. *Journal of Reproductive and Infant Psychology*, *29*(1), 43–55. doi:10.1080/02646838.2010.544295
Tolnay, S. E., & Guest, A. M. (1982). Childlessness in a transitional population: The United States at the turn of the century. *Journal of Family History*, *7*(2), 200–219.
Touleman, L. (1996). Very few couples remain voluntarily childless. *Population*, *8*, 1–27.
Umberson, D., Pudrovska, T., & Reczek, C. (2010). Parenthood, childlessness, and well-being: A life course perspective. *Journal of Marriage and Family*, *72*(3), 612–629.
Veevers, J. E. (1973a). Voluntary childless wives: An exploratory study. *Population Studies*, *57*(3), 356–366.
Veevers, J. E. (1973b). Voluntary childlessness: A neglected area of family study. *Family Coordinator*, *22*(2), 199–205.
Veevers, J. E. (1974). Voluntary childlessness and social policy: An alternative view. *Family Coordinator*, *23*(4), 397–406.
Veevers, J. E. (1975). The moral careers of voluntarily childless wives: Notes on the defence of a variant world view. *Family Coordinator*, *24*(4), 473–487.
Vinson, C. (2010). Perceptions of childfree women: The role of the perceivers' and targets' ethnicity. *Journal of Community & Applied Social Psychology*, *20*(5), 426–432.

Chapter 2

What Is It Like Being Involuntarily Childless? Searching for Ways of Understanding from a Psychological Perspective

Megumi Fieldsend

Abstract

Becoming a mother is a significant transition in adult development. For women who wanted to have children but found themselves unable to do so, life without the fulfilment of motherhood can affect meaning-making in everyday life. Although increasing numbers of studies concerning childlessness have been carried out, much of this research has tended to focus on infertility and issues around fertility treatments. Little is known, however, about the psychological impact childlessness can have on women in midlife and how they experience the absence of children. The aim of this chapter is to offer readers an overview of psychological understanding in current research trends by reviewing papers that focus on women in midlife who are involuntarily childless. Findings from the 40 most relevant papers will be discussed under one of four key features: (1) psychological distress: medical consequences of infertility, (2) childlessness: life-span perspectives, (3) involuntary childlessness: psychosocial perspectives and (4) coping: ways of building resilience. The findings point to the dominance of quantitative approaches in researching infertility, while confirming that little has been carried out that looks at lived experience of involuntary childlessness. I hope the findings shown here will point to the necessity of psychological research applying qualitative experiential approaches that can facilitate a deeper understanding of women facing this challenge.

Keywords: Involuntary childlessness; women; midlife; experiences; psychological; review

Introduction

Having children is a milestone in adult development bringing new meanings in one's life. Normatively, people will have had children by midlife, be involved in parental roles, and engaged in careers and/or social roles (Moen & Wethington, 1999; Staudinger & Bluck, 2001). Midlife is, therefore, dynamically transitional and experiential. While there are women who choose not to have children, for those who are involuntarily childless, life without the 'heartfelt wish' (Warnock, 2002, p. 27) of motherhood can affect them in various ways and degrees, and the meaning of life itself comes under question.

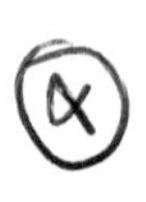

Research on childlessness tends to draw the researcher's attention to infertility and its association with medical treatments, hence its centrality can be heavily clinical. Though of importance, this may lack understanding of lived experience of involuntary childlessness, in particular, how women facing life without the children they hoped for reconstruct meanings in their lives, and how personal experiences impact on self and identity when, for example, friends and contemporaries pursue their lives with children.

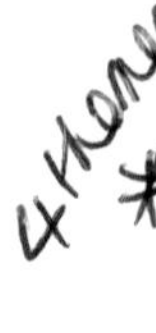

In this chapter, I will look at studies on childlessness, by reviewing papers that focus on women, involuntary childlessness and midlife. The findings from the papers reviewed here are gathered around themes, such as depression and distress, social expectations, long-term impact of the absence of children and ways of coping. Each theme that emerged is further clustered under one of the following features: (1) psychological distress: medical consequences of infertility, (2) childlessness: life-span perspectives, (3) involuntary childlessness: psychosocial perspectives and (4) coping: ways of building resilience. These key themes will be discussed individually from psychological perspectives. The aim is to offer readers an overview of psychological understanding in current research trends, and to point to the necessity of further psychological studies, considering the importance of women's personal accounts.

Involuntary Childlessness

According to the Office for National Statistics for England and Wales (2015), 'around 1 in 5 of women born in 1969' at the age of 45 are childless 'compared with 1 in 9' of their mothers' generation (born in 1942), clearly showing an increase in the number of childless women, and more understanding needs to be paid to a life without the experience of

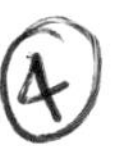

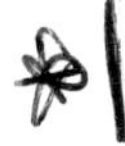

'one of the most universal, common and fundamental assumptions the majority of men and women make from an early age about their future' (Purewal & van den Akker, 2007, p. 79).

In order to view what is known in more recent research from psychological perspectives, a literature search was conducted covering publications after 1990. Five databases were used with the following search terms:

- Broader terms: midlife, involuntary childlessness and women;
- Narrower terms: mid*stage, mid*phase, mid*adulthood, unintentional, permanent, undesired, female; and
- Associated terms: years after, post-reproductive age, infertile, failed *in vitro* fertilisation (IVF).

The following results were obtained from each database:

> Sixty-two in PsychInfo/PsycARTICLES (EBISCO), 30 in Science Citation Index (Web of Science which includes Medline), 46 in Scopus (Elsevier), 19 in ScienceDirect (Elsevier) and 6 in JSTOR. Google Scholar and Discover were also used to locate additional nine papers during the search.

This initial search yielded 172 articles, excluding duplicated papers, which were further filtered down by looking at *age range* and *childless status*. The number of citations was also considered as a parameter in identifying research trends and relevance. Further, two articles published in late 1980 were also included, because they were highly cited peer-review papers and discussed key issues in understanding research on midlife and childlessness. Although titles of papers and abstracts may have seemed at first sight related to the topic, close readings revealed divergences in participants' age range and characteristics. Considering these aspects, the most relevant 40 papers were selected.

The main finding from each study reviewed was constellated, through inductive process rather than pre-defined categories, around themes that emerged. The themes were further clustered under the four broadly divided key psychological perspectives noted in the introduction, and each of these will now be discussed.

Psychological Distress: Medical Consequences of Infertility

Infertility 'has been defined variably as failure to conceive after frequent unprotected sexual intercourse for one or two years' (NICE, 2013,

p. 76). For infertile women, the development of assisted reproductive technologies (ARTs), since the first baby by IVF was born in 1978 (Warnock, 2002), has given them hope and alternative possible ways towards motherhood. However, emotional distress accompanied with fertility treatments has been found to be a strong reason for infertile couples to take the decision to cease trying to conceive (Gameiro, Boivin, Peronace, & Verhaak, 2012). Further, medical solutions provide no guarantee of success. In fact, success rates reported in the UK show a significant decrease from the age of 40–43 (13.6%) to 43–44 (5%), and less than 2% for women over 44 (see NHS UK Choices, 2016, IVF).

Sundby, Schmidt, Heldaas, Bugge, and Tanbo (2007) conducted a follow-up survey on 66 women in Norway who experienced IVF treatment 10 years prior to the study. The mean age of the participants at the time they underwent IVF was age 33 (age range: 25–40). The majority of these women had children (through IVF, spontaneous pregnancy or adoption) but 11 remained childless. The results from a questionnaire revealed that some degree of distress still existed, such as difficulty in talking about IVF experiences. However, most of the participants were found to be getting on with their everyday lives. The study indicates that infertility is a temporal life event rather than negatively affecting one's life for a long time. The paper makes a contribution to understanding the consequences of IVF experience years afterwards. However, the main issue seems to be that the quantified results are based on 82% (N = 55) of the women who succeeded in having children. This finding may undervalue the voices of women who experienced IVF and go through life without the children they hoped for.

Depression and Distress

Much previous research on infertility has tended to focus on issues around depression, anxiety and self-esteem, and questionnaires and scale measures have been used widely (Greil, 1997). The impact of infertility is, therefore, commonly evaluated with standardised measures.

For example, Demyttenaere, Nijs, Evers-Kiebooms, and Koninckx's (1991) study found higher levels of depression in infertile women than normative levels found in the general population. A study by Connolly, Edelmann, Cooke, and Robson (1992) on infertile couples reported higher mental distress in women than men. Both studies used state-trait anxiety inventory, depression inventory and health-related scales as a part of measuring distress levels.

In more recent years, Schwerdtfeger and Shreffler (2009) looked at mothers and involuntarily childless women (2,894 in total) who were at 'childbearing age (25–45)' (p. 215) to examine the psychological impact of their reproductive experiences. Data were drawn from the National Survey of Fertility Barriers conducted in the United States. A comparative study was carried out over the four sub-groups: mothers – without fertility issues (46%); mothers – experienced pregnancy loss (42%); childless – experienced pregnancy loss (4%) and childless – infertile/not yet conceived (8%). The time elapsed since those mothers and childless women who experienced pregnancy loss, and those childless women being infertile, was more than seven years. Depression levels across the groups were examined using a 10-item (e.g. 'I felt depressed', 'I was happy') self-report depression scale. Fertility-related distress was calculated by the participants' response rates (yes = 1, no = 0) to a series of questions given. The statistical analyses showed that regardless of motherhood status, a higher level of depression was found in women who experienced a pregnancy loss and/or infertility. In particular, women in both childless groups showed the lowest happiness levels compared with those in mothers' groups, and women in the childless-infertile group scored the highest on the item 'could not get going' (to indicate a depressive attitude) on the depression scales. This chapter reports the traumatic consequences that loss and infertility have on involuntary childlessness. It should be noted, however, that the findings are drawn from pre-selected items with scale measures, and outcomes of infertility are represented within these limitations.

Desire and Regret

The experience of infertility clearly indicates the need for research looking into the psychological implications, particularly for women whose desire to have biological children was disrupted. van Balen and Trimbos-Kemper (1995) looked at desire and motives to have children and examined 108 couples with an average of 8.6 years of infertility. The authors used 'the parenthood-motivation list' which consists of six categorised motives (well-being, happiness, identity, control, parenthood and continuity), and the levels of desire were also measured using a six-point Likert-scale. In their study, women showed a greater and more enduring desire than men to have their own children, with anticipated happiness as a motive. Similar results were found by Koropeckyj-Cox (2002), who used data from the National Survey (US) of Families and Households. The authors looked at parental status and attitude towards children to examine their influences on psychological well-being. The participants were 2,073 women and 1,259 men (age range: 50–84). The paper reports that childless women who showed the attitude of 'better to have a child' are more disposed to psychological distress (e.g. depression and loneliness) than childless people with 'OK to be childless' and parents irrespective of whether or not having 'excellent relationships' with their children existed. Considering the participants age range, the prolonged desire to have children still remains among childless women who seem to have ongoing self-discrepancies.

Regret also possibly induces distress. Jeffries and Konnert (2002) examined 'a child-related regret' among involuntarily childless women, voluntarily childless women and mothers. The authors interviewed 72 women (age range: 45–83) using a series of questions and self-rated measures. A question about 'reasons for having or not having children' was used to identity parental status and how women evaluate themselves in terms of their status, and their child-related perception were examined. A half (50%) of involuntarily childless women showed child-related regrets over the 'general absence of children' in comparison to 30% of voluntarily childless women. More than half of mothers showed regret over their attitude towards and time spending with their children, but no regret for having children. In terms of age differences, younger women (aged between 45 and 54) showed more regret than older women (age range: 55–83) in their study. The findings revealed that both involuntarily childless women and mothers have distress over their child-related regrets. There is an issue, however, in the division among childlessness women, in that instead of self-identified childless statuses, women were categorised as either involuntary or voluntary by the authors depending on their responses to the question on reasons given during the interviews. Although the authors acknowledge this point, women's personal perceptions towards childlessness in this regard may have been underestimated.

Greil, Slauson-Blevins, and McQuillan's (2010) review paper points out concerns about the dominant use of quantitative methods as well as 'clinical emphases' (p. 140) on infertility research. The authors argue for the need of more quantitative and qualitative integrations in research methods, while also acknowledging methodological progressions.

Childlessness: Life-span Perspectives

Existing literature has also reported prolonged mental health issues, such as persistence of anxiety, depression and stress (Cousineau & Domar, 2007; McQuillan, Greil, White, & Jacob, 2003) and profound grief (Kirkman, 2003). Infertility, therefore, could challenge women emotionally and psychologically over the course of their lives. More qualitatively oriented studies have tended to look at infertility or involuntary childlessness as part of life-span perspectives.

Long-term Impact of the Absence of Children

Johansson and Berg (2005) looked at the life-world of eight childless women (aged between 34 and 41) who stopped their IVF treatment two years prior to the study. All the participants had experienced difficulties in conceiving over a period of more than seven years. Of the eight women, one had a foster-child and was in the process of adopting another child at the time of interview. Data were gathered through interviews and analysed using Giorgi's descriptive phenomenological method. Five descriptive features presented are 'childlessness is a central part of life', 'IVF is a positive and important part of life', 'contact with other people is not important', 'hope of achieving a pregnancy still exists' and 'attempts to find other central values in life'. The paper describes 'life-grief' (p. 60) as the core structure of involuntary childlessness.

Daniluk (1996) interviewed 37 infertile women (aged between 25 and 44, mean age = 36) who had sought medical intervention. The duration attempting to conceive was from two to 15 years (average 6.4 years), but 'recently abandoned their efforts to bear a child' (p. 81). The data were analysed using Colaizzi's seven-step descriptive phenomenological method to examine lived experience of biological childlessness. Nine themes emerged that illustrate subjective meanings structure attached to a transitional process, such as 'sense of futility in continuing to pursue solutions to their infertility'; 'profound sense of loss and grief'; 'need for acceptance and support from significant others' and 'sense of relief at taking back their lives'. The findings suggest that infertility is not only a single event in life but is a long-term adaptation process. The paper presents cognitive involvement of 'reevaluation of their beliefs, needs, and priorities' (p. 95) as well as emotional preparation and social support to initiate identity and meaning reconstructions.

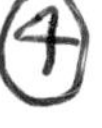

Another phenomenologically oriented paper by McCarthy (2008) examined lived experience of 22 women aged between 33 and 48 (mean age = 39.9) with an average of 3.9 years post-failed treatment. The mean years for the women who had undergone treatments was 4.1. The participants were interviewed and described the experience of their treatment. One thing of note here is that half of the participants who had adopted or had step-children identified themselves as infertile, and took part in talking about their fertility treatment experiences. The analysis revealed the women's contradictive sense over infertility, referring to their experiences as 'loss and opportunity', 'emptiness and gratitude' and infertility as a 'present absence'. The core structure of these experiences was illustrated as '[l]iving an existential paradox' (p. 321). The paper highlights temporal and qualitative experiences of infertility and suggests the need to understand the influences these have on women's life.

Ferland and Caron (2013) emphasise the lack of research considering the long-term influence infertility has on life for childless women who experienced failed fertility treatment. The authors interviewed 12 women aged between 46 and 59 (mean age = 54) who were postmenopausal. The duration participants pursued medical interventions was from two to 11 years (mean six years), indicating the long-term medical impact of infertility. The three main themes that emerged are presented into stages: 'finding out', 'living with it' and 'coming to terms'. For the participants, life is with an ongoing grieving process, referring to infertility as 'the death of child they [the participants] never had' (p. 187). The women recount feelings of an unjustifiable sense towards the loss of hope, shame and guilt 15–25 years after the treatments, illustrating the long-term impact of being involuntarily childless. The study also suggests the positive implication that caring for other children seems to help the women in alternating the lost meaning attached to the hope of becoming mothers. Although, it is difficult to see the exact process of analysis, because the authors refer to it with the general term 'established methods of qualitative inquiry' (p. 183), unlike survey studies, this paper shows insightful features the women are dealing with in everyday life.

Women living without the heartfelt children they wished for entails a passage towards non-motherhood. Infertility could become involuntary childlessness as life progresses through the childbearing phase into midlife and beyond. As Mynarska, Matysiak, Rybińska, Tocchioni, and Vignoli (2015) state, involuntary childlessness is a dynamic process 'influenced by the continuously changing context' (p. 35). Burns (1987) also points to the notion that 'infertility is involuntary childlessness' (p. 359), because although the children women hoped for are physically not present, they may be 'psychologically present' (p. 359) in the family-oriented social system.

Involuntary Childlessness: Psychosocial Perspectives

Matthews and Matthews's (1986) paper seems to be one of the earlier theoretical papers arguing the need for academic study on infertility and involuntary childlessness similar to that conducted on parenthood.

They argue that the development of ARTs led researchers to investigate fertility treatment and infertility, or medical causes of infertility. However, very little attention or investigation has been paid to social as well as psychological consequences of involuntary childlessness. The authors draw on symbolic interactionism and emphasise the importance of understanding passages infertile couples go through, the process that interplays between self, identity and social roles, and 'the often psychologically painful transition to nonparenthood' (p. 642).

Self and Identity

Letherby (2002) concurs with Matthews and Matthews's (1986) notion and draws necessary awareness of differences but also overlapping consequences of 'the biological condition of "infertility" and the social experience of "involuntary childlessness"' (Letherby, 2002, p. 277). The author points out that 'as the life course continues, "infertility" and "involuntary" childlessness may take on a different significance' (p. 285) and when medical or biological solutions are not achieved, the evaluation of experiences will become 'the social experience' (p. 282) of involuntary childlessness.

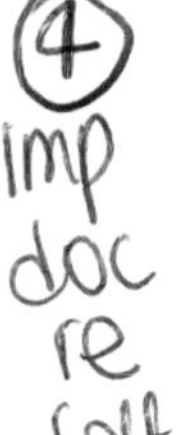

This notion was captured in Letherby's (1999) exploratory study on 65 self-identified infertile and/or involuntarily childless women, which shows a complex perceived sense of self and identity. The women who participated in the study include 12 biological (secondly infertile or children with ARTs) and eight social (e.g. through adoption, fostering or with step-children) mothers, and also women without children (e.g. failed medical attempts or unexplained infertility). Of the 65, data on 24 were gathered through interviews and 41 by correspondence, and a grounded theory (GT)-oriented analysis was conducted. All of the women (age range from early 20s to early 70s) – both mothers and non-mothers – shared a sense of being others and strangers in society. The paper reports on the influence that the dominant social discourse of motherhood has on expected motherhood and the participants' highly stigmatised sense of self.

The perception towards infertility shifts in various social and relational contexts. Todorova and Kotzeva (2006) used interview data of nine (eight primary and one secondary infertile, aged 22–41) women and investigated their 2–12 years of infertility and their treatment experiences. The study employed interpretative phenomenological analysis (IPA; Smith, Flowers, & Larkin, 2009), and four themes emerged which refer to the complex identity constructions drawing on both medical and social contexts. For example, the experience of fertility treatments exhibits incomplete sense of self with emptiness that needs to be fulfilled, and a self-governed identity is found as a determinant during the treatment. With this, the childless situation brings a separated sense of self from society, and further this influences relational connections between the self and other, and with a partner/husband. Although, the participants in their study still had hope for children, the paper highlights socially influential identity constructions that derive from 'separate, autonomous and agentic' (p. 136) experiences of infertility.

Relationships

Relationships with others and society are highlighted in existing literature typically by making comparisons between parents and childless individuals. Klaus and Schnettler (2016) used a longitudinal survey study examining social support and social networks among 5,782 individuals in Germany, of which 655 (11%) were childless. The authors were interested in looking at both men and women aged 40 and over in order to investigate social relationships happening in their mid and later lives. Their comparative study of parents revealed positive outcomes of childless adults, in that childless individuals tended to have greater stability among their 'friends and collateral kin' (p. 102) than those with parents. Further, childless individuals tended to receive more effective support from their friends and collateral kin compared with the support that parents received from their own children. The paper reports evidence that life without children does not always have negative social relationships, namely social isolation.

Albertini and Mencarini (2014) used the data of 33,759 individuals from the 2003 Italian Gender and Generation survey. The age range shown in the study was from 30s to 70s and beyond, with a mean age of 53.7. This was also a comparative study between childless individuals and parents (both genders included), investigating support given and received in their lives. The results agreed with the positive finding of Klaus and Schnettler (2016). However, the data further pointed to the notion that childless individuals, particularly those in their 50s and 60s showed a tendency to have fewer personal relationships with others. Though this was not identified as a factor leading to social isolation, the paper suggested the need of organisational or health professionals' involvement in supporting them in their later lives.

Although similar findings have been addressed in other studies, they seem to be drawn from sociological and demographical data available with their focus on aging and gerontological concerns (e.g. Dykstra & Hagestad, 2007a, 2007b; Wenger, Scott, & Patterson, 2000), neglecting the qualitative differences between voluntary and involuntary childlessness.

Social relationships often develop through online communities. Malik and Coulson (2013) specifically focused on women living with *permanent involuntary childlessness* and examined messages posted in one of the biggest and active online support communities. A total of 224 online messages (with 49 identified using unique names) was analysed using thematic analysis. This qualitative study revealed the importance of online communities as a safe platform for social connections. The analysis showed deeper levels of shared concerns as well as positive feelings accompanied with the feelings of belonging within this online community. The themes presented were 'feeling like an outsider', 'a whole lifetime of loss', 'coming to terms with childlessness' and 'finding a safe haven online'. The paper illustrates women's tendency to isolation in their everyday social contexts. A shortcoming of this, however, may be that online-message-base data collection lacks participants' homogeneity. As the author pointed out, it is difficult to obtain further information on individuals due to anonymity. In addition, and intuitively, there may be an online community discourse specific to this support group. If this is the case, there may be women who share involuntary childlessness but find difficulties in sharing their positions in the discourse; therefore, idiographic accounts for such women are potentially difficult to capture.

Social Expectations

Women living in their midlife without children are often viewed as career-oriented, non-normative people rather than family-oriented, normative people (Newton & Stewart, 2013). Riessman (2000) conducted fieldwork in southern India (Kerala) on infertility. The experiences of 31 married infertile women (aged 22–57) on their social interactions were examined using a Grounded Theory principle. The infertile women in her study were found to be facing and negotiating ways of dealing with normatively constructed beliefs and values, as well as social expectations. Reflecting on her research, she refers to the point that investigating life without children needs to take into account the importance of social influences on women rather than looking at their life as a consequence of infertility or a medically influenced life course.

Loftus and Andriot (2012) investigated psychosocial influences and the impact that 'a failed life course transition' (p. 241) had on women who were infertile. The authors interviewed 40 women aged between 25 and 46 (mean age = 33.8), and the data were examined using qualitative data analysis software. The emergent features the paper reports on include: 'Retreating to men', 'Rejection', 'Failure' and 'Exclusion'. Unable to have their own children, these women equate a sense of failure with that of meeting a social expectation. The impact of the loss of expected discourses with mothers was also reported. An inability to share this gendered status of womanhood was found to be a significant issue on social interactions, particularly difficulties in keeping positive relationships with other women with children.

Coping: Ways of Building Resilience

For childless women, being with mothers could be a constant reminder of what they could not have and their hardships. Everydayness in itself, therefore, could become a 'second-wave trigger of reflection' (Mälkki, 2012, p. 207).

Influences of Partner/Husband

Accounts of women as well as men embedded within everyday situations were captured by Peters, Jackson, and Rudge (2011). The authors conducted a narrative analysis on five heterosexual married couples who remained childless. Their desires to have children were lost when their fertility treatments ended unsuccessfully. The participants' struggles, especially women, over incompatibilities with social norms were evidenced through their life story narratives, such as 'on the edge of society' or 'sitting on a different side of the world'. The paper illustrated neatly the important role the couples' *dyadic* relationships played in everyday social and individual resilience.

Similarly, extended literature that looks at relationships among couples has evidenced the effect that close relationships has on successful coping to adverse situations. For example, in Sydsjö, Svanberg, Lampic, and Jablonowska's (2011) study, data were collected from the 206 couples (women with a mean age of 47, men with a mean age of 49) who had undergone the process of IVF more than 20 years ago. In order to measure individuals' evaluations on their marital relationships, the authors used the self-reported questionnaire ENRICH. The inventory covers different dimensions, such as 'conflict resolution', 'family and friends' and 'conception of life'. Although the majority of couples had more than one child (biological or adopted children) since their last IVF attempt, the overall findings suggest the effectiveness of couples' enduring relationships on their lives. In particular, the level of consolation with feelings of emotional sharing in the couples' relationships was found to be higher in childless couples than in those with children.

Coping and Social Connections

The construction of relational connections is complex and diverse, and it could play a role in the effect on individuals' coping styles. A cross-sectional study conducted by Lechner, Bolman, and van Dalen (2007) examined the association between satisfaction of psychosocial support received, coping styles (*active* or *passive*) and distress among 116 involuntarily childless individuals (87 women and 24 men) with a mean age of 39 (SD = 6.0). A series of scale base questionnaires was used for data collection. The results show that there is a tendency among women to use passive coping styles, such as 'withdrawing your[one]self completely from others'. With this characteristic, high levels of distress, such as depression and complicated grief, were found in women who felt the lack of support. The paper reports the necessity of continuous support with the suggestion that sufferers take active coping strategies. A criticism of using these questionnaires, however, is that one item shown in the passive coping styles assessment was 'escaping in fantasies'. This could be seen as a passive attitude. However, such a passive coping style could also, for some people, be of help in dealing with everyday life. This point will be addressed briefly in the following section.

Bergart (2000) presents the accounts of 10 married women (age range: 32–45) investigating how they 'viewed their lives' (p. 49) after failed fertility treatment. The data were gathered through interviews and analysed using Grounded Theory. The paper highlights the women's physical and emotional struggles during the process of having treatments and the extended influences this had on their lives. The women showed a sense of 'loss of control', having their lives in 'limbo', 'being seduced into false hope' and doctors' influences on their 'decision[s] to stop'. This paper is persuasive on the claim made for the need of better relationship establishment with social workers and medical professionals during and after treatments, which would further assist women to develop ways of coping. The relational deficits were viewed by the participants, suggesting the author illustrates structural accounts of the women's lives.

Theoretical Perspectives on Coping

Several papers discuss theoretical perspectives on ways of coping. The following are brief overviews of three key papers that help in understanding different aspects in coping styles.

(1) Psychosocial influences on cognitive coping strategies

Folkman and Lazarus (1980) defined coping as 'the cognitive and behavioral efforts made to master, tolerate, or reduce external and internal demands and conflicts among them' (p. 223). Making efforts can be influenced by an individual's appraisal to a stressful event encounter. According to the authors, a stressful situation can be evaluated in three forms, either 'feels harmed, threatened, or challenged' (p. 223). Based on this evaluation, a person makes an effort to manage or alter the stressor itself (problem-focused coping) and/or regulate emotion (emotion-focused coping): the transactional model of stress and coping (Lazarus & Folkman, 1984).

For women, going through fertility treatment, the problem is one of conceiving. Under this circumstance, although emotion-focused coping may also be involved, a woman may make an effort to manage the situation by trying a different type of fertility treatment as a way of problem-focused coping. For permanently involuntarily childless people, coping resources for managing their childless situations may be limited. Chochovski, Moss, and Charman (2013) emphasise the importance psychosocial influences have on coping strategies in such situations. The authors were interested in the impact of resilience and the quality of relationships that a partner/husband has on women's cognitive coping strategies. In their study, data were collected from 184 childless women (age range: 21–29 = 19%, 30–39 = 64% and 40–49 = 17%) who all 'had unsuccessfully completed IVF treatment' (p. 123). In the study, more than 70% of the participants ended their last IVF within the past '0–6 months'. The study used self-reported scale-based questionnaires examining resilience, relationship quality and depression (level of stress). The results revealed that women who showed a high level of resilience, reappraised their feelings positively and regulated their emotions. However, the effect this had on coping tended to be temporary, whereas, relationship quality with partner/husband seemed to provide *a secure attachment* as the time following IVF progressed. This seemed to result in developing positive coping to the situation. The paper suggests the necessities of looking at psychosocial factors that can help in reducing emotional demands and facilitate positive coping.

(2) Life longings: a self-regulatory strategy

An underpinning of self-regulation involves conscious control to change the self, and '[t]he capacity to self-regulate in order to manage complex social relationships constitutes an essential skill that holds families, groups, and even whole societies together' (Forgas, Baumeister, & Tice, 2009, p. 3). Broadly, there seem to be five features in self-regulating processes: 'controlling one's thoughts', 'controlling emotions and moods', 'confining impulses (automatic responses) by behavioural changes', 'regulating motivation' and 'regulating performances' (Forgas et al., 2009).

Kotter-Grühn, Scheibe, Blanchard-Fields, and Baltes (2009) introduced the concept of 'life longings' (p. 634) that have six underlying characteristics: 'feelings of incompleteness', 'dealing with utopian conceptions of life that are not fully attainable', 'tritime focus – from the past and anticipated meaningful experiences in the present and future', 'reflection and evaluation – comparing actual situations with ideal ones', 'ambivalent emotions' and 'symbolically rich in emotional and mental meaning – for the object of longing'. The authors applied a quasi-experimental questionnaire design to examine whether having children for childless women represents a goal or arises as a life longing, and how the experience of life longing has been an influence on their lives. Data were collected from 168 middle-aged (age range: 33–53, mean age = 45.2) childless women, of which the main findings were drawn from 102 involuntarily childless women.

The hope to have one's own children for involuntarily childless women was found to be an unaccomplished goal that resulted in a significant loss in their lives, and because the intensity of the wish was strong, it appeared to be difficult to let go of the desire. The findings refer to this point as:

> When a goal was unsuccessfully pursued over a long time, women might finally disengage from active goal pursuit (i.e., they withdraw effort) but continue pursuing it at the level of imagination (i.e., they remain cognitively and emotionally committed). (Kotter-Grühn et al., 2009, p. 641)

This indicates that having children is not merely a failed goal but it influences on tritime (temporal continuity), as well as on self-regulation. For the participants who are still unable to adjust the goal, the experience of life longing seems to provide them with a way of dealing with loss by replacing it with 'meaningful fantasies that persons can engage in to feel more complete' (p. 635). This appears to be accompanied by having controllability over the life longing situation. The overall results suggest a potential functionality over the experience of life longing as 'a loss-based compensatory strategy' (p. 635) – another way that self-regulation operates.

(3) Empathic activism

Nouel (2007) presented the concept of 'empathic activism' (p. 236), a compassionate and transformative coping strategy.

> It requires that a person move toward grasping others' experiences and be moved to act on their behalf, as well as to address the conditions from which these situations may arise. (Nouel, 2007, p. 239)

The author goes on to explain that this process takes a 'Buddhist conception' (p. 239) and 'a way of bridging a duality common in [our] Western thinking of action and relationship' (p. 240).

Employing this as a conceptual framework, the author interviewed four mothers who lost their children through tragedies. Although the instances are different from the invisible losses of involuntary childlessness, it might be possible to refer to the concept of understanding ways of dealing with the physically absent but the psychologically present childless situation (Boss, 2006; Burns, 1987). Data were examined through existential and phenomenological lenses. The women's shared accounts are illustrated as a form of narrative. The processes emerging are reactions to what happened with emotional struggles; recollective accounts that speak of their hidden sense of loss and a sense of isolation from the world around. However, the mothers appear to find connections with other women who had similar experiences and are able to share or support each other. Through these new connections, the women seem to regain their sense of usefulness by making use of their own experience.

> Helping others also helps her in return by giving her a sense that she is making a difference. She becomes aware that the knowledge and compassion gained from her experience can make a difference for others. (Nouel, 2007, p. 243)

The author emphasises that dealing with a loss 'does not necessarily require letting go' (p. 254) of the sadness, but transforming it by actively and empathically engaging in helping others. In other words, empathic activism could facilitate in transforming relationships with attached symbolic features of loss into a gradual, and psychologically and socially involved, coping strategy.

Concluding Discussion

The first feature of involuntary childlessness was discussed from clinical viewpoints. Issues around infertility and the experiences of having ARTs were the main concerns. The studies report that the impact of infertility could be temporary. However, they also show the great psychological distress among infertile women, particularly, that of depression and anxiety. The second theme described a continuous sense of loss and grief that further seemed to entail a passage towards non-motherhood. The prolonged desire to have children and regrets over children not being present appear as sources underpinning such distress. When women stop their fertility treatments, the medical consequences of infertility can become tritime experiences, and the influences of childlessness over one's life course were discussed. The third aspect pointed to the psychosocial experiences of involuntary childlessness. The studies around self and identity, relationships with others and society and social expectations have shown the relational impact these have on women. Here, it appears that the complexities of gendered discourse and stigmatised women's accounts highlight the legitimacy of biologically childless women and the challenges they face in their everyday lives. The final theme elucidated women's ways of dealing with life. The influences of partner/husband on coping have been evidenced in several studies. Three studies that capture coping strategies were also discussed looking at different aspects of coping styles.

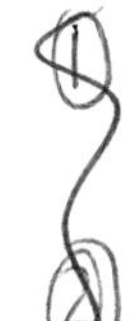
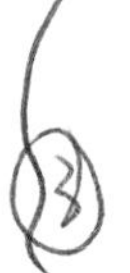
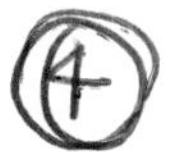
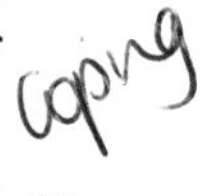

This chapter has shown the disparate issues existing among involuntarily childless women, and papers reviewed here have revealed the intricate nature of the psychological impact that childlessness has on women and their lives. While many studies have focused on infertility and its treatment experiences, little is known about what it is actually like being involuntarily childless, in that research explicitly trying to get at experiences of women after they stopped pursuing motherhood seems to have been neglected. In addition, women who are involuntarily childless, but have not experienced medical interventions, appear to have been of less concern.

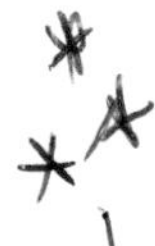

Methodologically, much existing literature has tended to employ questionnaires and been evaluated with standardised measures. The dominance of quantitative approaches is noticeable, particularly in

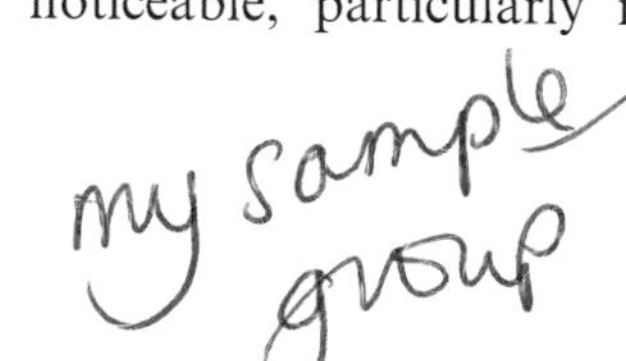

studies looking at infertility from medical viewpoints. Quantitative research is useful to examine, for example, the levels of depression childless women might have when compared nomothetically with other women with children. However, it can undervalue a personal account or feeling associated with depression, which is caused by the absence of children.

In contrast, more qualitatively oriented methods have appeared to be used in investigating involuntary childlessness from life-span perspectives. These often accompany psychosocial inquiries. Increasing numbers of phenomenologically oriented studies have also been identified with their focus on experiences. However, they seem to try to investigate core structures of experiences rather than looking into the process of what individuals are experiencing as they live. It has also been noticed that extant literature examining qualitative aspects of life without children appears to emphasise socially constructed viewpoints, and intrapersonal features of involuntary childlessness appear to be less focused on.

The diverse themes that emerged from the literature reviewed in itself tells us that experiences of childlessness cannot be quantified under a one dimensional focus. Both intrapersonal and interpersonal processes can also be considered qualitatively in order to gain rich data. Childlessness is increasing. Midlife develops dynamically. Research that can raise social awareness of involuntary childlessness, as well as a deeper psychological understanding of women living with involuntary childlessness, is clearly needed.

Acknowledgements

I would like to thank Professor Jonathan A. Smith and an anonymous reviewer for their helpful comments on an earlier draft of this chapter. Thanks also to Dr Natalie Sappleton, the editor, who gave me the opportunity to submit my work.

References

Albertini, M., & Mencarini, L. (2014). Childlessness and support networks in later life: New pressures on familistic welfare states? *Journal of Family Issues*, *35*(3), 331–357.

Bergart, A. M. (2000). The experience of women in unsuccessful infertility treatment: What do patients need when medical intervention fails? *Social Work in Health Care*, *30*(4), 45–70.

Boss, P. (2006). *Loss, trauma, and resilience: Therapeutic work with ambiguous loss*. New York, NY: Norton.

Burns, L. H. (1987). Infertility as boundary ambiguity: One theoretical perspective. *Family Process*, *26*(3), 359–372. doi:10.1111/j.1545-5300.1987.00359.x

Chochovski, J., Moss, S. A., & Charman, D. P. (2013). Recovery after unsuccessful in vitro fertilization: The complex role of resilience and marital relationships. *Journal of Psychosomatic Obstetrics & Gynaecology*, *34*(3), 122–128. doi:10.3109/0167482X.2013.829034

Connolly, K. J., Edelmann, R. J., Cooke, I. D., & Robson, J. (1992). The impact of infertility on psychological functioning. *Journal of Psychosomatic Research*, *36*(5), 459–468.

Cousineau, T. M., & Domar, A. D. (2007). Psychological impact of infertility. *Best Practice & Research Clinical Obstetrics & Gynaecology*, *21*(2), 293–308.

Daniluk, J. C. (1996). When treatment fails: The transition to biological childlessness for infertile women. *Women & Therapy*, *19*(2), 81–98.

Demyttenaere, K., Nijs, P., Evers-Kiebooms, G., & Koninckx, P. R. (1991). Coping, ineffectiveness of coping and the psychoendocrinological stress responses during in-vitro fertilization. *Journal of Psychosomatic Research*, *35*, 231–243.

Dykstra, P. A., & Hagestad, G. O. (2007a). Roads less taken: Developing a nuanced view of older adults without children. *Journal of Family Issues*, *28*(10), 1275–1310.

Dykstra, P. A., & Hagestad, G. O. (2007b). Childlessness and parenthood in two centuries: Different roads – Different maps? *Journal of Family Issues*, *28*(11), 1518–1532.

Ferland, P., & Caron, S. L. (2013). Exploring the long-term impact of female infertility: A qualitative analysis of interviews with postmenopausal women who remained childless. *The Family Journal*, *21*(2), 180–188. doi:10.1177/1066480712466813

Folkman, S., & Lazarus, R. S. (1980). An analysis of coping in middle-aged community sample. *Journal of Health and Social Behavior*, *21*(3), 219–239.

Forgas, J. P., Baumeister, R. F., & Tice, D. M. (2009). The psychology of self-regulation: An introductory review. In J. P. Forgas, R. F. Baumeister, & D. M. Tice (Eds.), *Psychology of self-regulation: Cognitive, affective, and motivational processes* (pp. 1–17). New York, NY: Psychology Press.

Gameiro, S., Boivin, J., Peronace, L., & Verhaak, C. M. (2012). Why do patients discontinue fertility treatment? A systematic review of reasons and predictors of discontinuation in fertility treatment. *Human Reproduction Update*, *18*(6), 652–669.

Greil, A. L. (1997). Infertility and psychological distress: A critical review of the literature. *Social Science & Medicine*, *45*(11), 1679–1704. doi:10.1016/S0277-9536(97)00102-0

Greil, A. L., Slauson-Blevins, K., & McQuillan, J. (2010). The experience of infertility: A review of recent literature. *Sociology of Health & Illness*, *32*(1), 140–162. doi:10.1111/j.1467-9566.2009.01213.x

Jeffries, S., & Konnert, C. (2002). Regret and psychological well-being among voluntarily and involuntarily childless women and mothers. *International Journal of Aging and Human Development*, *54*(2), 89–106.

Johansson, M., & Berg, M. (2005). Women's experiences of childlessness 2 years after the end of in vitro fertilization treatment. *Scandinavian Journal of Caring Sciences*, *19*(1), 58–63. doi:10.1111/j.1471-6712.2005.00319.x

Kirkman, M. (2003). Infertile women and the narrative work of mourning: Barriers to the revision of autobiographical narratives of motherhood. *Narrative Inquiry*, *13*(1), 243–262. doi:10.1075/ni.13.1.09kir

Klaus, D., & Schnettler, S. (2016). Social networks and support for parents and childless adults in the second half of life: Convergence, divergence, or stability? *Advances in Life Course Research*, *29*, 95–105. doi:10.1016/j.alcr.2015.12.004

Koropeckyj-Cox, T. (2002). Beyond parental status: Psychological well-being in middle and old age. *Journal of Marriage and Family*, *64*(4), 957–971. Retrieved from http://www.jstor.org/stable/3599995

Kotter-Grühn, D., Scheibe, S., Blanchard-Fields, F., & Baltes, P. B. (2009). Developmental emergence and functionality of Sehnsucht (life longings): The sample case of involuntary childlessness in middle-aged women. *Psychology and Aging*, *24*(3), 634–644. doi:10.1037/a0016359

Lazarus, R. S., & Folkman, S. (1984). *Stress, appraisal, and coping*. New York, NY: Springer.

Lechner, L., Bolman, C., & van Dalen, A. (2007). Definite involuntary childlessness: Associations between coping, social support and psychological distress. *Human Reproduction*, *22*(1), 288–294. doi:10.1093/humrep/del327

Letherby, G. (1999). Other than mother and mothers as others: The experience of motherhood and non-motherhood in relation to 'infertility' and 'involuntary childlessness'. *Women's Studies International Forum*, *22*(3), 359–372.

Letherby, G. (2002). Challenging dominant discourses: Identity and change and the experience of 'infertility' and 'involuntary childlessness'. *Journal of Gender Studies*, *11*(3), 277–288. doi:10.1080/0958923022000002124

Loftus, J., & Andriot, A. L. (2012). That's what makes a woman: Infertility and coping with a failed life course transition. *Sociological Spectrum*, *32*(3), 226–243.

Malik, S. H., & Coulson, N. S. (2013). Coming to terms with permanent involuntary childlessness: A phenomenological analysis of bulletin board postings. *Europe's Journal of Psychology*, *9*(1), 77–92. doi:10.5964/ejop.v9i1.534

Mälkki, K. (2012). Rethinking disorienting dilemmas within real-life crises: The role of reflection in negotiating emotionally chaotic experiences. *Adult Education Quarterly*, *62*(3), 207–229. doi:10.1177/0741713611402047

Matthews, R., & Matthews, A. M. (1986). Infertility and involuntary childlessness: The transition to nonparenthood. *Journal of Marriage and Family*, *48*(3), 641–649.

McCarthy, M. P. (2008). Women's lived experience of infertility after unsuccessful medical intervention. *Journal of Midwifery & Women's Health*, *53*(4), 319–324. doi:10.1016/j.jmwh.2007.11.004

McQuillan, J., Greil, A. L., White, L., & Jacob, M. C. (2003). Frustrated fertility: Infertility and psychological distress among women. *Journal of Marriage and Family*, *65*(4), 1007–1018. doi:10.1111/j.1741-3737.2003.01007.x

Moen, P., & Wethington, E. (1999). Midlife development in a life course context. In S. L. Willis & J. D. Reid (Eds.), *Life in the middle: Psychological and social development in middle age* (pp. 3–23). San Diego, CA: Academic Press.

Mynarska, M., Matysiak, A., Rybińska, A., Tocchioni, V., & Vignoli, D. (2015). Diverse paths into childlessness over the life course. *Advances in Life Course Research*, *25*, 35–48. doi:10.1016/j.alcr.2015.05.003

NHS UK choices. (2016). *IVF: Chances of success*. Retrieved from http://www.nhs.uk/Conditions/IVF/Pages/Introduction.aspx

National Institute of Clinical Excellence (NICE). (2013). *Fertility: Assessment and treatment for people with fertility problems*. Retrieved from https://www.nice.org.uk/guidance/cg156/evidence/full-guideline-188539453

Newton, N. J., & Stewart, A. J. (2013). The road not taken: Women's life paths and gender-linked personality traits. *Journal of Research in Personality*, *47*(4), 306–316. doi:10.1016/j.jrp.2013.02.003

Nouel, G. (2007). Construction of meaning in the face of mortality. In A. Tomer, G. T. Eliason, & P. T. P. Wong (Eds.), *Existential and spiritual issues in death attitudes* (pp. 235–255). Mahwah, NJ: Lawrence Erlbaum Associates.

Office for National Statistics. (2015). *Childbearing for women born in different years, England and Wales: 2014*. Retrieved from http://www.ons.gov.uk/peoplepopulationandcommunity/birthsdeathsandmarriages/conceptionandfertilityrates/bulletins/childbearingforwomenbornindifferentyearsenglandandwales/2015-11-10

Peters, K., Jackson, D., & Rudge, T. (2011). Surviving the adversity of childlessness: Fostering resilience in couples. *Contemporary Nurse*, *40*(1), 130–140. doi:10.5172/conu.2011.40.1.130

Purewal, S., & van den Akker, O. (2007). The socio-cultural and biological meaning of parenthood. *Journal of Psychosomatic Obstetrics & Gynaecology*, *28*(2), 79–86. doi:10.1080/01674820701409918

Riessman, C. K. (2000). Stigma and everyday resistance practices: Childless women in South India. *Gender & Society*, *14*(1), 111–135. doi:10.1177/0891243000 14001007

Schwerdtfeger, K. L., & Shreffler, K. M. (2009). Trauma of pregnancy loss and infertility among mothers and involuntarily childless women in the United States. *Journal of Loss and Trauma*, *14*(3), 211–227. doi:10.1080/153250208 02537468

Smith, J. A., Flowers, P., & Larkin, M. (2009). *Interpretative phenomenological analysis: Theory, method and research*. London: Sage.

Staudinger, U. M., & Bluck, S. (2001). A view of midlife development from life-span theory. In M. Lachman (Ed.), *Handbook of midlife development* (pp. 3–39). New York, NY: Wiley.

Sundby, J., Schmidt, L., Heldaas, K., Bugge, S., & Tanbo, T. (2007). Consequences of IVF among women: 10 years post-treatment. *Journal of Psychosomatic Obstetrics & Gynecology*, *28*(2), 115–120.

Sydsjö, G., Svanberg, A. S., Lampic, C., & Jablonowska, B. (2011). Relationships in IVF couples 20 years after treatment. *Human Reproduction*, *26*(7), 1836–1842. doi:10.1093/humrep/der131

Todorova, I. L. G., & Kotzeva, T. (2006). Contextual shifts in Bulgarian women's identity in the face of infertility. *Psychology and Health*, *21*(1), 123–141.

van Balen, F., & Trimbos-Kemper, T. C. M. (1995). Involuntarily childless couples: Their desire to have children and their motives. *Journal of Psychosomatic Obstetrics & Gynecology*, *16*, 137–144.

Warnock, M. (2002). *Making babies. Is there a right to have children?* Oxford: Oxford University Press.

Wenger, G. C., Scott, A., & Patterson, N. (2000). How important is parenthood? Childlessness and support in old age in England. *Ageing and Society*, *20*, 161–182.

Chapter 3

Wanting to Want: Constructing the Ambivalent Childless Self

Anna Gotlib

Abstract

In this chapter, I consider how voluntarily childless (VC) women can respond not just to master narratives of mandatory motherhood, but to their own internalised narratives of wantonness – of not desiring something they ought, or of being ambivalent about motherhood altogether. This chapter, then, is about the practices of choosing and endorsing one's desires, however clear or ambiguous, about intentional childlessness, and in the process, of learning to hold oneself as a valued moral agent, as a dissident, but non-wanton, self. Secondarily, it is also about challenging Frankfurt's claims that the formation and maintenance of moral identities require a kind of wholeheartedness that admits of no doubts. First, I begin with a personal story of my struggles with desiring my choices – of coming to endorse, however not-wholeheartedly, my non-wanting of motherhood, and thus rejecting the pronatalist narratives that marked my first-order desires as mistaken, and my second-order ones as deviant. Second, I offer an overview of voluntary childlessness as experienced by women most pressured to reproduce in the context of the bad moral luck of pronatalism. I note that my approach, grounded in philosophical feminist value theory, is focused on women who are not involuntarily childless or infertile, and who, because of social, economic and other privilege find themselves to be the targets of pronatalist narratives of 'desirable' motherhood. Finally, I conclude with a discussion of the dissident practices of identity-creation through which women can embrace both their certainties and ambiguities about their VC status by offering counterstories in response to accusations of wanton-hood, or of improperly, unnaturally or heretically motivated wills.

Keywords: Voluntary childlessness; pronatalism; narrative; counterstories; feminist value theory; Frankfurt; identity

Introduction

In 'Freedom of the Will and the Concept of a Person', Harry Frankfurt offers a novel way of thinking about free will. It is unique to adult human beings, he argues, who, unlike animals or children, are able to reflect on first-order desires and beliefs while also developing second-order desires and judgements (Frankfurt, 1971). For example, I may have first-order desires to avoid work responsibilities, but at the same time, I also have second-order desires not to be ruled by these desires, because I wish to be the kind of person who is responsible and not easily given over to whims. But simply having second-order desires is insufficient for the kind of freedom that Frankfurt argues only true moral agency can grant: What is required is a second-order volition – that is a second-order desire that a particular first-order desire motivates me to act. In other words, my moral agency requires that I have a desire about the efficacy of my desire, which suggests that I care about how my will, and thus identity, are constituted. But this is merely theory. Concerns about our identity-constituting desires are not only academic, but also quite personal. Indeed, as a voluntarily childless (hereinafter VC) woman, the validity, stability, authenticity and thus moral status of my motherhood-related desires are routinely tested and policed: Am I really sure? How do I know I am not just selfish? How will I deal with nearly certain regret? How can I not bring myself to desire that which is most desirable? and so on. While I have argued previously about the prevalence of pronatalist essentialising and gaslighting of women (Gotlib, 2016), I want here to consider how VC women can respond not just to master narratives of mandatory motherhood, but to their own internalised narratives of wantonness – of not desiring something they ought, or of being ambivalent about motherhood altogether. This chapter, then, is about the practices of choosing and endorsing one's desires, however clear or ambiguous, about intentional childlessness, and in the process of learning to hold oneself as a valued moral agent, as a dissident, but non-wanton, self (Lindemann, 2014). Secondarily, it is also about challenging Frankfurt's claims that the formation and maintenance of moral identities require a kind of wholeheartedness that admits of no doubts. First, I begin with a personal story of my struggles with desiring my choices – of coming to endorse, however not-wholeheartedly, my non-wanting of motherhood, and thus rejecting the pronatalist narratives that marked my first-order desires as mistaken and my second-order ones as deviant. Second, I offer an overview of voluntary childlessness as experienced by women most pressured to reproduce in the context of the bad moral luck of pronatalism. I note that my approach, grounded in philosophical feminist value theory, is focused on women who are not involuntarily childless or infertile, and who, because of social, economic and other privilege find themselves to be the targets of pronatalist narratives of 'desirable' motherhood. Finally, I conclude with a discussion of the dissident practices of identity-creation through which women can embrace both their certainties and ambiguities about their VC status by offering counterstories in response to accusations of wanton-hood, or of improperly, unnaturally or heretically motivated wills.

Wanting to Want

In many ways, this is a difficult paper to write. On the one hand, as an academic who has been grappling with the reality of pronatalism and totalising motherhood, it is somewhat familiar ground (Gotlib, 2016). On the other, as a VC woman, the dilemmas remain all too real, the self-doubt all too familiar and the external pressures often unrelenting. In part to make the abstract vivid, and in part to situate myself among those who might find themselves in my words, I begin with my story – a story of an uneasy, anxiety-filled and often surprising coming to not only know, but (somewhat) endorse myself as a VC woman who, for all her ongoing doubts, no longer stories her potential non-motherhood as 'maybe', 'for now' or 'not yet'.

As a young girl, I never played with dolls in the 'usual' way – while other children's dolls had tea parties and played dress-up, mine, along with my sizeable family of stuffed animals, held 'meetings', went to war and generally refused to behave. It was not that I rejected playing at motherhood, or thought it odd or foreign – other options were just that much more appealing. As I grew older and my attention shifted to the wider world, I continued not to share my friends' sometimes singular focus on marriage and children. In fact, while I craved the excitement and romance of a serious relationship, I saw it as an end-in-itself – not a means to growing a family – and even began to view my friends' developing desires for domestic bliss as not only disappointing, but claustrophobic and limiting: not altogether awful or impossible, but again, something that lacked that singular attraction.

After meeting, and eventually marrying, my partner, I became a classic postponer, the *not now* person: not now – not while we are not more economically secure, not until we travel more; not now – I have a dissertation to write; not now – I am looking for a job; not now – I am trying to earn tenure. *Not now*. I wanted to want – to want to have a child *for certain*, or to want not to have a child *for certain*. But neither certainty came. Not helping matters was my partner's relaxed, non-committal attitude towards parenthood. Quite content to be childless, he never pushed one way or the other. The only thing he wanted was for me to be finally settled, and to able to live with, my choices.

But the process of choosing my choices does not exist in a vacuum. Unlike in the case of women who desire, but cannot have, children and who often receive both pity and sympathy, attempts at normative uptake from others in the case of being VC tends to fail (Park, 2005). Like many VC or VC-tending women, the assumption is often that if one is not infertile, then one is simply too selfish or too unfocused (and will eventually get around to it when she 'grows up' and the baby fever takes hold). Otherwise, a woman cannot just *decide* not to procreate (Overall, 2012, p. 2). And thus a VC woman often hears that surely, if she was more 'adult' and 'knew her own mind', she would re-think her choices through, be less 'deficient', and more attuned to the 'real world' (Gillespie, 2000, p. 228; Rich, Taket, Graham, & Shelley, 2011, p. 235). Indeed,

> [c]ompared to the involuntarily childless and to parents, the voluntarily childless are seen as less socially desirable, less well-adjusted, less nurturant, and less mature, as well as more materialistic, more selfish, and more individualistic. Childfree women's lives have been seen as less rewarding than those of mothers of any number of children, and they have been judged to be less happy in the near future and in their elderly years than have mothers Callan (1985), Ganong, Coleman, and Mapes (1990), Houseknecht, (1987), Mueller and Yoder (1997), Polit (1978) and Veevers (1980). (Park, 2005, p. 376)

In other words, the VC woman becomes in many ways liminal, marginalised. If we take pronatalism to be a kind of an ideology – a set of intersecting master narratives about woman-as-mother that direct not only political, but social, economic and medical discourses – then the answer has to do with a need for control of not only the central message of mandatory motherhood, but also of the boundaries of how women are constituted. Thus,

> [w]omen who transgress discourses of what constitutes suitable 'normal' behavior for women come to be constructed as selfish, deviant and ultimately unfeminine (Butler, 1990; DiLapi, 1987; Ireland, 1993). As Morell (1994) has argued, the normalising of motherhood has been perpetuated through discourses that deprecate childless women. Thus, women who choose to remain childless have been 'called upon to account for themselves' in ways that women who become mothers have not (Morell, 1994). Dyson (1993) has emphasized that chosen childlessness is often incomprehensible to others who feel the need to express their bewilderment. (Gillespie, 2000, p. 230)

Yet ways to 'account for myself' – to family, friends, colleagues and even to curious acquaintances and strangers – were elusive. In part, I was not able to settle on what I imagined a reasonable narrative of being VC would be like. In fact, everything about my circumstances seemed to point to a sensible, secure motherhood – or at least did not offer strong arguments against it: I was neither an early articulator (Kelly, 2009) who knew with absolute certainty that children were not in her future, nor was I convinced that I would not be a decent mother. I was not suffering from any medical conditions that would make childbearing overwhelmingly difficult or impossible. I was a tenure-track academic with a partner who was also gainfully employed. I enjoyed spending time with my friends' children (even though I noted that I perhaps enjoyed a bit more returning them to their parents). Aside from professional ambitions and a desire to travel, I did not have any grandiose plans for my future that would necessarily exclude children. With the benefit of hindsight, I was that odd creature, somewhere in the middle: a lukewarm, ambivalent potential parent with no particular desires or plans to become one. Or, put another way, were I to become a mother, I would not bemoan my fate, but drop anchor and embrace this new turn in my life. And yet my vague preference was to remain as

I was – untethered by parenthood and unmoored among the rapidly growing families of so many of my friends and colleagues. But what I really desired was *to be sure* either way, to be so confident that being VC was my agential choice, or to be committed enough to potential motherhood as something other than a default, I-can-cope-with-it position. Indeed, I wanted truly, honestly, unapologetically to either desire parenthood for reasons that I could formulate internally and make intelligible to others, or with equal conviction reject it. I wanted to want – or to not want, wholeheartedly. What I did not want was to be ambivalent about this most important of choices. I wanted to care more about my motherhood status – and I certainly did not want to become Frankfurt's wanton.

Non-wholehearted Childlessness as Wanton-hood

Harry Frankfurt's rather influential theory of free will has as its goal the explanation of why persons value free will, and why and how free will is a uniquely human capacity. Yet not being a human wanton is no easy task. Frankfurt famously argues that what we, as human beings, ought to want to be is free, and this requires a particular attunement to one's desires (Frankfurt, 1971). Specifically, for a desire to be truly one's own, one has to possess a higher-order (second-order) desire about the initial desire. Indeed, one must have a second-order volition that the initial desire be controlling – it must be the desire that fully (wholeheartedly) satisfies the agent, that becomes her active will. Only in this way is the agent's will free and her actions truly autonomous (Frankfurt, 1971). A wanton, however, is none of these things. Although she possesses first-order desires, she does not care about which of them is the strongest, or which one of them happens to control her actions. A wanton does not care about the contents of her will – she does not care what does, or does not, move her, and why. Neither is she wholehearted about her resulting beliefs and actions, and is thus not a person in the fullest sense of the term. For example, in the first instance, I desire that my second-order volition to exercise (rather than to sit on the couch) be controlling, and thus I exercise – I am a free moral agent. In the second instance (perhaps as a compromised moral agent), I am the kind of person who is lazy and loathe to exercise, and thus remain on the couch while at the same time wanting the desire to exercise to override my laziness. Thus I am not a wanton, but am simply powerless to reify my second-order volition. In the third instance where

I am in fact a wanton, I might be moved (or unmoved) by my desires without necessarily wanting to be so moved (or unmoved) – I just do not care about how, or by what, my will and my actions are controlled. The free moral agent and the non-wanton possess free will in that their second-order volitions are (successfully or unsuccessfully) endorsed. And, I would add, the more significant or identity-constituting the desire, the more crucial the demand that one act as a wholehearted agent – not an ambivalently motivated one.

Thus, on Frankfurt's account, as an ambivalent VC woman, I am arguably not a wanton in the sense that I care about the kinds of desires control my choices, and which actions subsequently follow. It matters to me how and why I am motivated, and where those motivations lead. But I am also not a properly wholehearted individual whose will is unambiguously on one side of a dilemma, and thus free. I am exactly that ambivalently motivated, non-wholehearted individual who falls in between categories of personhood. And if I were to take Frankfurt's highly influential views on board, how am I to view myself as a moral agent? In order to be free, must I wholeheartedly desire, or not desire, motherhood? How am I to work through the multiple layers of personal, moral and socio-political ambiguities that seem to form and define my deliberative spaces as an ambivalently voluntary non-parent?

Although there have been a number of responses to Frankfurt's claims, I am going to focus on just one – the implications of his views on wholeheartedness that I take to apply rather well to ambivalent (non)motherhood. Specifically, this critique has to do with the worries about Frankfurt's requirement of an agential wholeheartedness as a kind of alienation from self. In 'Identification and Identity', David Velleman argues that while Frankfurt's 'well constituted self' requires resolution of ambiguities and calls for wholeheartedness, such a stance amounts to defensively denying (or hiding from) our undesired emotions, and does not effectively make them not-ours (Velleman, 2002). Yet, as Frankfurt puts it:

> In order for a conflict [...] to be resolved [...] Resolution requires only that the person become finally and unequivocally clear as to which side of the conflict he is on. The forces mobilized on the other side may then persist with as much intensity as before; but as soon as he has definitely established just where he himself stands, his will is no longer divided and his ambivalence is therefore gone. He has placed himself wholeheartedly behind one of the

> conflicting impulses, and not at all behind the other. (Frankfurt, 2004, p. 91)

This makes it clear that for Frankfurt, an agent's failure to wholeheartedly integrate his or her unstable and incoherent will into a state of semi-permanent ambivalence is something to be avoided, since instability and incoherence are not – and cannot be – ideal ways to be constituted as an agent. Such resolution, however, is not possible for an ambivalent agent. Wholeheartedness requires clarity, a choosing of sides – and to be behind one's action-guiding choices unequivocally, while quite possibly alienating oneself from one's unendorsed motives. Thus, we have two options in regard to Frankfurt's insistence on wholeheartedness: first, we can either accept the view that it is just better for one to be wholehearted about one's desires, decisions and actions, and thus strive for such a state. Alternatively, we can admit to possessing conflicting impulses, and argue for a position with regard to motherhood that is an agent's own, freely endorsed – and ambivalent.

While I take the second option as the more fruitful direction in examining VC ambivalence as a kind of agency, I suspect that the story is much more complicated: we are neither as transparent to ourselves as Frankfurt takes us to be, nor as able to simply resolve to choose among conflicting, identity-defining desires through wholehearted acts of will. And since I take Frankfurt to be more concerned with the kinds of choices that speak to agency and character (rather than, say, to taste and manners), the story matters that much more because the stakes are nothing short of our moral lives and identities.

What Frankfurt also misses in his assessment of our moral selves is what Lisa Tessman, in *Moral Failure: On the Impossible Demands of Morality*, gets right: the inescapable tragedy of our moral lives and choices. Her claim is that despite the fact that some actions are morally required (or morally non-negotiable), we cannot attend to them all (or even perhaps to most of them) – and that this inability neither excuses nor justifies our moral failures (Tessman, 2015). We are the kinds of creatures who, despite all our efforts to be the right kind of moral actor, remain torn by impossible demands, and inevitably fail. It is difficult to imagine how Frankfurt's insistence on wholeheartedness would play out in a dilemmatic situation such as one presented in William Styron's novel *Sophie's Choice*, where a mother must choose whether to give up her son or daughter to Nazis and certain death. What would it mean for her to be 'wholehearted' about her desires and decisions in this case – and would it not, in the end, require a kind of a monstrous dedication to non-ambivalence over all the other concerns that constitute our moral lives?

Even though most cases of contradictory choices and desires are not nearly as existentially dramatic as Sophie's, we can still put significant pressure on the demand for wholeheartedness and commitment to resolution as clarity of desire. And in moving beyond Tessman's poignant evocation of the worst moral dilemmas a human being might face, how are we to think about our choices, our actions and our moral requirements in the quotidian demandingness of our ordinary lives? Specifically, how are women to evaluate their own uncertain desires in regard to (non) motherhood? It seems that, at the very least (and *pace* Frankfurt), ought does not always imply can, moral contexts can be contradictory or simply irresolvable and can lead to if not always tragedy, then certainly confusion, ambiguity and uncertainty.

The Intelligibility of Choice

Before continuing any further, a small, but vital, clarification is needed. The case of the non-wholehearted mother differs, of course, from the kinds of required-but-unthinkable choices noted by Tessman. Indeed, one might believe that I am greatly overstating the dilemma – after all, I can choose to become a mother wholeheartedly, or I can be quite alienated from my decision, and neither of these eventualities are morally tragic. The uncertain mother's sense of herself is not that of a wanton (unless she truly does not care about the contents of her will or her actions); she can be wholehearted and fully resolved, or not; she can proclaim her will as divided between the longing for motherhood on the one hand and for greater personal and career options on the other. But she is not Styron's Sophie, for her choice, however unsettled internally, is not one that is morally unthinkable, although in some cases troubling, wanting or otherwise problematic. The mother-as-moral-agent – wholehearted or not – seems to remain (mostly) both morally intelligible to herself and to others. Indeed, she can, in most cases, make decisions of which she is not fully certain, but which nevertheless are not psychologically or morally destructive of herself, and do not rise to the level of moral failure.

But things change rather dramatically when the question is not how one becomes a mother, but how one declines entering motherhood altogether. Specifically, the moral status of an ambivalent VC woman is not granted the non-wholehearted-yet-still acceptable narrative of the uncertain mother. Nor can her choice be properly viewed through Tessman's lens of dilemmatic tragic choices. Indeed, she faces a problem not of moral failure due to impossible moral demands, but of perceived moral failure due to a lack of intelligibility. While the temporary ambivalence of a VC woman is often assumed, for a largely pronatalist society has a difficult time envisioning a woman who wholeheartedly could reject desiring children (she will always have children *eventually!*), the kind of permanent ambivalence that I have in mind often receives no uptake: it simply *cannot be* the case that a woman who: (1) can (physically) have children, (2) is choosing not to have them and (3) is ambivalent rather than militantly 'childfree' (because while an unambiguously VC woman presents a direct, yet intelligible, challenge to pronatalism, ambivalence presents something odd and confusing). While I will not explore this issue much further, it is helpful to note here that childless women – whether involuntarily so, unambivalently VC, or ambivalently VC – have internalised the pronatalist pressure to identify their womanhood in relation to their childbearing choices. Thus the battles rage over whether one is 'childless', 'childfree' or some other version of 'child' with a number of VC women all too eager to declare themselves unambivalently 'childfree' to both distance themselves from the misfortune of the 'childless', and from the ambiguities of those somewhere in the middle (Blackstone, 2014). It is this language of 'childless' and 'childfree' that is often a point of contention, with those who are VC at pains to distinguish themselves as 'free' (rather than 'less') from those who are desperate to have children, and are therefore indeed 'less' without them.[1] So those women who, like me, do not desire to be mothers, nor are unable to be mothers, nor are militarily VC ('childfree') are left somewhat liminal, in pronatalist moral spaces that do not allow our narratives to find a home.

The difference among all three 'child—' positions lies both in the perception of 'choice' and intelligibility: the childlessness *happened* to the involuntarily childless; the voluntarily childfree 'selfishly' intended, caused, but *owned*, their decision; and the ambivalent VC are just that – between moral categories, at the margins of moral spaces. And thus women who are not desiring motherhood, but who are at the same time

[1]For further discussions about the distinctions between childlessness 'voluntary childlessness' and 'childfreedom', see Shapiro (2014), Blackstone and Stewart (2012), Hara (2008), Iwasawa (2004), Merlo and Rowland (2000), Chancey and Dumais (2009), Park (2005), Basten (2009) and McAllister and Clarke (1998).

conflicted, non-wholehearted and ambivalent *want to want*, having internalised the narratives of how 'wrong' they are for not wanting, and especially for not declining motherhood clearly enough (Gotlib, 2016). They are gaslighted as a matter of course (Harding, 2009).

And yet, there are many of these ambivalent VC women who, as Mardy Ireland notes, are 'becoming childless' in a long, often complicated process 'involving the tension between living one's life and giving one's life particular meaning' (Wager, 2000, p. 393, citing Ireland, 1993, p. 44). Carolyn Morell notes that VC women

> speak about being 'wistful' about not being a mother, or having unsettling 'rumblings', 'musings', 'twinges' or 'passing thoughts' about the path not taken. It is common for even the most dedicated intentional not-mother to have her temporary moments of wavering. For example, Cynthia Minden (1996), in her essay 'Other than Mother' [...] concludes that it is 'impossible to sail through your fertile years without at least a tiny pondering, a momentary musing about "what if". Societal messages are so pervasive that we seldom recognize the subtle ways in which we have been influenced and directed' (1996, p. 257). (Morell, 2000, pp. 316–317)

The reasons for this lack of uptake of VC women's narratives, whether of certainty or especially of ambivalence, are complex, and come burdened with centuries of misogyny and social control of women's bodies – indeed, this story is much too long for my purposes here. I must note, however, that the VC narratives themselves are not static, but multidimensional, intersectional and reflective of a woman's changing and evolving life course.[2] For example, while younger VC women often find themselves struggling with both external uptake and internal validation of their choices, older VC women, having spent a large part of their lives justifying and defending their choices, tend to 'score higher on perceived autonomy and environmental mastery which entails exerting control over external circumstances' (Jeffries & Konnert, 2002, p. 101), as '[t]hey appear to be accustomed to charting their own destiny rather than letting others dictate or at least influence the course of their lives' (Jeffries & Konnert, 2002, p. 102). The ageing

[2]I am grateful to an anonymous reviewer for this insight.

process, therefore, seems to both build resilience to external pressures and, as a result, to reduce anxieties and consolidate decisions to remain VC – in other words, to desire one's desires, and to be unafraid of making them public, clear and no longer open to third-party debate. Yet while age might grant women a certain degree of self-trust and confidence with regard to their parenting choices, the stigmas prevalent in the ongoing master narratives of cis/heteronormativity (not to mention race, economic security and so on) can result in 'the internalisation of anti-homosexual prejudice [...]' that 'may constitute barriers to the parental projects of lesbians and gay men' (Gato, Santos, & Fontaine, 2017, p. 319), regardless of their choices. My point here is this: one's age, gender, race and other aspects of one's identity matter when considering whether, how and why life-altering parenting choices are made. Who we are, and who we are perceived to be, are thus often functions of the master narratives that form, control and sometimes determine not only parenthood decisions, but our very reasons for making them in the first place.

Much more remains to be said on the intersectional factors that at work in the decision to remain childless. However, for now, I want to focus on one particular aspect of women's experiences with motherhood that, especially in the Global North, has been instrumental in contributing to the gaslighting of the VC: the growing power and influence of pronatalism itself and its attendant narratives of mandatory motherhood. In the next section, I argue that it is the bad moral luck of pronatalism's current rise that is storying many VC women's choices as moral failure. I now turn to this task.

The (Bad) Moral Luck of Pronatalism

Moral Luck

Sometimes we have good luck, and sometimes our luck changes. However, what is intended by *moral* luck is not simply a description of events, but a moral claim that a particular set of circumstances, understood as one's luck, makes a difference in how we perceive, and evaluate, one's actions. And even though our intuitions about accidents and control over circumstances might protest against judging Donna, who was not paying attention and hit a dog with her car (bad moral luck), versus Dan, who was similarly not paying attention and did not hit the dog as he managed to run across the street faster (good moral luck) differently based just on this luck, we nevertheless tend to do so, placing their moral standing on the scales of that judgement (Nagel, 1993; Williams, 1982).

But the story does not end there. Perhaps Donna was not paying attention because she worked the night shift, and Dan, on the other hand, was returning from a party a bit inebriated. And yet however aware or unaware of these moral-luck-constituting facts, we still tend to judge them as similarly morally responsible for the outcomes of their actions. Still, we might heed Margaret Walker's reminder that moral luck begins when our 'responsibilities' have 'outrun [our] control' (Nelkin, 2013, citing Walker, 1991). We might also consider Lisa Tessman's claim that moral luck impacts agents 'systemically', through 'circumstances that are [...] arranged and that tend to affect people as members of social groups' (Tessman, 2005, p. 13) – and that this differs from 'natural' or 'accidental' luck (Tessman, 2005).

Another way of viewing systematic moral luck is through the lens of agency:[3] given that agency in its broadest outlines involves a modicum of self-direction and self-definition (although always within a cultural or circumstantial context, for ideal-theory agency is not what is at issue here), what one does (and why) as an agent can be poorly and incorrectly interpreted by those who may not know (or care) about the constraining effects of bad moral luck on one's choices. Thus, moral luck in this case acts as an often-invisible factor in how one is viewed, and importantly, assessed as a moral agent. In other words, through conditions not of our making, some of us happen to find ourselves on the wrong side of these deliberately (or negligently) arranged, bad-luck-making (social, political and economic) systems – and are subsequently judged for our 'moral failings'. In the next section, I will consider pronatalism as precisely this kind of systemic arrangement – this design – that dominates, shapes and defines motherhood and that places a heavy burden on (especially ambivalent) VC women who happen to defy its dictates.

Pronatalism and the VC Woman

A brief explanatory note before proceeding:[4] although my focus here is on women's experiences with voluntary childlessness in a pronatalist

---

[3]I am grateful to an anonymous reviewer for suggesting that agency ought to be noted as a part of the discussion of moral luck.

[4]Again, I am grateful to an anonymous reviewer for pointing out that this is an issue that requires noting.

society, I by no means intend to silence their partners (if they indeed have one) by suggesting that these partners either never share in the decision-making process, nor are themselves not deeply affected by the choice to remain childless. In fact, partners of VC women fall all along the spectrum of roles and reactions to voluntary childlessness, and the complex and important conversations about their agency in childbearing and childrearing decisions deserve their own space among the various discourses around (non)parenthood. However, this is not my focus here. My reasons for centring on the (non)mother has to do with the unique moral jeopardy in which her decision places her in a society which defines her primarily by her childbearing functions. In fact, as Park noted,

> While the rhetoric of committed fatherhood dominates today, research continues to discover the greater importance of the parent identity and role for women than for men, even when men perceive themselves as very invested in their children (Hochschild, 1989; McMahon, 1995). Although findings are not entirely consistent, child-free women appear to be more stigmatized for their childlessness than do their male counterparts (Goetting, 1986; Houseknecht, 1987). This finding makes sense as motherhood is seen as the very essence of femininity and healthy, mature womanhood, whereas masculinity continues to be defined fundamentally by occupational achievement. In addition, women generally may be more likely than men to be labeled as norm violators (Schur, 1983). (Park, 2002, p. 26)

So what is this systemic bad moral luck that I think creates the unique difficulties and vulnerabilities of VC women? To put it quite simply, wholeheartedness about not desiring children is often precluded by the bad, non-accidental moral luck of pronatalism's social dominance. Those women who are decidedly VC face constant, oppressive backlash via pronatalist master narratives, while those who are already ambivalent are made more vulnerable by the repeated messages that undermine their self-trust. By pronatalism, I mean an attitude that favours and encourages childbearing, as well as supports policies and practices that construe and venerate motherhood as the *sine qua non* of womanhood. Women, pronatalism claims, must be led, motivated or, if necessary, compelled towards the realisation of motherhood as not only a social good, but, importantly, as something that is essentially in their own best interests as women. It is, in short, it is a claim about who women essentially are (Gotlib, 2016; Parry, 2005; Ulrich & Weatherall, 2000).

Thus, women who happen to live within the Global North in the latter part of the twentieth century, and the beginning of the twenty-first, find themselves facing powerful social narratives about the necessary relationship between 'woman' and 'mother' that place significant decisional and justificatory burdens on those who decide to counter them. It is important to note that the kinds of pronatalist pressures addressed here, while affecting all women in numerous ways, are not necessarily similar in their goals: while the middle-class, cis/heteronormative, and often white women fall under the motherhood mandate, there is a significant number of women who are members of the LGBTQ communities, too old, too poor, non-white, disabled and so on who are systematically excluded from the ranks of desirable motherhood, and in fact are often discouraged, and punished, for embracing parenthood (Hirsch, 2002). While I take pronatalism, among other things, to be responsible for this sorting of women into 'desirable' and 'undesirable' motherhoods, I do not delve into these distinctions here. I only note these disparities as not to give the false impression that I am painting all women, and their relationships to pronatalism, with a single brush. This chapter, then, mostly focuses on those whose confrontation with pronatalism intersects with the presence of significant social, gender and racial privilege (May, 1995).

The reasons for the hegemony of pronatalism are historical, social, economic and fundamentally reactive: nationalism, fears about the shrinking workforce, the narratives of VC 'coldness' as a rejection of 'natural' womanhood itself – or else an act of such decadence, laziness and selfish unreasonableness made by otherwise successful women who have 'opted out' of motherhood (Basten, 2009; Gotlib, 2016). As I and others have argued elsewhere (Gotlib, 2016; Kukla, 2005), some of the most powerful social forces – popular culture, the legal and political system and the biomedical institution itself – have assumed alarmingly pronatalist positions, using their very public voices to weave narratives of womanhood as mandatory motherhood on one side, and failure and liminality on the other.

To take just one example, the release of a *Time* magazine article charting the rise of voluntary childlessness resulted in cries of 'childfree propaganda', and charges that the article itself was a paean to adult immaturity born of thoughtlessness and a lack of direction, conviction and will (Sandler & Witteman, 2013; Walshe, 2013). Importantly, what the resulting backlash emphasised was the inevitability of a too-late realisation of personal emptiness and wasted potential for a truly fulfilling life – of a fundamental, tragic mistake. No woman who proclaims herself to be VC, the response suggested, can *really, knowingly* endorse her actions. At best, she is – confused – and if she is at all ambivalent, she should hope that someone, or something, will direct her towards motherhood. When not warning of personal regret, pronatalist narratives are often cloaked in the guise of scientifically grounded worries about a childless woman's well-being: thus, *The Atlantic* proclaims that 'Childless Men and Women May Die Sooner' (Abrams, 2012). The suggestion, as always, is that no reasonable person – and certainly no reasonable woman – would subject herself to not only the emotional, but ostensibly *scientifically certain, medically assured* suffering if she really considered her childbearing decisions.

The world of law and politics similarly insists that the VC woman is mistaken at best (if not dangerously selfish and self-regarding). Focusing specifically on the American pronatalist narrative, policies restricting the availability of abortion and other birth-control measures tend to predominate. The Guttmacher Institute notes that 14 states introduced laws seeking to ban abortion before viability; 10 states have introduced laws to ban all, or nearly all, abortions; eight states have passed 'personhood' laws; and eight states have also introduced laws to limit 'the morning after' pill (Gotlib, 2016; The Guttmacher Institute, 2014). Moreover, some political theorists have focused on a low-childbirth-precipitated shrinking population of future workers, fomenting fears of political, economic and for some, moral collapse. For instance, Phillip Longman claims that: (1) modern medicine and reduced fertility may lead to a collapse of world population, (2) as a result, the world markets will be negatively impacted, (3) an aging population will lead to a collapse of the American healthcare system and thus (4) the state must provide economic and other incentives for young families to continue growing – to shift those who are ambivalent about parenthood with a narrative of the necessity of other-regarding, selfless acts of societal rescue (Gotlib, 2016; Longman, 2004). And while it would be overstating the case to suggest that such unambiguously pronatalist narratives are alone sufficient to introduce undermining doubt into a VC woman's reasoning, neither can repeated exposure to such narratives be rejected as inconsequential. Thus, VC women are undermined in their confidence, while any existing ambivalence that they might have for their own (non-pronatalism-caused) reasons is routinely and enthusiastically exploited.

But perhaps the most powerful pronatalist force facing VC women is the biomedical establishment itself. Let's begin by noting that pregnancy and childbearing have become largely medicalised and monitored rituals of well-woman visits, testing and ever-growing lists of requirements and dangers (Kukla, 2005). The female body (and especially within the for-profit medical climate within the United States) has largely been medically storied as 'pre': pre-menstrual, pre-pregnant, pre-menopausal and more broadly, always pre-disease (Kukla, 2005). Female bodies have become morally contested, regulated spaces, both fragile and on the brink of abnormality that required correction. In fact, in 2006, the *Washington Post* introduced the term 'pre-pregnant' in the course of reporting on a recommendation from the Centers for Disease Control and Prevention (CDC) that all American women of childbearing age begin addressing their 'pre-conception' health: from the time of their first menstrual period until menopause, they are to take folic acid supplements, not smoke, not 'misuse' alcohol, maintain a healthy weight, refrain from drug use, avoid 'high-risk' sexual behaviour, and never miss a 'well-woman' check. In other words,

> [t]he CDC was asking women to behave as if they were already pregnant, even if they had no intention of conceiving in the near – or distant – future. For the first time, a U.S. government institution was explicitly saying what social norms had always hinted at: All women, regardless of whether they have or want children, are moms-in-waiting. Telling women that what is best for a pregnancy is automatically best for them defines motherhood as a woman prioritizing the needs of a child, real or hypothetical, over her own. (Valenti, 2012, ¶6)

Thus, regardless of desire or intent to enter motherhood, the biomedical establishment marks all pre-menopausal women as always necessarily pre-pregnant (Kukla, 2005). And the possibility that pregnancy is, by choice, not in a woman's future is not only resisted through policy, but within actual practice. That is, while the decision to have children is not (usually) subject to demands for wholehearted assurance and justification – after all, it is 'normal' and 'natural' for a woman to desire motherhood – VC-motivated requests for sterilisation are met with demands for reasons, scorn and often rejection

(Gillespie, 2000; Vesper, 2008, p. 228). For example, Annily Campbell's study of 23 childfree women who chose sterilisation

> described encounters with (mostly male) doctors in which they were put in the position of explaining their desire to become sterilized and convincing the doctors that their decision was well thought out and not whimsical and 'spur of the moment'. Many reported 'being laughed out of the surgery', meaning the doctor would not take them seriously and dismissed them as foolhardy. (Vesper, 2008, p. 19)

Indeed, childless women making sterilisation requests are often turned away by physicians insisting that their (relative) youth both pointed towards the possibility of changed minds and rash decisions (Campbell, 1999; Gillespie, 2000). The message is clear: a choice to voluntarily forego motherhood cannot be rational, and the VC woman who, at least according to her biological clock, *still has time to change her mind* has to be viewed as irrational in her rush. She thus must be denied in her desire to bring her childbearing potential to a 'premature' conclusion.

So where does that leave the VC woman? Out of these disparate elements, clothed in social, political and even medical language, emerge the stories of physical, psychological and moral failure, self-doubt, and liminality that leave her with two stances towards her decision: on the one hand, a defiant, 'childfree' wholeheartedness that marks her as socially suspect and open to pronatalist attack. On the other, there is that second group – those harbouring ambivalence about their VC choices. And because the ambivalent may not always reach that unequivocal clarity about motivations and desires that allows for wholeheartedness (and thus fully join their proudly 'childfree' sisters), they remain doubly liminal: first, in relation to the clearly VC; second, in relation to the hegemonic pronatalism within which they keep searching for the kinds of moral spaces that would grant uptake to their particular stories of coming to (mostly) not want.

Counterstories: Wholehearted, Half-hearted and Ambivalent

I began this chapter with worries about wanting to want – wanting to want to be a mother, or, alternatively, wanting to know with certainty that motherhood is not what is desired. In short, I began (and end) with worries about certainty, and its lack. And even though in the previous section

I left things in a rather grim state, I want to conclude by pointing to two possible responses to the moral dilemmas of the ambivalent VC woman.

The first response is to the worry about whether VC ambivalence, such as my own, inevitably leads to a weak will, or worse – to wantonhood. I think that a case can be made that it is in fact quite all right – morally speaking – to be ambivalent (perhaps permanently so) about one's identity-constituting desires, such as one's status as a (non)parent. As a VC woman, the first move towards rescuing one's agency is to recognise the bad moral luck of having to make such decisions amid the master narratives of powerful pronatalist forces, and that these forces effect all women, regardless of childbearing status. Such recognition is not easy – and, I suggest, requires the solidarity of others. Turning away from the messages of the motherhood mandate and offering other, better stories calls for the kind of solidarity with VC and non-VC-women who, together, can create counternarratives that

> don't try to free one group by oppressing another [...] They are credible because they offer the best available explanation of who the group members are [...]. By pulling apart the master narratives that construct a damaged identity and replacing them with a more credible less morally degrading narrative, counterstories serve as *practical* tools for reidentifying persons. They serve to repair the damaged identity. (Lindemann, 2001, pp. 183–186)

These alternative stories, by granting mutual uptake and thus strengthening a sense of moral agency through solidarity, can allow the ambivalent VC woman to see that she, unlike a wanton, just might be responsive to valid reasons to be, and to remain, ambivalent about motherhood. In fact, through her participation in these counternarratives – counterstories to the pronatalist messages of her failure, her weak will, her selfishness – she might endorse *her own good reasons* to be ambivalent, and accept that ambivalence, that complexity, that sense of not everything *ever* being quite settled. She might also come to view her lack of wholeheartedness about non-motherhood as neither a sign of a weak-willed person nor of a wanton. Instead, she may come to know and recognise that her own struggles with internal and external pronatalist pressures, the gravity of her decision, and the shifting valences of reasons regarding her childbearing decision are anything but indicative of not caring about her will, or being helpless against desire. It is in, and through, such engagement with her own and others' counterstories that she can begin repairing herself as an agent by telling her narrative not as a means of justification or excuse, but as a matter of mutual moral intelligibility. The already-fragile identities of (ambivalent) VC women are thus not further damaged by hiding the complexities of their choices. Indeed, quite the opposite: VC women, by embracing their often-ambivalent relationship to their status, through narratives of credibility and solidarity, might very well overcome the damaging narratives of pronatalist, and mutual, mistrust and emerge as complex agents, capable of defining and defending, their choices, decisions and selves.

The second response is to the more global worry about wholeheartedness as a requirement of motherhood – or its lack. I suggest that demanding that women – those who are VC, those desiring motherhood, or those who are already mothers – be wholehearted about their choices is yet another version of pronatalist oppression that concerns *all* women. Just as socially 'desirable' mothers are queried (and often not trusted) about their VC choices, the less 'desirable' ones are pushed for justifications of their parental desires – are they *really sure* that they want to bring a child into the world, given their class, gender expression, and so on? And any answer short of 'absolutely yes' is sure to merit cascades of suspicious, doubt, further –questions – as if a woman's entire identity rests with her relationship to motherhood, and specifically to the wholehearted kind. Yet the choice of whether or not to become a mother is not one that creates or undoes one's moral agency, nor does it create or undo womanhood itself. What can destroy both are unyielding moral demands – wholeheartedness about complicated, personal decisions from theorists like Frankfurt; mandatory motherhood (for some; non-motherhood for others) from a culture of pronatalism. Thus, the kind of solidarity that I have in mind is one that not only challenges these demands, but does so by giving voice to differing, perhaps dissident, phenomenologies of motherhood (and non-motherhood) such that they all come to legitimately constitute the moral spaces of women's experiences. And it is when these agents – these *women* – begin to share their dissident counterstories of resistance not just to pronatalism, but to demands that they *choose sides*, often in opposition to each other, then perhaps they can redefine their complex and ambivalent childbearing choices as meaningful, dynamic and intelligible, reclaiming their experiences and their lives.

References

Abrams, L. (2012). Study: Becoming a parent significantly decreases risk of premature death. *The Atlantic Monthly*, December 6. Retrieved from http://www.theatlantic.com/health/archive/2012/12/study-becoming-a-parent-significantly-decreases-risk-of-premature-death/265959/

Basten, S. (2009). *Voluntary childlessness and being childfree*. Oxford & Vienna Institute of Demography. Retrieved from https://www.spi.ox.ac.uk/fileadmin/documents/PDF/Childlessness_-_Number_5.pdf

Blackstone, A. (2014). Childless...or childfree? *Contexts*, *13*, 68–70.

Blackstone, A., & Stewart, M. D. (2012). Choosing to be childfree: Research on the decision not to parent. *Sociology Compass*, *6*(9), 718–727.

Callan, V. J. (1985). Perceptions of parents, the voluntarily, and involuntarily childless: A multidimensional scaling analysis. *Journal of Marriage and the Family*, *47*, 1045–1050.

Campbell, A. (1999). *Childfree and sterilized*. London: Cassell.

Chancey, L., & Dumais, S. A. (2009). Voluntary childlessness in marriage and family textbooks, 1950–2000. *Journal of Family History*, *34*(2), 206–223.

Frankfurt, H. G. (1971). Freedom of the will and the concept of a person. *Journal of Philosophy*, *68*(1), 5–20.

Frankfurt, H. G. (2004). *The reasons of love*. Princeton, NJ: Princeton University Press.

Ganong, L. H., Coleman, M., & Mapes, D. (1990). A meta-analytic review of family structure stereotypes. *Journal of Marriage and the Family*, *52*, 287–297.

Gato, J., Santos, S., & Fontaine, A. M. (2017). To have or not to have children? That is the question. Factors influencing parental decisions among lesbians and gay men. *Sexuality Research and Social Policy*, *14*, 310–323.

Gillespie, R. (2000). When no means no: Disbelief, disregard and deviance as discourses of voluntary childlessness. *Women's Studies International Forum*, *23*(2), 223–234.

Gotlib, A. (2016). 'But you would be the best mother': Unwomen, counterstories, and the motherhood mandate. *Journal of Bioethical Inquiry*, *13*(2), 327–347.

Hara, T. (2008). Increasing childlessness in Germany and Japan: Toward a childless society? *International Journal of Japanese Sociology*, *17*(1), 42–62.

Harding, K. (2009). Voluntary childlessness 'unnatural and evil'. *Salon*. Retrieved from http://www.salon.com/2009/06/15/childless_by_choice/

Hirsch, C. M. (2002). When the war on poverty became the war on poor, pregnant women: Political rhetoric, the unconstitutional conditions doctrine, and the family cap restrictions. *William & Mary Journal of Women and the Law*, *8*, 335–356.

Houseknecht, S. K. (1987). Voluntary Childlessness. In M. B. Sussman & S. K. Steinmetz (Eds.), *Handbook of marriage and the family* (pp. 369–395). New York, NY: Plenum Press.

Ireland, M. S. (1993). *Reconceiving women: Separating motherhood from female identity*. New York, NY: The Guilford Press.

Iwasawa, M. (2004). Partnership transition in contemporary Japan: Prevalence of childless non cohabiting couples. *The Japanese Journal of Population*, *2*(1), 76–92.

Jeffries, S., & Konnert, C. (2002). Regret and psychological well-being among voluntarily and involuntarily childless women and mothers. *International Journal of Aging and Human Development, 54*(2), 89–106.

Kelly, M. (2009). Women's voluntary childlessness: A radical rejection of motherhood? *WSQ: Women's Studies Quarterly, 37*(3/4), 157–172.

Kukla, R. (2005). *Mass hysteria: Medicine, culture, and mothers' bodies.* Oxford: Rowman & Littlefield Publishers.

Lindemann, H. (2001). *Damaged identities, narrative repair.* Ithaca, NY: Cornell University Press.

Lindemann, H. (2014). *Holding and letting go: The social practice of personal identities.* New York, NY: Oxford University Press.

Longman, P. (2004). *The empty cradle: How falling birthrates threaten world prosperity and what to do about it.* New York, NY: Basic Books.

May, E. T. (1995). *Barren in the promised land: Childless Americans and the pursuit of happiness.* Cambridge, MA: Harvard University Press.

Merlo, R., & Rowland, D. (2000). The prevalence of childlessness in Australia. *People and Place, 8*(2), 21–32.

McAllister, F., & Clark, L. (1998). *A study of childlessness in Britain.* Family Policy Studies Centre, Joseph Rowntree Foundation. Retrieved from http://www.jrf.org.uk/publications/studychildlessness-britain. Accessed on December 15, 2014.

Morell, C. (2000). Saying no: Women's experiences with reproductive refusal. *Feminism & Psychology, 10*(3), 313–322.

Mueller, K. A., & Yoder, J. D. (1997). Gendered norms for family size, employment and occupation: Are there personal costs for violating them? *Sex Roles, 36*, 207–220.

Nagel, T. (1993). Moral luck. In D. Statman (Ed.), *Moral luck* (pp. 57–71). Albany, NY: State University of New York Press.

Nelkin, D. K. (2013). Moral luck. In E. N. Zalta (Ed.), *The Stanford encyclopedia of philosophy.* Retrieved from https://plato.stanford.edu/archives/win2013/entries/moral-luck/

Overall, C. (2012). *Why have children? The ethical debate.* Cambridge, MA: The MIT Press.

Park, K. (2002). Stigma management among the voluntarily childless. *Sociological Perspectives, 45*(1), 21–45.

Park, K. (2005). Choosing childlessness: Weber's typology of action and motives of the voluntarily childless. *Sociological Inquiry, 75* (3), 372–402.

Parry, D. C. (2005). Women's leisure as resistance to pronatalist ideology. *Journal of Leisure, 37*(2), 135–151.

Polit, D. F. (1978). Stereotypes relating to family-size status. *Journal of Marriage and the Family, 40*, 105–114.

Rich, S., Taket, A., M. Graham, & Shelley, J. (2011). 'Unnatural', 'unwomanly', 'uncreditable' and 'undervalued': The significance of being a childless woman in Australian society. *Gender Issues, 28*, 226–247.

Sandler, L., & Witteman, K. (2013). None is enough. *Time*, August 12.

Schur, E. M. (1983). *Labeling women deviant.* Philadelphia, PA: Temple University Press.

Shapiro, G. (2014). Voluntary childlessness: A critical review of the literature. *Studies in the Maternal*, *6*(1). Retrieved from http://www.mamsie.bbk.ac.uk/documents/Shapiro_SiM_6(1)2014.pdf

Tessman, L. (2005). *Burdened virtues: Virtue ethics for liberatory struggles*. New York, NY: Oxford University Press.

Tessman, L. (2015). *Moral failure: On the impossible demands of morality*. New York, NY: Oxford University Press.

The Guttmacher Institute. (2014). *State policies in brief*. Retrieved from https://www.guttmacher.org/statecenter/spibs/spib_RFU.pdf

Ulrich, M., & Weatherall, A. (2000). Motherhood and infertility: Viewing motherhood through the lens of infertility. *Feminism & Psychology*, *10*, 323–336.

Valenti, J. (2012). Are all women born to be mothers? *The Washington Post*. August 31. Retrieved from http://www.washingtonpost.com/opinions/are-all-women-born-to-be-mothers/2012/08/31/b5df2f0e-f2b1–11e1-adc6–87dfa8eff430_story.html

Veevers, J. E. (1980). *Childless by choice*. Toronto: Butterworths.

Velleman, J. D. (2002). Identification and identity. In S. Buss & L. Overton (Eds.), *The contours of agency: Essays on themes from Harry Frankfurt* (pp. 91–123). Cambridge, MA: MIT Press.

Vesper, P. A. (2008). *No to children, yes to childfreedom: Pronatalism and the perspectives and experiences of childfree women*. M.A. thesis, Rutgers University, Camden.

Wager, M. (2000). Childless by choice? Ambivalence and the female identity. *Feminism & Psychology*, *10*(3), 389–395.

Walker, M. U. (1991). Moral luck and the virtues of impure agency. *Metaphilosophy*, *22*, 14–27.

Walshe, S. (2013). Should we care that smart women aren't having kids? *The Guardian*, August 7. Retrieved from http://www.theguardian.com/commentisfree/2013/aug/07/smart-women-not-having-kids

Williams, B. (1982). *Moral luck*. Cambridge: Cambridge University Press.

Further reading

Callan, V. J. (1986). Single women, voluntary childlessness and perceptions about life and marriage. *Journal of Biosocial Science*, *18*, 479–487.

Gillespie, R. (2003). Childfree and feminine: Understanding the gender identity of voluntarily childless women. *Gender and Society*, *17*(1), 122–136.

Paul, P. (2001). Childless by choice. *Advertising Age*, November 1. Retrieved from http://adage.com/article/american-demographics/childless-choice/44381/

Roberts, D. (1998). *Killing the black body: Race, reproduction, and the meaning of liberty*. New York, NY: Vintage.

Roberts, D. E. (1992). Racism and patriarchy in the meaning of motherhood. *The American University Journal of Gender, Social Policy & the Law*, *1*(1), 1–38.

Shaw, R. L. (2011). Women's experiential journey toward voluntary childlessness: An interpretative phenomenological analysis. *Journal of Community & Applied Social Psychology*, *21*, 151–163.

Shriver, L. (2005). No kids please, we're selfish. *The Guardian*, September 16. Retrieved from http://www.theguardian.com/books/2005/sep/17/society#box

Veevers, J. E. (1973). Voluntarily childless wives: An exploratory study. *Sociology and Social Research*, *57*(3), 356–366.

SECTION II
STRUCTURE, AGENCY AND CHILDLESSNESS

Chapter 4

Capital in Pronatalist Fields: Exploring the Influence of Economic, Social, Cultural and Symbolic Capital on Childbearing Habitus

Alyssa Mullins

Abstract

Explanations for voluntary or intentional childlessness range from macro-level forces, such as feminism and access to contraceptives, to micro-level or individual preferences, such as the prioritisation of leisure time over childrearing. However, some researchers contend that the decision (not) to have children is likely impacted by overlapping factors rather than a dichotomised characterisation of internal or external factors. This debate similarly reflects Pierre Bourdieu's 'third way' theoretical and methodological orientation. Bourdieu argued against a false dichotomy between the influence of structure over an individual and the ability for individuals to make active, free choices. He instead claimed that the social world consists of a complex interplay of both individual and structural factors, which he conceptualised as habitus, capital and fields. This chapter initiates the link between current understandings of childbearing preferences with Bourdieu's concepts of habitus (our taken-for-granted, internalised ideologies or identities), capital (economic, social, cultural and symbolic resources) and fields (the external social structures or institutions in which we interact) and proposes quantitative measures of childbearing habitus and capital.

This chapter consists of an exploratory comparison of characteristics of non-parents in relation to childbearing preferences, suggesting measures to identify deeply rooted childbearing habitus and the relationship between access to various forms of capital and the habitus. This study utilises survey responses from a sample of 972 childless men and women between 25 and 40 years of age, assessing measures of social support, cultural norms and economic resources in relation to participants' preference to have or not to have children in the future. A multivariate nested logistic regression was conducted to explore the odds of identifying as voluntarily childless (VC) (not wanting or probably not wanting, to have children in the future) based on socio-demographic factors, as well as various measures of social, economic, cultural and symbolic capital. Findings indicate several variations in significant factors contributing to a preference to remain childfree. Measures of cultural capital, including gender ideologies and pronatalist ideologies, appeared to be the greatest predictors of childbearing habitus. These findings support research suggesting that VC adults are more egalitarian and less traditional in gender relations as well as pronatalist assumptions.

Keywords: Childfreedom; voluntary childlessness; Bourdieu; habitus; capital; pronatalism

Introduction

On average, men and women are having fewer children and having them later in life. Further, voluntary childlessness,[1] defined here as the preference or intent to have no children, has received increased attention. Some researchers emphasise the impact of *subjective* realities, socialisation patterns and family experiences on individuals' childbearing preferences (Christoffersen & Lausten, 2009; Houseknecht, 1979). Others attribute voluntary childlessness to *structural* factors, including feminism, contraceptives and women's pursuit of higher education and careers. However, despite the widespread impact of social and structural changes, voluntary childlessness remains atypical (Livingston & Cohn, 2010; Newport & Wilke, 2013), arguably in part due to pronatalist ideologies deeply rooted within American culture. These ideologies view childbearing as normative and desirable, and permeate several

[1]More recently, researchers, members and activists prefer the term *childfree* (Bulcroft & Teachman, 2004; Cain, 2001), to emphasise intent rather than an absence of something (Gillespie, 2003; Scott, 2009). However, *childfree* is also potentially problematic as it may imply 'motives – such as a dislike of children – that may not apply ...' (Scott, 2009, p. 19). I use *voluntarily childless* and *childfree* synonymously to avoid endorsing either term (Scott, 2009).

institutions, including religion, government, media and communities (Scott, 2009). However, while pronatalist perspectives remain the cultural and behavioural norm in the United States, attitudes towards voluntary childlessness – much like divorce, non-marital childbearing, extramarital sex and cohabitation – are becoming less negative (Koropeckyj-Cox & Pendell, 2007; Thornton & Young-DeMarco, 2001).

Furthermore, some researchers consider the importance of the combined effect of structural and interpersonal factors (Heaton, Jacobson, & Holland, 1999) as contributing to a childfree lifestyle. While academic efforts to explain voluntary childlessness among men remain scarce (Waren & Pals, 2013), numerous attempts have been made to explain women's reasons to remain childfree. For instance, women may be pulled towards childfreedom to enjoy personal autonomy associated with non-motherhood, including travel, hobbies, individual identities and relationships with partners and other adults (Gillespie, 2003). Other factors may push women away from parenthood, including the perceived inability to balance competing work and family roles (Andrade & Bould, 2012), or preferences to pursue personal fulfilment, upward mobility or economic stability (Christoffersen & Lausten, 2009).

This chapter builds on the perspective that delaying or forgoing childrearing is an ongoing process impacted by overlapping factors rather than structural or internal explanations (Mason, 1997). I consider a Bourdieusian theoretical approach and the concepts habitus and capital (Bourdieu, 1990) to initiate a discussion of voluntary childlessness as a complex interplay of structural and individual-level factors carried out in practice. Here, childbearing preferences are considered habitus, or deeply rooted dispositions which shape and are shaped by the external world. Habitus also shape and become shaped by access to various forms of capital. For instance, individuals who support cultural pronatalist ideologies may select relationships or careers that are compatible with childrearing. On the other hand, access to quality and affordable health care may contribute to individuals internalising childrearing as more of an active and personal choice.

Literature Review

Contributions to the Decision (Not) to Become a Parent

Changes in childbearing preferences and behaviours have been attributed to historical economic and social patterns and changing cultural norms (Lisle, 1996; Mintz, 2009). Importantly, the birth control pill and advancements in contraceptive health have afforded men and women an unprecedented ability to control the timing or forgoing of childbearing. Access to birth control has also been directly and indirectly linked to women's expanding labour force participation and economic autonomy, decreasing teen pregnancy and abortion, changing family dynamics and access to social arenas (Ananat & Hungerman, 2012; Bailey, 2006; Cain, 2001).

Many young adults identify professional achievement as a goal prior to, or instead of, having children (Mahaffey & Ward, 2001; Waren & Pals, 2013). While there are some similarities among men and women's preferences to remain childless, there are also gendered educational and financial distinctions (Mahaffey & Ward, 2001; Waren & Pals, 2013). For instance, a perceived inability to balance work and family or a preference for economic stability may push some adults away from childbearing (Andrade & Bould, 2012; Xu, 2013). Competitive advancement and success oftentimes requires complete dedication, especially during reproductive years, which negatively impacts women more directly than men (Budig, Misra, & Boeckmann, 2012).

Women also experience a unique 'double bind' that pits pronatalist obligations for motherhood against standards for the 'ideal worker' (Hays, 1996) which has a disproportionately negative impact on mothers' employability and wages compared to childless women and men (Budig et al., 2012). In the United States, motherhood is characterised by a culture of 'intensive mothering', or the belief that mothers are responsible for the primary caretaking of children and this task should take priority over all other interests and desires (Hays, 1996). Cultural and structural transformations have made most families reliant on the economic contribution of wives and mothers (Skolnick & Skolnick, 2009), yet motherhood ideologies have not caught up to this reality (Hays, 1996; Kricheli-Katz, 2012). Meanwhile, popular conceptions about fatherhood are shifting towards an ideology of the involved father that not only provides for, but also spends quality time with his children (Wall & Arnold, 2007). While fathers do spend more time with their children than fathers of previous generations, this time spent seems to be affiliated with leisure and mentorship (Townsend, 2009; Wall & Arnold, 2007), rather than the intensive and tedious caretaking associated with motherhood. However, childfreedom research is particularly limited in the consideration of men's experiences, overall. Thus, more information is needed on men's experiences and childbearing preferences to further highlight similarities and differences among and between men and women.

Prevalence and Demographics

Voluntary childlessness is often defined as individuals who have never had a child, do not expect or want any, but are biologically capable of doing so (Posten, 1976). However, this phenomenon can be complex and multidimensional (Mosher & Bachrach, 1982). Women who are incapable of bearing children but also do not want to have any may consider themselves childfree, while those who postponed childbearing beyond reproductive years may not. Similarly, some adults may not have biological children but assume the role of adoptive, foster or step-parent (Kelly, 2009). Sociological research remains divided on sample inclusion based on these complex criteria, so significant gaps in the literature remain regarding differences among the childfree (Mosher & Bachrach, 1982).

Childlessness as an active choice is most prevalent among the middle class. Working class and poor adults are more likely to experience higher rates of unplanned pregnancies early in life, limited access to reproductive preventative technologies, and socialisation which elevates childbearing as one's most important life accomplishment (Edin & Kefalas, 2005; Edin & Nelson, 2013). On the other hand, middle- and upper-class populations have greater access to health care and effective reproductive technologies, higher education and professional arenas and leisure time, granting them more autonomy in childbearing decisions (Abma & Martinez, 2006; Gillespie, 2003).

However, certain social disadvantages also contribute to the likelihood of remaining childless. Delayed childbearing among women who become mothers has been associated with stable family backgrounds and higher education, but unstable family background, including family discord, parental divorce, poverty and parental unemployment have also been identified as precursors for the preference to remain childless among some adults (Cain, 2001; Christoffersen & Lausten, 2009; Wallerstein, Lewis, & Blakeslee, 2000). These contrasting links provide insight into the complexities of a childfree identity outside of the perspective of autonomous, career or hobby-driven and middle-class adults.

Childfreedom is commonly considered most prevalent among white Americans. However, limitations within literature indicate that little is known about the true prevalence or experiences of childlessness among women of colour (Kelly, 2009). (Non-)childbearing preferences may also be shaped by or shape marital status. Some unattached individuals may consider their opportunities limited by 'social norms and the absence of a partner' (Mosher & Bachrach, 1982, p. 521). Others may select or avoid partners based on the compatibility of parenting preferences. Religion and religiosity also play important roles in childbearing preferences and behaviours. Childfree adults have the lowest rates of religiosity while the most religiously devout tend to have the most children (Frejka & Westoff, 2008; Hayford & Morgan, 2008; Mosher & Bachrach, 1982). Religious activities can be a source of cultural and social support, or social sanctions, in favour of pronatalist norms (Abma & Martinez, 2006; Zhang, 2008).

In short, studies have found that voluntarily childless (VC) adults tend to be more educated, have higher incomes and careers in professional or leadership positions and indicate less conventional gender role ideologies and religiosity compared to parents (Abma & Martinez, 2006; Frejka & Westoff, 2008; Park, 2005). Leisure time, personal autonomy and a prioritisation of adult relationships may 'pull' some adults towards a childfree lifestyle (Gillespie, 2003), while career or educational plans, becoming ready for the 'parenting lifestyle' (Sassler & Miller, 2014), or personal hardships (Cain, 2001; Christoffersen & Lausten, 2009) may also push some adults away from (or delay) childbearing. Taken together, individual, interpersonal and structural barriers and advantages provide insight into the complex interplay between an individual's personal preference for childbearing and the factors that contribute to this decision. These patterns support the claim that childbearing decisions are likely rooted in class-based habitus, influenced by access to resources and cultural identities in various fields or social arenas.

Theoretical Orientation

Contrasting explanations within literature regarding macro and micro contributors to childfreedom reflects Bourdieu's (1990) critique of an ideological debate within sociology. He argued that sociology falsely dichotomises the influence of structure over an individual and the ability for individuals to make active, free choices. Instead, he claimed that the social world consists of a complex interplay of individual and structural factors and described this theory of practice using the terms 'habitus', 'capital' and 'field'. Habitus include our subjective identities, or durable dispositions deeply rooted within individuals (Bourdieu, 1990). Habitus are shaped by the social world, yet contain individuals' freedom to perceive the social world in varied ways and shape their actions towards that world. Essentially, 'individuals are able to exercise choices within the limits of a specified social structure' (Bourdieu, 1990, p. 53). Habitus may be 'shared' among groups, based on similar experiences, cultural norms and interactions among individuals in shared social arenas (Bourdieu, 1990).

I conceptualise the preference to remain childless as the *habitus* to identify individuals' childbearing identities in relation to personal preferences and external norms and expectations (Gillespie, 2003; Hays, 1996; Mosher & Bachrach, 1982). Bourdieu posed that class-based tastes, preferences and practices are influenced by an interaction between habitus and a configuration of capital. Bourdieu supported Marx's claim that economic capital – money and objects used to produce goods and services – remain important while interacting with additional forms of capital (Bourdieu, 1984, 1990). Childfree adults often report higher incomes, on average, than those that intend to (or do) have children (Park, 2005; Sassler & Miller, 2014). This negative relationship may seem counterintuitive with the average cost of raising a child in the United States exceeding $245,000 (Lino, 2014), but exemplifies the potential interplay between forces. For example, someone with a high-status job may make more money but find balancing their career and childcare more difficult, or even less desirable. Additionally, greater access to quality and affordable health care provides greater agency over reproductive health to delay or prevent childbearing to pursue other interests.

Bourdieu added the importance of social capital, or social groupings and ability to network to gain status or material goods. Family, friends and relationship support networks may encourage and/or contribute to a chosen lifestyle, like the decision (not) to have children. Likewise, Bourdieu considered the importance of cultural capital, or class-based interpersonal skills or knowledge of styles and practices valued by society. This relates to the cultural ideology of pronatalism, which 'condemns those who do not reproduce' (Cain, 2001, p. 19). Subscribing to this culturally valued ideology may correlate with access to other forms of capital, such as a wider social support network and fewer experiences of shame and stereotyping.

Lastly, Bourdieu discusses symbolic capital in relation to prestige and reputation. Symbolic capital also refers to the process of transforming economic, social and/or cultural capital within social fields. In this chapter, I define symbolic capital as social contribution, or 'the belief that one is a vital member of society, with something of value to give to the world' (Keyes, 1998, p. 122) in support of the pronatalist principle that having children corresponds with greater social value (Edin & Kefalas, 2005; Livingston & Parker, 2011).

Some feminists argue that Bourdieu's theoretical perspective prioritises social class over sex/gender, race and sexuality (Lovell, 2000; McCall, 1992). Despite these critiques, Bourdieu's approach remains useful in this study, as childbearing preferences and behaviours are linked to social class in complex ways (Christoffersen & Lausten, 2009; Sassler & Miller, 2014), while limiting childfreedom literature through an exclusively gendered lens may further perpetuate a fragmented understanding of childbearing preferences, ignoring structural and subjective similarities and differences among men and among women. Bourdieu's sociology provides an important lens within this field of study, for which 'we should defend his achievements by putting his theories to work in fresh ways, yet … with a critical gaze' (Fowler, 2010, p. 487). The purpose of this study is to introduce a Bourdieusian outlook regarding the interplay between structure and agency in the study of voluntary childlessness rather than contribute to a particular worldview of *why* people remain childfree. However, this perspective should also be supplemented with feminist insights to further provide critical assessments of the concepts of structure and identities (Lovell, 2000).

Understanding voluntary childlessness as a complex and recurring interplay between structural forces and active agents may shed light on factors contributing to and resulting from the decision (not) to become a parent, as well as how these factors co-exist in a recurring and evolving manner. This research is the first step in this shift by utilising elements of the Bourdieusian theoretical perspective. This shift may provide a more complete view of the complex interplay between individual childbearing preferences and structural influences of social arenas in which we interact.

The Current Study

I intend to contribute to the limited use of Bourdieu's concepts in quantitative studies (Edgerton, Roberts, & Peter, 2013) and the growing body of research on childfreedom by providing quantitative measures of childbearing habitus and capital in support of a shift towards a more complex understanding of voluntary childlessness. This underutilised theoretical paradigm may assist researchers in resolving the complexities of the structural and subjective forces seemingly at odds in existing literature (Gillespie, 2003).

This chapter should be viewed as an initial discussion of the ways access to capital correlates with personal childrearing preferences, although measuring the full complexity of this interplay is beyond the scope of my analysis. This research derives from a larger exploration of distinct habitus between adults who are temporarily childless (TC), including those that want (or probably want) children in the future, and childfree (VC), those that do not (or probably do not) want children. Initial analyses identified significant motivational and personality differences between groups (Mullins, 2016) consistent with patterns in existing childfreedom literature (Scott, 2009). For instance, VC respondents indicated greater agreement with motivations such as 'I do not want to take on the responsibility of raising a child' and 'the costs outweigh the benefits of having a child …'. On the other hand, TC participants expressed greater agreement with statements such as 'I believe I have a maternal/paternal instinct' and 'I want to pass my genes/family name to the next generation'.

Sample and Methods

In November 2015, an online questionnaire was distributed to childless men and women between the ages of 25 and 40 (McQuillan et al., 2012) residing in the United States using non-representative, purposive and convenience sampling. VC adults were oversampled to ensure a comparable distribution of intended parents and the childfree. Efforts were also made to recruit male participants to address the gap in understanding men's experiences of childfreedom (Waren & Pals, 2013). I recruited participants from community forums (see Mullins, 2016 for details), including childfree communities and some targeting *future* parents, as well as more broad interest groups whose moderators would be amenable to the sharing of a survey of this sort.

Some researchers oppose including adults of childbearing ages in cross-sectional studies of childlessness, as intentions may change over time (Christoffersen & Lausten, 2009). However, while intentions, plans and behaviours can shift, intent at any point in time is important to understand this identity (Rovi, 1994). Bivariate analyses and a nested logistic regression were used to identify patterns between the childfree and adults that intend to have children. Additionally, a brief exploration into the interaction between gender and significant measures of capital was conducted to initiate the need for further investigation into the potential for difference in differences between groups.

Variables and Measures

Childlessness Habitus. Childlessness was defined as having no biological, adopted or step children that participants consider 'like their own', including those who are pregnant/expecting. Respondents were categorised into one of two habitus groups based on whether they want children in the future. Those that want or probably want children were considered TC, and those who do not or *probably* do not want children were considered VC.

Economic capital includes annual household income, measured using a nine-point scale ranging from 'Less than \$20,000' to '\$160,000 or more', each recoded to its midpoint. Health care coverage, satisfaction with spending money and a composite measure of economic hardship (α = 0.88) (Shreffler, Griel, Mitchell, & McQuillan, 2015) were also included. Scores on the composite measure ranged from 3 to 15, with higher values indicating more frequent financial hardship in the past 12 months.

Social capital includes satisfaction with leisure time, frequency of time spent with friends, number of friends with children, perceptions of having things in common with friends that have children and a composite measure of perceived social support (α = 0.75) including statements such as 'I get the emotional help and support I need from my family' (Sarason & Sarason, 1985; Zimet, Powell, Farley, Werkman, & Berkoff, 1990). Scores on the composite measure ranged from 4 to 20. Higher values indicated greater social support.

Cultural capital includes two broad categories, cultural gender ideologies and pronatalism. Measures of gender ideologies assessed agreement with traditional and egalitarian ideologies such as, 'It is much better for everyone if the man earns the main living and the woman takes care of the home and family' and 'If a husband and a wife both work full-time, they should share household tasks equally' (McQuillan, Griel, Shreffler, & Bedrous, 2015). Due to low reliability (α = 0.55) and significantly independent effects, a composite measure was not used. The second measure of cultural capital includes a composite measure of the importance of becoming a parent and commitment to pronatalist ideologies (α = 0.94) (McQuillan et al., 2015). Scores range from 4 to 20 with higher scores representing more positive pronatalist views.

Symbolic capital includes a composite variable of three aspects of social contribution (Keyes, 1998) and a fourth measure assessing overall feelings of value within society ($\alpha = 0.75$). Scores ranged from 4 to 20. Higher values indicate greater perceived social value.

Demographic measures include race/ethnicity, age, gender, relationship status, educational attainment, hours worked per week, income and religious affiliation.

Results

Sample Characteristics

Approximately 59% of the sample were VC (see Table 1). The average age was 29.7 years and the sample was predominantly white (88.6%). Approximately 82% were women, although there was more gender and sexuality diversity among VC respondents. Men and non-binary participants represented 21% of the VC sample, compared to 14.5% of the TC. Approximately 86% of the TC identified as heterosexual, compared to 73% of the childfree. TC participants were almost twice as likely to be married (66%) compared to VC participants (36%). However, 26% of the childfree were either cohabitating with an unmarried partner or in a long-term relationship. TC participants had a higher median income ($70,000) than VC participants ($50,000). A greater proportion of the TC group (82.5%) had at least a four-year degree compared to the childfree (70%). Lastly, Atheist respondents were disproportionately represented among both groups (35% of TC, 51% of VC) although TC participants were more likely to identify as Christian (13%) or Catholic (8%) compared to VC participants (7% and 3%, respectively).

Bivariate Results

Bivariate analyses of several measures of capital revealed statistical, but not substantial, differences between groups. For instance, childfree participants were statistically more likely to have trouble paying bills ($p < 0.05$), buying necessities ($p < 0.01$) and paying for medical care ($p < 0.01$). They also had statistically lower income ($p < 0.001$) and were more likely to rely on public health insurance (9%) or have no insurance (9%). VC respondents also reported statistically, but not substantially, less social capital. For instance, TC participants reported greater emotional help

Table 1. Sample Characteristics of Temporarily and Voluntarily Childless Adults ($N = 972$).

	All	Childbearing Preference	
		Temporary	**Voluntary**
	$N = 972$ **%**	**$N = 399$** **%**	**$N = 573$** **%**
Gender			
Women	81.8	85.5	79.2
Men	16.8	14.0	18.7
Other	1.4	0.5	2.1
Average Age[a]	29.7 (4.1)	29.0 (3.3)	30.1 (4.5)
Race/Ethnicity[b]			
Black or African American	1.9	0.5	2.8
Asian	3.1	3.0	3.1
White (Caucasian)	88.6	89.7	87.8
Hispanic or Latino	6.3	4.3	7.7
Bi- or Multi-racial	4.0	3.3	4.5
Other	2.5	2.8	2.6
Sexual orientation			
Heterosexual/Straight	78.7	86.5	73.3
LGBTQA +	21.1	12.8	26.7

Relationship status			
Single, never married	17.9	10.0	23.4
Unmarried, living with a partner	13.6	10.5	15.7
Divorced or separated	1.4	0.5	2.1
Married	48.1	65.7	35.8
In a long-term relationship	15.4	10.8	18.7
Dating one or more partners	3.3	1.8	4.4
Average total annual income	US$61,479.17 (US$40,951.91)	US$66,997.46 (US$40,300.43)	US$57,654.32 (US$40,998.58)
Highest level of education			
Some high school, no degree	0.3	0.3	0.4
High school diploma/GED	2.7	2.0	3.1
Some college, no degree	14.0	8.0	18.2
Associate's (two-year) degree	7.9	6.8	8.7
Bachelor's (four-year) degree	44.3	45.9	43.3
Master's degree or equivalent	22.8	28.8	18.7
Doctorate degree (PhD, MD, etc.)	7.6	7.8	7.5

Table 1. (*Continued*)

	All	Childbearing Preference	
		Temporary	Voluntary
	$N = 972$ %	$N = 399$ %	$N = 573$ %
Currently enrolled/attending school	22.9	22.3	23.4
Average number of hours worked[c]	39.7	40.4 (13.3)	39.2 (14.9)
Religious preference			
Christian	9.5	13.3	6.8
Catholic	4.8	8.0	2.6
Jewish	1.1	1.8	0.7
Muslim	0.2	0.3	0.2
Agnostic	21.7	22.8	20.9
Atheist	44.1	34.8	50.6
Spiritual but not religious	10.4	11.0	10.0
Other	7.1	6.7	7.5

[a]Reported as mean (standard deviation).
[b]Sum will not equal 100% as respondents were able to select more than one option.
[c]Reported as mean (standard deviation).

and support from family ($p < 0.001$), support for major life decisions ($p < 0.05$), and had people to count on during difficult times ($p < 0.05$). On the other hand, childfree respondents were significantly, while not substantially, more satisfied with the amount of leisure time they have ($M = 3.7$) compared to TC ($M = 3.5$), on average ($p < 0.01$). Both groups' cultural gender ideologies were relatively egalitarian, while average responses among the childfree were statistically more egalitarian. TC adults were slightly more likely to agree that mothers should prioritise their children above all else ($M = 2.7$), compared to VC participants ($M = 1.9$) ($p < 0.001$). TC respondents were also statistically, but not substantially, more likely to agree that 'fathers should play an active role in raising children' ($M = 4.4$ and 4.3 respectively, $p < 0.05$).

Measures of pronatalist cultural capital revealed the most substantial bivariate difference between groups. TC respondents were substantially more likely to agree that having children is important to feeling complete as a woman/man ($M = 3.1$) ($p < 0.001$), have always thought they'd be a parent ($M = 3.9$) ($p < 0.001$), and would consider their lives more fulfilling with children ($M = 3.8$) ($p < 0.001$). Additionally, TC participants reported substantially greater agreement that it is important for them to have children ($M = 3.9$, $p < 0.001$) VC participants strongly disagreed with each of these statements, on average.

There were no significant differences in the composite symbolic capital measure between groups. On average, respondents moderately agreed that they have something valuable to contribute to society.

Multivariate Results

The multivariate model consisted of a nested logistic regression exploring the odds of not (or probably not) wanting children in the future based on socio-demographic factors (Model 1), social (Model 2), economic (Model 3), cultural (Model 4) and symbolic (Model 5) capital. Each model of the nested regression was statistically significant. Model 5 ($\chi^2 = 981.70$, $p < 0.001$). incorporated all measures of capital and socio-demographic variables. In Model 5, identification as Hispanic/Latino or bi- or multi-racial ($p < 0.05$) increased the odds of voluntary childlessness, however small sample sizes resulted in large standard errors for these factors. Marriage decreased the odds of voluntary childlessness ($p < 0.01$), controlling for all other factors. Increased time spent with friends also independently decreased the odds of childfreedom ($p < 0.05$). Compared to employer-based private insurance, having public or some other type of insurance increased the odds of being VC by 8.5 times ($p < 0.01$), controlling for all other variables. Higher income was also a significant predictor of childfreedom ($p < 0.05$), independent of other factors. Increased support for an egalitarian division of household labour increased the odds of voluntary childlessness by 2.2 times ($p < 0.01$), while increased support for fathers being more active in childcare decreased the odds of voluntarily childlessness ($p < 0.01$), independent of all other factors. Lastly, increased support of pronatalist cultural capital ideologies ($p < 0.001$) decreased the odds of voluntary childlessness, controlling for all other variables. Gender, age, sexual orientation, education attainment, student status, average hours worked and identification as Atheist were not significant socio-demographic factors in Model 5. Financial hardship, satisfaction with spending money and private/individual or no insurance were also not significant in the full model. Support for traditional gender ideologies and symbolic capital also did not independently predict childfreedom (Table 2).

Interaction Effects

Interaction effects were briefly explored to identify potential relationships between gender and measures of capital. Gender significantly interacted with time spent with friends ($p < 0.05$). In this sample, the more time women spent with friends, the less likely they were to identify as childfree, meanwhile the interaction had the opposite effect for men. Additionally, higher income increased the probability of identifying as childfree more sharply for men than women ($p < 0.001$). Models considering the interaction between gender and marriage, the importance of parenthood, egalitarian ideologies and the belief that fathers should play a more active role in childrearing were not significant.

Discussion

Several sample characteristics were consistent with existing profiles of childless adults. The sample was disproportionately white (Abma & Martinez, 2006; Rovi, 1994). TC respondents were almost twice as likely to be married compared to the VC while childfree respondents were more than twice as likely to be single (never married), indicating the

Table 2. Nested Logistic Regression: Odds Ratios of Voluntarily Childlessness, Demographic and Capital Predictors.

	Respondents Who Do Not Want (or Probably Do Not Want) Children				
	Model 1	**Model 2**	**Model 3**	**Model 4**	**Model 5[e]**
Socio-demographics					
Male	0.12/1.12 (0.24)	0.17/1.18 (0.26)	0.17/1.18 (0.26)	0.87/2.39 (1.23)	1.02/2.77 (1.47)
Black	0.94/2.57 (2.19)	1.24/3.46 (2.94)	1.34/3.81 (3.23)	−0.68/0.50 (0.68)	−0.91/0.40 (0.54)
Asian	0.31/1.37 (0.83)	0.19/1.21 (0.76)	0.22/1.25 (0.81)	1.59/4.93 (6.65)	1.73/5.64 (7.78)
Hispanic/Latino	0.05/1.05 (0.43)	−0.00/1.00	−0.17/0.85 (0.36)	2.62/13.71 (15.71)*	2.52/12.41 (14.24)*
Bi- or Multi-racial	0.53/1.70 (0.50)	0.60/1.83 (0.55)*	0.58/1.78 (0.54)	1.98/7.23 (5.68)*	1.85/6.38 (5.05)*
Other Race/ethnicity	−0.31/0.73 (0.55)	−0.34/0.71 (0.58)	−0.42/0.66 (0.54)	0.79/2.20 (4.96)	0.41/1.51 (3.33)
Age	0.13/1.14 (0.02)***	0.15/1.17 (0.03)***	0.16/1.18 (0.03) ***	0.08/1.08 (0.06)	0.08/1.08 (0.06)
Non-heterosexual	0.77/2.17 (0.45)***	0.77 / 2.16 (0.46) ***	0.75/2.11 (0.46) ***	−0.77/0.46 (0.24)	−0.75/0.47 (0.24)
Married[a]	−1.36/0.26 (0.04)***	−1.38/0.25 (0.04)***	−1.35/0.26 (0.05) ***	−1.17/0.31 (0.15)*	−1.25/0.29 (0.14)**

Table 2. (*Continued*)

	Respondents Who Do Not Want (or Probably Do Not Want) Children				
	Model 1	**Model 2**	**Model 3**	**Model 4**	**Model 5[e]**
Education attainment[b]	−0.26/0.77 (0.05)***	−0.28/0.76 (0.05)***	−0.27 / 0.76 (0.06) ***	−0.27/0.77 (0.15)	−0.29/0.75 (0.15)
Student	0.04/1.04 (0.19)	0.06/1.06 (0.20)	−0.00/1.00 (0.20)	−0.31/0.73 (0.32)	−0.27/0.76 (0.33)
Avg. hours worked	−0.00/1.00 (0.01)	−0.00/1.00 (0.01)	0.00/1.00 (0.01)	0.00/1.00 (0.02)	0.00/1.00 (0.02)
Atheist[c]	0.74/2.09 (0.32)***	0.72/2.05 (0.33)***	0.69/1.99 (0.32) ***	−0.29/0.75 (0.30)	−0.27/0.76 (0.31)
Social capital					
Social support		−0.05/0.95 (0.03)	−0.04/0.96 (0.03)	0.16/1.17 (0.08)*	0.12/1.13 (.08)
Time spent with friends		0.26/1.29 (0.15)*	0.24/1.27 (0.16)*	−0.49/0.61 (0.17)	−0.57/0.57 (0.16)*
# friends with children		−0.12/0.89 (0.07)	−0.14/0.87 (0.07)	0.18/1.20 (0.25)	0.14/1.15 (0.24)
Less in common, friends with kids		0.40/1.49 (0.11)***	0.40/1.50 (0.12) ***	0.07/1.08 (0.20)	0.06/1.07 (0.20)
Leisure time satisfaction		0.14/1.15 (0.08)*	0.08/1.08 (0.08)	0.25/1.29 (0.22)	0.24/1.27 (0.22)

Economic capital			
Financial troubles (12 months)	0.02/1.02 (0.05)	0.06/1.06 (0.11)	0.06/1.06 (0.11)
Spending money satisfaction	0.21/1.23 (0.09) **	−0.10/0.90 (0.16)	−0.08/0.92 (0.17)
Insurance[d]			
Private, individual	0.37/1.44 (0.37)	0.13/1.14 (0.68)	0.09/1.10 (0.66)
Public or other	0.80/2.23 (0.70)*	2.10/8.16 (6.55)**	2.14/8.48 (6.98)**
No insurance	0.58/1.78 (0.67)	0.61/1.84 (1.36)	0.69/1.99 (1.49)
Income	−6.61e-07/1.00 (2.54e-06)	0.00/1.00 (6.99e-06)*	0.00/1.00 (6.97e-06)*
Cultural capital			
Separation of spheres		−0.39/0.68 (0.19)	−0.37/0.69 (0.20)
Egalitarian division of housework		0.85/2.34 (0.67)**	0.79/2.21 (0.64)**
Women's place is the home		−0.21/0.81 (0.35)	−0.22/0.80 (0.34)
Fathers should be more active		−0.91/0.40 (0.12)**	−0.94/0.39 (0.12)**

Table 2. (*Continued*)

	Respondents Who Do Not Want (or Probably Do Not Want) Children				
	Model 1	**Model 2**	**Model 3**	**Model 4**	**Model 5[e]**
Mothers should prioritise children above all				0.12/1.13 (0.20)	0.12/1.13 (0.21)
Importance of parenthood				−1.08/0.34 (0.04)***	−1.08/0.34 (0.04)***
Symbolic capital					
Perceived social value					0.11 / 1.12 (0.07)
Sample size (*N*)	882	882	882	882	882
χ^2	181.56***	221.54***	239.37***	978.92***	981.70***
df	13	18	24	30	31

Entries are given as logistic regression coefficient/odds ratio (OR) with the OR standard error in parentheses.
[a]All other relationship statuses combined as reference group.
[b]Higher values indicate greater educational attainment.
[c]All other religious preferences combined as reference group.
[d]Private, employer insurance as reference group.*$p < 0.05$; **$p < 0.01$; ***$p < 0.001$.

potential for preferences to change based on future partnerships (Mosher & Bachrach, 1982). VC respondents were also more likely to be divorced, cohabitating or in unmarried, long-term relationships and were more likely to identify as a non-binary gender or non-heterosexual orientation. Overall, this diversity supports the importance of exploring the interplay between childbearing preferences and various ideologies, identities and changing structural patterns.

Atheists were vastly overrepresented in the sample, particularly among the childfree. While Atheists account for approximately 4–5% of the US population (Central Intelligence Agency, n.d.), approximately 50% of VC participants considered themselves Atheist. This disproportionate representation may be a result of a web-based sample selection (Pew Research Center, 2015). However, there is likely an interaction between the active effort of delaying or forgoing childbearing among non-parents and reduced rates of religiosity (Frejka & Westoff, 2008; Hayford & Morgan, 2008; McQuillan, Griel, Shreffler, & Tichenor, 2008; Mosher & Bachrach, 1982) The link between religiosity and childbearing preferences among non-parents should be explored in greater detail among a more representative sample in future research.

Childbearing Preferences and Capital

This chapter contributes to existing childfreedom literature by using the Bourdieusian concepts habitus and capital to explore relationships between childbearing preference and correlated factors. Findings include preliminary support for a more nuanced understanding of the interplay between structural, interpersonal and individual factors relating to childbearing preferences. Subtle and substantial differences identified raise additional questions about the ways in which childbearing preferences can be an outcome as well as a contributing factor to access to different types of capital.

Economic capital was an important, yet multifaceted correlate of childlessness. Delaying and forgoing childbearing are often linked to economic advantage, including prioritising professional or economic pursuits (Xu, 2013), the incompatibility of high-status careers and childrearing (Keizer, Dykstra, & Jansen, 2008) or structural barriers and ideological preferences which more frequently lead the working class or poor into parenthood early in life (Edin & Kefalas, 2005; Edin & Nelson, 2013; Livingston, 2015b). In this sample, both groups were among a slightly more advantaged middle class (DeNavas-Walt & Proctor, 2015), on average, although VC respondents indicated greater economic hardship in the last 12 months, were less likely to have employer-based health coverage, and twice as likely to have no health insurance. Similarly, the significant difference between income and men and women's probability of being childfree should be explored in greater detail. The particularly greater odds of childfreedom among higher-earning men may relate to career demands and/or a preference to focus on work, prioritising finances for travel and leisure, or the disproportionate burden men experience to prioritise work above all else.

These findings support the overlap and inconsistencies in existing literature regarding the economic status of childless adults. While some studies suggest that the childfree typically have higher incomes and education attainment compared to parents (Livingston, 2015a; Park, 2005; Rovi, 1994), others have found links between structural disadvantage and the preference to forgo childbearing (Christoffersen & Lausten, 2009). Additional research is needed to further characterise these differences to alleviate inconsistencies. However, economic factors alone do not provide a coherent enough distinction among childless adults. Instead, much like Bourdieu's (1990) call for a deeper understanding of capital beyond economic measures, the decision to remain childless among individuals is not likely a strictly economic evaluation of the costs of raising a child (McQuillan et al., 2008).

Social capital, or support networks, are important contributors to the ability to balance demands of childrearing and other responsibilities. Leisure time and relationships with other adults are often cited as contributors to the decision (not) to have children (Gillespie, 2003; McQuillan et al., 2015). Bivariate findings indicated statistically greater levels of social support among those that wish to have children in the future. In the multivariate model, time spent with friends was a significant predictor of childfreedom, and further highlights interactions between multiple characteristics. The significant, opposite effect of gender on the probability of childfreedom for men and women highlights the importance of considering gendered socialisation. For instance, are men socialised by friends to be more independent while women are socialised to become mothers?

Measures of cultural capital were important predictors of childbearing habitus, supporting claims that VC adults are more egalitarian and less traditional in gender relations and pronatalist assumptions. However, both groups were relatively egalitarian overall. The most substantial bivariate difference was in response to the statement 'a mother should prioritise her children above all else'. TC participants reported moderate average agreement while VC participants were more likely to disagree. This finding supports the culture of 'intensive mothering' (Hays, 1996) among those that want to have children in the future, but raises additional questions about why this relationship exists. Have external cultural pressures influenced those with a pro-childbearing habitus that to be a good mother a woman must prioritise their children above all else? Has disagreement with this ideology, but a perceived lack of alternate options, influenced the decision to remain childless among the childfree?

While there are statistical differences between groups regarding differential access to forms of capital, the greatest and seemingly most obvious, difference between the TC and the VC relates to the support for pronatalism. However, despite the strong association between measures of pronatalism and childbearing habitus, the current model cannot answer whether the increased importance of parenthood causes more pronatalist fertility intentions or whether decreased intentions result in a reassessment of cultural attitudes regarding importance of parenthood (McQuillan et al., 2008). A more detailed exploration into this substantial difference may further expose the complex interplay between pronatalism as capital, childbearing preferences as a deeply rooted habitus, and the influence of (or onto) various social arenas.

The limited substantial differences in several of the measures of capital, and various similarities between groups identified in a more detailed analysis (Mullins, 2016), also provide grounds for a more nuanced discussion of childbearing habitus among non-parents. For instance, there were no significant differences between groups' symbolic capital, measured here as perceived social value (Keyes, 1998). While identity making through childbearing is particularly common among working class and poor parents and parents-to-be (Edin & Kefalas, 2005; Livingston & Parker, 2011; Sassler & Miller, 2014), the respondents in this sample did not indicate a shortage of life purpose or successes outside of their desire to become a parent, on average. This class-based distinction may highlight differences among parents-to-be, where those delaying or actively planning childbearing may, in some ways, be more similar to the childfree than to others who will or have become parents.

Limitations/Future Research

As a preliminary exploration, this research is not without limitations. Findings should not be generalised to a broader population beyond identifying emerging themes as the sample is not nationally representative of the US population. Oversampling and convenience sampling techniques were used to increase variance among the childfree and provide a robust comparative sample.

Fertility was intentionally overlooked in this analysis to emphasise preference regardless of biological capability. However, differences in parenting preferences and the importance of parenthood among those facing biological barriers may provide further indication of the relationship between childrearing and access to forms of capital. Since the measures of the importance of parenthood were substantially significant, researchers should continue exploring processes through which parenthood comes to be valued and how this might vary among those facing fertility barriers (McQuillan et al., 2015).

The sample is also limited to mostly white, heterosexual and middle-class respondents, limiting the ability to identify childbearing preferences and capital among non-parents of marginalised groups. The lack of diversity in samples of childless adults is common in existing literature (Kelly, 2009) and should be explored in greater detail to fill in the many gaps that remain regarding the intersection between race, class and meanings of parenthood (Clark, 2012). While these measures of capital provide useful substantial and significant comparisons between the two groups in this sample, the significant gendered interactions highlight the need for additional explorations of the interrelatedness of characteristics, while continuing to incorporate both structural and agentic factors. Future research should explore the intersection of capital(s) and habitus, and, more importantly, consider the aspects of race, gender, sexuality and embodied capital (Lovell, 2000) not addressed here.

References

Abma, J. C., & Martinez, G. M. (2006). Childlessness among older women in the United States: Trends and profiles. *Journal of Marriage and Family*, *68*, 1045–1056.

Ananat, E. O., & Hungerman, D. M. (2012). The power of the pill for the next generation: Oral contraception's effects on fertility, abortion, and maternal and child characteristics. *Review of Economics and Statistics*, *94*, 37–51.

Andrade, C., & Bould, S. (2012). Child-care burden and intentions to have a second child: Effects of perceived justice in the division of child-care. *International Review of Sociology: Revue Internationale de Sociologie*, *22*, 25–37.

Bailey, M. J. (2006). More power to the pill: The impact of contraceptive freedom on women's life cycle labor supply. *Quarterly Journal of Economics, 121*, 289–320.

Bourdieu, P. (1984). *Distinction: A social critique of the judgment of taste*. Cambridge, MA: Harvard University Press.

Bourdieu, P. (1990). *The logic of practice*. Stanford, CA: Stanford University Press.

Budig, M. J., Misra, J., & Boeckmann, I. (2012). The motherhood penalty in cross-national perspective: The importance of work-family policies and cultural attitudes. *Social Politics, 19*, 163–193.

Bulcroft, R., & Teachman, J. (2004). Ambiguous constructions: Development of a childless or child-free life course. In M. Coleman & L. H. Ganong (Eds.), *Handbook of contemporary families: Considering the past, contemplating the future* (pp. 116–135). London: Sage Publications.

Cain, M. (2001). *The childless revolution: What it means to be childless today*. Cambridge, MA: Perseus Publishing.

Central Intelligence Agency. (n.d.). *The world factbook*. Retrieved from https://www.cia.gov/library/publications/the-world-factbook/geos/us.html. Accessed on May 10, 2016.

Christoffersen, M. N., & Lausten, N. (2009). Early and late motherhood: Economic, family background and social conditions. *Finnish Yearbook of Population Research*, 79–95.

Clark, A. M. (2012). *A phenomenology of the meaning of motherhood for African American and Hispanic women who do not have children in the United States*. Master's thesis, Department of Sociology, University of Nebraska.

DeNavas-Walt, C., & Proctor, B. D. (2015). Income and poverty in the United States: 2014. *United States Census Bureau Current Population Reports*, September.

Edgerton, J. D., Roberts, L. W., & Peter, T. (2013). Disparities in academic achievement: Assessing the role of habitus and practice. *Social Indicators Research, 114*, 303–322.

Edin, K., & Kefalas, M. (2005). *Promises I can keep: Why poor women put motherhood before marriage*. Los Angeles, CA: University of California Press.

Edin, K., & Nelson, T. J. (2013). *Doing the best I can: Fatherhood in the inner city*. Los Angeles, CA: University of California Press.

Fowler, B. (2010). Reading Pierre Bourdieu's masculine domination: Notes toward an intersectional analysis of gender, culture, and class. *Cultural Studies, 17*, 468–494.

Frejka, T., & Westoff, C. F. (2008). Religion, religiousness and fertility in the US and in Europe. *European Journal of Population, 24*, 5–31.

Gillespie, R. (2003). Childfree and feminine: Understanding the gender identity of voluntarily childless women. *Gender & Society, 17*, 122–136.

Hayford, S. R., & Morgan, S. P. (2008). Religiosity and fertility in the United States: The role of fertility intentions. *Social Forces, 86*, 1163–1188.

Hays, S. (1996). *The cultural contradictions of motherhood*. New Haven, CT: Yale University Press.

Heaton, T. B., Jacobson, C. K., & Holland, K. (1999). Persistence and change in decisions to remain childless. *Journal of Marriage and the Family*, *61*, 531–539.
Houseknecht, S. K. (1979). Timing of decision to remain voluntarily childless: Evidence for continuous socialization. *Psychology of Women Quarterly*, *4*, 81–96.
Keizer, R., Dykstra, P. A., & Jansen, M. D. (2008). Pathways into childlessness: Evidence of gendered life course dynamics. *Journal of Biosocial. Science*, *40*, 863–878.
Kelly, M. (2009). Women's voluntary childlessness: A radical rejection of motherhood? *WSQ: Women's Studies Quarterly*, *37*, 157–172.
Keyes, C. L. M. (1998). Social well-being. *Social Psychology Quarterly*, *61*, 121–140.
Koropeckyj-Cox, T., & Pendell, G. (2007). Attitudes about childlessness in the United States: Correlates of positive, neural, and negative responses. *Journal of Family Issues*, *28*, 1054–1082.
Kricheli-Katz, T. (2012). Choice, discrimination, and the motherhood penalty. *Law & Society Review*, *46*, 557–587.
Lino, M. (2014). *Expenditures on children by families, 2013*. U.S. Department of Agriculture, Center for Nutrition Policy and Promotion. Retrieved from http://www.cnpp.usda.gov/sites/default/files/expenditures_on_children_by_families/crc2013.pdf. Accessed on May 10, 2016.
Lisle, L. (1996). *Without child: Challenging the stigma of childlessness*. New York, NY: Routledge.
Livingston, G. (2015a). *Childlessness*. Pew Research Center, May 7. Retrieved from http://www.pewsocialtrends.org/2015/05/07/childlessness-falls-family-size-grows-among-highly-educated-women/. Accessed on July 10, 2015.
Livingston, G. (2015b). *For most highly educated women, motherhood doesn't start until the 30s*. Pew Research Center, January 15. Retrieved from http://www.pewresearch.org/fact-tank/2015/01/15/for-most-highly-educated-women-motherhood-doesnt-start-until-the-30s/. Accessed on May 10, 2016.
Livingston, G., & Cohn, D. (2010). *Childlessness up among all women; Down among women with advanced degrees*. Pew Research Center, June 25. Retrieved from http://www.pewsocialtrends.org/2010/06/25/childlessness-up-among-all-women-down-among-women-with-advanced-degrees/. Accessed on June 5, 2015.
Livingston, G., & Parker, K. (2011). *Attitudes about fatherhood*. Pew Research Center, June 15. Retrieved from http://www.pewsocialtrends.org/2011/06/15/chapter-2-attitudes-about-fatherhood/. Accessed on June 5, 2015.
Lovell, T. (2000). Thinking feminism with and against Bourdieu. *Feminist Theory*, *1*, 11–32.
Mahaffey, K. A., & Ward, S. K. (2001). The gendering of adolescents' childbearing and educational plans: Reciprocal effects and the influence of social context. *Sex Roles*, *46*, 403–417.
Mason, K. O. (1997). Explaining fertility transitions. *Demography*, *34*, 443–454.
McCall, L. (1992). Does gender fit? Bourdieu, feminism, and conceptions of social order. *Theory and Society*, *21*, 837–867.

McQuillan, J., Griel, A. L., Shreffler, K. M., & Bedrous, A. V. (2015). The importance of motherhood and fertility intentions among US women. *Sociological Perspectives*, *58*, 1–16.

McQuillan, J., Griel, A. L., Shreffler, K. M., & Tichenor, V. (2008). The importance of motherhood among women in the contemporary United States. *Gender & Society*, *22*, 477–496.

McQuillan, J., Greil, A. L., Shreffler, K. M., Wonch-Hill, P. A., Gentzler, K. C., & Hathcoat, J. D. (2012). Does the reason matter? Variations in childlessness concerns among U.S. women. *Journal of Marriage and Family*, *74*, 1161–1181.

Mintz, S. (2009). Beyond sentimentality: American childhood as a social and cultural construct. In A. S. Skolnick & J. H. Skolnick (Eds.), *Family in transition* (15th ed., pp. 293–306). New York, NY: Pearson Education, Inc.

Mosher, W. D., & Bachrach, C. A. (1982). Childlessness in the United States: Estimates from the national survey of family growth. *Journal of Family Issues*, *3*, 517–543.

Mullins, A. R. (2016). *'I kid you not, I am asked a question about children at least once a week': Exploring differences in childbearing habitus in pronatalist fields.* Unpublished doctoral dissertation, University of Central Florida, Orlando, FL.

Newport, F., & Wilke, J. (2013). Desire for children still norm in U.S. *Gallup*, September, 25. Retrieved from http://www.gallup.com/poll/164618/desire-children-norm.aspx. Accessed on June 4, 2015.

Park, K. (2005). Choosing childlessness: Weber's typology of action and motives of the voluntarily childless. *Sociological Inquiry*, *75*, 372–402.

Pew Research Center. (2015). *Coverage error in internet surveys: Who web-only surveys miss and how that affects results.* Pew Research Center, September 22. Retrieved from http://www.pewresearch.org/2015/09/22/coverage-error-in-internet-surveys/. Accessed on May 10, 2016.

Posten, D. L. (1976). Characteristics of voluntarily and involuntarily childless wives. *Social Biology*, *23*, 296–307.

Rovi, S. (1994). Taking 'no' for an answer: Using negative reproductive intentions to study the childless/childfree. *Population Research and Policy Review*, *13*, 343–365.

Sarason, I. G., & Sarason, B. R. (1985). *Social support: Theory, research and applications.* The Hague: Martinus Niijhoff.

Sassler, S., & Miller, A. J. (2014). 'We're very careful…': The fertility desires and contraceptive behaviors of cohabitating couples. *Family Relations*, *63*, 538–553.

Scott, L. S. (2009). *Two is enough: A couple's guide to living childless by choice.* Berkeley, CA: Seal Press.

Shreffler, K. M., Griel, A. L., Mitchell, K. S., & McQuillan, J. (2015). Variation in pregnancy intendedness across U.S. women's pregnancies. *Maternal Child Health Journal*, *19*, 932–938.

Skolnick, A. S., & Skolnick, J. H. (2009). *Family in transition* (15th ed.). New York, NY: Pearson Education, Inc.

Thornton, A., & Young-DeMarco, L. (2001). Four decades of trends in attitudes toward family issues in the United States: The 1960s through the 1990s. *Journal of Marriage and Family*, *63*, 1009–1037.

Townsend, N. (2009). The four facets of fatherhood. In A. S. Skolnick & J. H. Skolnick (Eds.), *Family in transition* (15th ed., pp. 283–293). New York, NY: Pearson Education, Inc.

Wall, G., & Arnold, S. (2007). How involved is involved fathering? An exploration of the contemporary culture of fatherhood. *Gender & Society*, *21*, 508–527.

Wallerstein, J. S., Lewis, J. M., & Blakeslee, S. (2000). *The unexpected legacy of divorce: A 25 year landmark study*. New York, NY: Hachette Books.

Waren, W., & Pals, H. (2013). Comparing characteristics of voluntarily childless men and women. *Journal of Population Research*, *30*, 151–170.

Xu, Q. (2013). Absent or ambivalent mothers and avoidant children – An evolutionary reading of Zhang Kangkang's motherhood stories. *Finnish Yearbook of Population Research*, *XLVIII*, 147–168.

Zhang, L. (2008). Religious affiliation, religiosity, and male and female fertility. *Demographic Research*, *18*, 233–261.

Zimet, G., Powell, S. S., Farley, G. K., Werkman, S., & Berkoff, K. A. (1990). Psychometric characteristic of the multidimensional scale of perceived social support. *Journal of Personality Assessment*, *55*, 610–617.

Chapter 5

Social Inclusion, Connectedness and Support: Experiences of Women without Children in a Pronatalist Society

Melissa Graham, Beth Turnbull, Hayley McKenzie and Ann Taket

Abstract

Women's reproductive circumstances and choices have consequences for their experiences of social connectedness, inclusion and support across the life-course. Australia is a pronatalist country and women's social identity remains strongly linked to motherhood. Yet the number of women foregoing motherhood is increasing. Despite this, women without children are perceived as failing to achieve womanhood as expected by pronatalist ideologies that assume all women are or will be mothers. Defying socially determined norms of motherhood exposes women without children to negative stereotyping and stigma, which has consequences for their social connectedness, inclusion and support. This chapter examines theories of social connectedness, inclusion and support, drawing on Australian empirical data to explore how women without children experience social connectedness, inclusion and support in a pronatalist society within their daily lives.

Keywords: Social inclusion; social connectedness; social support; social exclusion; women without children; Australia

Introduction

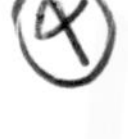

A woman's decision to have or not have children is dependent on a diversity of factors, circumstances and decisions which have consequences for her experiences of social inclusion, connectedness and support across the life course. Yet these personal circumstances and choices

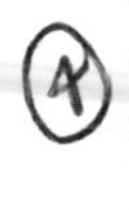
are subject to public gaze and scrutiny. Most societies and cultures situate women as mothers and as such women's social identity remains strongly linked to motherhood (Anderson, 2007; Dever, 2005; Graham & Rich, 2012a; Graham & Rich, 2012b; Heard, 2006; Jackson & Casey, 2009; McQuillan et al., 2012; Morrell, 2000). Pervasive pronatalist ideologies are evident in Australia (Anderson, 2007; Dever, 2005; Heard, 2006; Jackson & Casey, 2009). However, the number of women without children is increasing. Australian 2011 census data indicates 31% of all women aged 15 years and over do not have children (Australian Bureau of Statistics, 2012a), which was a 3% increase from 2006 (Australian Bureau of Statistics, 2012b). Australia is not unique; other countries have also observed similar patterns of increasing numbers of women not having children (Miettinen, Rotkirch, Szalma, Donno, & Tanturri, 2015). It has been posited that these trends are 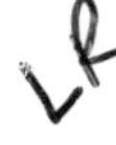 attributable to the rise of feminism; affording women broader access to contraception and reproductive choice, and increasing workforce participation (Gillespie, 2003; Seccombe, 1991).

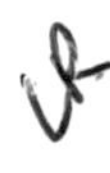
Despite the increasing number of women not having children and the achievements of feminist movements, women without children continued to be stigmatised, negatively stereotyped and subsequently socially excluded. This chapter draws on Australian empirical mixed-methods data from the *Life as a woman with no children in Australian society: resources, opportunities and participation* study with 1,070 women with no children aged 25–64, to examine the exclusion of women without children from social participation at: the societal level, where mothers are constructed as insiders and women without children are outsiders; the community level, where women without children are stereotyped and stigmatised; and the individual level within families and friendship groups. Throughout this chapter, illustrative quotes are drawn from open-ended questions in the self-administered online questionnaire. In this chapter, pronatalism is considered first, followed by an exploration of stigma and negative stereotyping in relation to the social exclusion of women without children. Finally, social inclusion, connectedness and support are discussed, providing a picture of the everyday experiences in a pronatalist society of women without children.

Prevailing and Pervasive Pronatalism

> I have made a choice knowingly. There is nothing wrong with me, I am not strange and I am happy. Do not assume

> that because you have children that I share your dream of having them. Accept me for who I am, not who you think I should be. I don't criticise you for wanting/having children so why do you do the reverse to me? (ID 33; voluntarily childless; aged 45).

Pronatalism, a prevailing characteristic of Australian culture and society, encourages procreation. Furthermore, pronatalism assumes and expects all women *want*, *can*, and *will* be mothers; constructing motherhood as natural (Shapiro, 2014), an obligatory rite in the path to female fulfilment (Dux & Simic, 2008) and a requirement for the achievement of a woman's feminine identity (Gillespie, 2000; Hird & Abshoff, 2000). Consequently, pronatalism disempowers and marginalises women who do not meet pronatalist norms of stereotypical femininity – motherhood (Gotlib, 2016; Mumtaz, Shahid, & Levay, 2013).

> Motherhood discourses can be seen to be drawn from, and enmeshed in powerful, hegemonic ideological doctrines. Experts and opinion formers constitute powerful elites who have been able to privilege their accounts of the natural inevitability of a desire for motherhood in women; of motherhood as women's principal social role; and crucially, the centrality of motherhood to understandings of feminine identity. (Gillespie, 2000, p. 225)

Heitlinger (1991) argues pronatalism occurs culturally, ideologically, psychologically, at the cohort level and in relation to population-level policy. Gotlib (2016) further suggests pronatalism stipulates who and what women are, and pronatalist discourse is supported through policies. Social-cultural norms shape and influence the importance of role identities (McQuillan et al., 2012) and tie womanhood to motherhood (Arendall, 2000; Turnbull, Graham, & Taket, 2016b), with motherhood being central to a woman's identity (Gillespie, 1999, 2000, 2003; Heitlinger, 1991). Women without children fail to achieve social-cultural constructions of womanhood and are viewed as incomplete. Analysis of Australian policy in relation to women's reproductive choices and their consequences found policies perpetuate socially, culturally and ideologically stereotypical positions, promoting and positioning women's roles in society as mothers and carers, thereby conserving the notion of traditional gender roles within families (Graham, McKenzie, & Lamaro, 2018; Graham & Rich, 2012a).

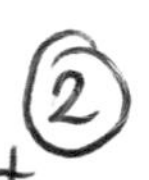

Women without children continue to be characterised as unconventional, undesirable, maladjusted, socially deviant and less feminine than women with children (Çopur & Koropeckyj-Cox, 2010; Doyle, Pooley, & Breen, 2013; Gillespie, 1999, 2000; LaMastro, 2001; Letherby, 1999; Morell, 1994; Park, 2002; Rich, Taket, Graham, & Shelley, 2011) as they fail to achieve womanhood, being motherhood, as expected by pronatalist ideologies.

> I recently posted on a Facebook thread that I was happy not having children and I felt that decision has brought me happiness. About half a dozen people, most[ly] men had negative replies for my comment. One said something like, 'it's women like you who are wrong with this world. It's your sacred role and purpose to be a mother. I hope you enjoy all of your money'. (ID 482; voluntarily childless; aged 40)

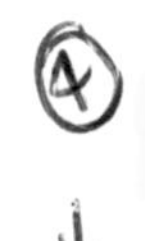

The private nature of mothering and childbearing is in the public realm where it is up for comment and debate, as evident in social norms and policy inclusion positions. A feminist approach recognises the connection of the public and private where the 'personal is political' (Campbell & Wasco, 2000; Laakso & Drevdahl, 2006; Smith, 1987; Watson, 1995), drawing attention to the '*political meanings and imperatives'* of women's daily lived experiences (Hughes, 2002, p. 152). As such, the personal and private nature of women's decision to have or not have children is done so within the context of the pronatalist environment, whereby the rhetoric of childbearing is directed and promoted to women. For example, research mapping policies specific to women's reproductive choices and consequences found policies promoted motherhood. The policies aimed to assist women who had made the decision to have children, rather than assist women in the decision-making process. The inherent assumption underlying these policies is that all women will become mothers, and therefore support women to become mothers. Demonstrating this is Australia's Paid Parental Leave Scheme, whereby women, not men, are assumed to be the primary caregivers of children (Graham, McKenzie, Lamaro, & Klein, 2016). It is this policy assumption which then impacts the norms of motherhood and the assumption that this is what all women want, and therefore, will do.

> The number of times I have [been] personally stigmatised is countless but I tend to view prevailing community perceptions such as public policy as an indicator of how child-free women are viewed as public policy is, arguably, shaped by prevailing public opinion. (ID 223; voluntarily childless; aged 45)

By defying the socially determined norms of motherhood, women without children are subject to negative stereotyping (Mueller & Yoder, 1997, 1999) and stigmatisation (Culley & Hudson, 2005; Park, 2002; Rich et al., 2011), and consequently social exclusion (Graham, Hill, Shelley, & Taket, 2013; Hinton, Kurinczuk, & Ziebland, 2010; Letherby & Williams, 1999; Turnbull, Graham, & Taket, 2016a; Turnbull et al., 2016b; Turnbull, Graham, & Taket, 2016c), situating them as a population group from which people seek social distance (Gillespie, 2000; Park, 2002; Turnbull et al., 2016b; Veevers, 1974). This social distance has consequences for the social inclusion, connectedness and support of women without children. The following section explores stigma, stereotyping and social exclusion.

Stigma, Stereotyping and Social Exclusion

> There have been so many judgements made in social situations over the years, so many strangers giving pitying or uncomfortable looks after asking the all-invading question 'do you have children?'. (ID 203; circumstantially childless; aged 50)

Social exclusion allows insight into the processes whereby individuals are denied full social participation due to their incongruence with societal rules and norms. Due to normative pronatalist ideology and discourses, women who do not have children challenge dominant social norms and moral rules (Carey, Graham, & Shelley, 2009), resulting in negative stereotyping and stigmatisation. Stigma is a discrediting attribute that devalues an individual (Goffman, 1963) and these attributes become associated with discrediting dispositions which become the basis for social exclusion of those individuals 'marked' with the discrediting disposition (Major & O'Brien, 2005). Being a woman without children is a stigmatised position within Australia's pronatalist society; a society where not mothering is deviant and motherhood is privileged (Carey et al., 2009; Rich, et al., 2011). Within the context of prevailing and pervasive pronatalist discourses, not mothering is non-normative social behaviour and thus a discrediting and stigmatising attribute constructing a population group that is stigmatised (Gillespie, 2000; Lampman & Dowling-Guyer, 1995; Letherby, 1994, 2000; Letherby & Williams, 1999; Miall, 1986; Park, 2002; Rich et al., 2011; Riessman, 2000). Women without children are often devalued, discredited, overlooked, ignored, invisible and not recognised as a stigmatised population group within society.

> I'm upper middle class, highly educated and working in a professional environment. The clear sense I get from some people that women without children are inferior human beings is a niggle for me. For women who don't have anywhere near the advantages I do, I imagine it does them some real personal damage. (ID 566; circumstantially childless; aged 35)

> A former friend once told me my position on a foreign political matter was less valid than hers because I didn't have kids and she did. It was hurtful and made me realise the level of bias against childless/childfree people. (ID 202; involuntarily childless; age 46)

> The government marginalises childless women. I felt my needs were invisible to the political debate. (ID 181; voluntarily childless; aged 53)

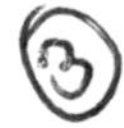

Research has consistently highlighted the negative stereotyping and stigmatisation of women without children. For example, involuntarily childless women; that is, women who wish to have biological children but are unable to achieve a viable pregnancy, have been labelled as sad, pitiful, suffering, desperate, 'victims' of childlessness and sympathy-worthy (Bays, 2017; Graham & Rich, 2012a; Letherby, 2002a). In contrast, voluntarily childless women who have freely chosen not to have children are depicted as individualistic, selfish, irresponsible, self-centred, materialistic, career-focused, abnormal, immature, unfeminine, less caring and less socially desirable (Gillespie, 2000; Ireland, 1993; Letherby, 2002a; Letherby, 2002b; Park, 2002; Somers, 1993; Veevers, 1974). These negative evaluations of women without children can make them particularly vulnerable to being stigmatised because they disrupt dominant constructions of feminine identity to which motherhood is central, particularly voluntarily childless women (Hird & Abshoff, 2000; Shapiro, 2014).

> An elderly woman asked me if I had children and I said no. I told her that I did not want to have children. She was very shocked and kept telling me that I had to and that children are everything. That it is not natural not to want children. I listened to her because I did not want to offend her. But I was so angry for her to judge me like that. (ID 233; voluntarily childless; aged 34)

> I have been stigmatised many times. I have been called 'weird', 'selfish', 'strange', 'unnatural' 'numerous times'. (ID 254; voluntarily childless; aged 53)

Women without children have reported a need to justify their non-motherhood (Doyle et al., 2013; Graham et al., 2013; Maher & Saugeres, 2007; Rich et al., 2011; Simpson, 2007; Tietjens-Meyers, 2001; Turnbull et al., 2016a) to subvert attention away from this discrediting attribute (Graham et al., 2013; Park, 2005). Letherby (1999, 2002b) found voluntarily childless women felt it was easier to say that they had not made a decision, and keep their 'status' and experiences hidden, while Morell (1994) suggests women must undertake subversive action to hide their non-mother identity. Morison, Macleod, Lynch, Mijas, and Shivakumar (2016) found two contradictory rhetorics of choice which allowed voluntarily childless women to resist and challenge stigmatising identities by drawing on the 'childfree-by-choice' or the 'disavowal of choice' script.

> When people ask me if I have children I lie and say I have because I feel like they will think I am lesser if I admit I don't. (ID 589; involuntarily childless; aged 42)

Our study found one in five women reported stigma consciousness, including experiences of being stereotyped, judged, seen as different and treated differently, due to having no children, with women who intended to be mothers in the future reporting the least stigma consciousness and involuntarily childless women reporting the most stigma consciousness. Almost one-third (31.4%) of the women reported experiencing negative stereotyping, that they were viewed negatively in relation to a number of characteristics, such as being selfish, immature, unnatural, non-nurturing and abnormal, due to having no children.

Women who identified as intended future mothers reported the least perceived negative stereotyping, followed by circumstantially childless women (those who are unable to have children due to life circumstances), women who had not yet decided whether to have children, and involuntarily childless women. Voluntarily childless women reported the most negative stereotyping due to having no children. It is posited that the greater negative stereotyping experienced and reported by voluntarily childless women is a consequence of these women's deviance from the traditional ascribed gender role of woman as mother.

> Returning to Australia after living overseas I really felt the isolation of being a woman who was childless and maybe not married. It seems to be a well-worn path here in Australia, in that you 'should' be married, with a mortgage and children. Without these I have felt disconnected [from] my friends (with kids) and also my country. I think a lot of this is the perceived societal role of women here in Australia, which is highly conservative and traditional. (ID 463; circumstantially childless; aged 40)

Stigma consciousness and negative stereotyping due to having no children decreased with older age, with women aged 30–44 years experiencing the most stigma consciousness and women aged 30–49 years the most negative stereotyping.

> At a younger age most definitely [felt she was stereotyped or stigmatised due to not having children], as I chose to not have children I feel most women found that rather confronting. Now that I am older I feel the stigma has dropped off but I still get women in particular who feel sorry for me. (ID 56; voluntarily childless; aged 45)

> Yes [experienced stereotyping and stigma due to not having children] very much when my friends all had babies. Some women completely excluded me on the basis of my childlessness. (ID 160; circumstantially childless; aged 57)

The stigma and negative stereotyping attached to being a woman without children can result in social exclusion; a dynamic and contingent process driven by unequal power relationships. As a result, individuals experience exclusion in different ways in different places, times and contexts depending on the domains of life as well as their socio-demographic characteristics. Further, one's life-choices and circumstances can be conceptualised as both pathways to, and outcomes of, social exclusion. Exclusion interacts across the economic, political, social and cultural domains, and at the individual, community and societal level (Popay et al., 2008; Taket et al., 2009). Social exclusion is '*influenced by societal beliefs and structures which act to "exclude" individuals based on personal characteristics*' (Taket et al., 2009, p. 16), such as the discrediting attribute of being a woman who does not have children. The process of exclusion may be voluntary or involuntary (Burchardt, Le Grand, & Piachaud, 1999). The latter refers to the 'othering' of individuals, which is particularly the case for women without children due to non-conformity with pronatalist ideologies and social norms in Australia. However, equally, women without children may voluntarily exclude themselves due to the stigma and negative stereotyping surrounding their non-mothering position. Importantly, social exclusion is not a dichotomy whereby individuals are either included or excluded. Rather, individuals are positioned along a continuum from absolute inclusion to absolute exclusion in relation to specific contexts.

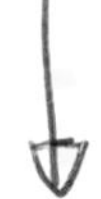

> As a church member being the age of 38 and being unmarried and childless it feels like people believe you are a failure. I often feel very ostracised at women's events as I feel I can't contribute to discussions as I am neither a married woman nor a mother, therefore an outsider. (ID 198; involuntarily childless; aged 38)

Due to dominant pronatalist ideologies and being 'marked' with a discrediting attribute, women without children may be considered to have little social value and subsequently excluded from full social participation. Findings from our study suggest women without children perceived exclusion due to having no children from: social participation including participating in social and leisure activities such as going out to restaurants, cinemas and sports events (43.2%); interactions including frequency of spending time with and talking to friends and family (47.2%) and support meaning the frequency of receiving instrumental and affective social support, such as practical help, advice in a crisis and being listened to (43.8%).

> [I] have missed out on invites to parties and functions with friends because they were concerned I wouldn't 'fit in' or that I would feel 'uncomfortable' dining with couples who had children. I have felt hurt and embarrassed on numerous occasions once I found out I had been deliberately excluded. (ID 189, circumstantially childless; aged 45)

In contrast, some women did not feel excluded from social interactions, participation and support. Social networks may change over time and women without children's friendship circles may shift towards other women without children and those who they believe will provide support in their older age.

> Not with my close friends or they wouldn't be my close friends. (ID 213; voluntarily childless; aged 50)

There were some differences between the types of women with no children and their experiences of exclusion, with women who had not decided whether to have children and women who intend to be mothers experiencing less perceived exclusion in relation to social participation, interactions and support. Social participation, interactions and support can be considered as indicators of exclusion within one's social domain of life. Perceived exclusion from social participation, interactions and support varied with age, with younger women (25–29 years of age) perceiving less exclusion from social participation, interactions and support than older women.

> One friend grew distant after she had children and realised I wasn't going to change my mind. Our friendship ended, I felt she was no longer interested in me as a person because I didn't fit with her expectations or 'wasn't like her' anymore. (ID 59; voluntarily childless; aged 56)

> Sitting in a room with about five girlfriends. I was the only one without children. I had no ability to participate in the conversation for about 2 hours as all they spoke of was their children and the common experiences they had with them. Afterwards they told me I was really quiet and was I all right. (ID 167; circumstantially childless; aged 50)

> A close friend announced she was pregnant. Unknown to her, I have been having trouble conceiving. I am (slightly)

> older than her, and always thought I would be pregnant before she was. It was the first time my difficulties conceiving had really hit home – it was hard to be excited for her, I almost cried! I can't tell her (or anyone else really, except my partner) about the conception difficulties. I don't know why – she would be sympathetic and understanding – I just can't. (ID 755; involuntarily childless; aged 31)

Having considered the influence of negative stereotyping and stigma on social exclusion, the following section explores social inclusion, connectedness and support of women without children.

Social Inclusion, Connectedness and Support

> Losing several very good friends to the world of 'mummyhood', even when you make all sorts of efforts to keep the relationship close, it dies. Because they can never spend time with you away from their kids. When you do finally get to see them all they do is moan and complain (or boast) about how hard it is being a mother, and you have less and less in common as the years roll by. I feel these relationships would probably have survived and grown if I too had chosen to have children. (ID 119; voluntarily childless; aged 36)

Pronatalist societies position normative nuclear families, and most especially mothers, as central to participation in, and contribution to, community and social embeddedness. In this way, social inclusion, connectedness and support are achieved through family networks which bridge the individual and society (Albertini & Mencarini, 2011). By positioning traditional patriarchal families (father, mother and children) as central to social embeddedness, societies, communities and individuals create structural and social-cultural barriers to the social inclusion of women without children, as well as other groups of women such as single mothers, and thereby their social connectedness and support. The pervasiveness of this normative understanding of family creates barriers to inclusion for multiple groups of women. Social inclusion, a process of improving capacity and resources to enable participation and voice in society (Taket et al., 2014), is of particular significance to women without children, who are often silenced or invisible in pronatalist

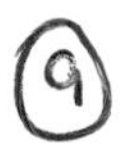

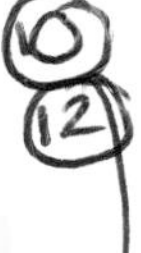

societies. Here, we consider social inclusion in relation to connectedness and support.

Social connectedness is an important resource. It provides people with a sense of belonging, access to reciprocal support, and a sense that they have a place and role within the society in which they live (Breheny & Stephens, 2009; Cohen, 2004). Social connectedness influences opportunities for social inclusion and support. An examination of social connectedness research suggests, compared with parents, non-parents have more limited social network supports (Wenger, Dykstra, Melkas, & Knipscheer, 2007), fewer potential supports to draw on (Schnettler & Wöhler, 2016) and smaller social networks (Lang, Wagner, Wrzus, & Neyer, 2013; Schnettler & Wöhler, 2016; Wenger, Scott, & Patterson, 2000). Women without children have smaller social networks and less support than women with children (Albertini & Mencarini, 2011; Dykstra, 2006; Ishii-Kuntz & Seccombe, 1989).

Few women in our study reported impaired social interactions, and most did not feel excluded by family due to having no children. However, some women did describe experiencing exclusion by family members, such as being treated as less important by their parents than siblings with children.

> My mum visits my sister every month because she has a child. My mum has visited me once this year. (ID 302; involuntarily childless; aged 32)

Women experienced feeling unwelcomed or excluded by friends and this was associated with age, with younger women feeling more exclusion from friendship circles. The older women also commented on losing friends over the years due to having no children.

> When I get together with my friends, they always talk about their children, and I sit there and have very minimal to say/input. I then tune out and feel lonely and very depressed. (ID 333; involuntarily childless; aged 36)

> My former best friend (from when we were 12 years old) recently confessed to me that she had deliberately broken off contact with me because I did not have or want children. (ID 229; voluntarily childless; aged 45)

> Being excluded from social circles as friends began to have children. (ID 105; involuntarily childless; aged 50)

In contrast, previous research has suggested that, while women without children have less contact with parents or relatives, they were more likely to have frequent contact with friends compared with mothers (Bachrach, 1980; Wenger et al., 2007). Similarly, Albertini, and Kohli (2009) posit the support networks of non-parents aged 50 years or older are more diverse, with stronger links to extended family members and friends. One quarter of the women in our study reported impaired social networks, with circumstantially childless women reporting the smallest social networks followed by voluntarily childless women. Social network impairment worsened with age, with older women reporting poorer social interactions within their networks compared with younger women.

> Not having children was devastating and I cried for years but the discrimination and exclusion is extraordinary. Nothing can prepare you for how downright mean people are. Nothing. If you lose a baby people are kind to you but if you have complex grief related to infertility, you are not allowed to talk about it ever. The constant message is that you are not an adult like parents are adults and that you don't know what love is. I don't see many friends with kids anymore, they feel too self-conscious as I do about how some people got to be lucky and others didn't. (ID 50; involuntarily childless; aged 48)

These findings are indicative of a trend towards declining social networks and interactions in older age (Baron, 2009). For example, Lang et al. (2013) found non-parents aged 60–86 years had statistically significantly smaller social networks than parents, and Vikström et al. (2011) found older non-parents aged 85 years or more have social networks with less support potential than parents.

Social support includes a diversity of ways in which individuals and communities give and receive tangible support (Berkman, 1984; Berkman & Glass, 2000; Sherbourne & Stewart, 1991). Social support can be categorised into four types: emotional support is the provision of reassurance, empathy and encouragement of the expression of feelings; informational support is the offering of advice, information and feedback to help one better understand an event, or provide resources and coping strategies; affirmational or appraisal support is the validation, acceptance and confirmation of the feelings, experiences and behaviour of another person; and instrumental support is the provision of tangible

assistance through goods and services (House, 1981; Langford, Bowsher, Maloney, & Lillis, 1997; Pearson, 1986; Sherbourne & Stewart, 1991). Central to social support is reciprocal exchange.

> [A] friend once told me I could never give her help, support or advice about children because I wasn't a mother. (ID 521; voluntarily childless; aged 44)

Women without children are often perceived as deficient and of little social value and consequently viewed as having no means to give back, excluding them from full participation in social relations. Compared to married parents, married couples without children have weaker social supports across the life-course (Ishii-Kuntz & Seccombe, 1989). When considering actual supports, non-parents report receiving less informal support than parents (Kohli & Albertini, 2009; Larsson & Silverstein, 2004). However, married non-parents are more likely to report access to instrumental support and emotional support from people not living with them compared with parents (Penning & Wu, 2014). A review of the perceived social support literature suggests involuntarily (infertile) childless women received more social support from family and friends, than involuntarily childless men (Moafi, Dolatian, & Alimoradi, 2014). Further to this, direct disclosure of infertility by involuntarily childless women has been positively associated with perceived quality of social support received (Steuber & High, 2015). However, women who are voluntarily childless report more reciprocal social relationships compared with the involuntarily childless (Wagner, Wrzus, Neyer, & Lang, 2015).

> Many of my friends also do not have children so we can talk together about our struggles with this. (ID 88; involuntarily childless; aged 45)

While only a small proportion (5.8%) of women in our study reported impaired social support (described as how often instrumental and affective support were available when needed), 46.2% of the women reported impaired subjective social support, that being, their satisfaction with their relationships, and the support provided to and by, friends and family. Social support varied by the types of women without children, with circumstantially childless women reporting the lowest levels of social support, followed by women who were undecided about whether they would have children, involuntarily and voluntarily childless women. Women who identified as future intended mothers and women who were undecided about whether they would have children reported better subjective social support than involuntarily, voluntarily and circumstantially childless women. Women who intended to become mothers in the future reported the highest levels of social support. Social support and subjective social support decreased with age, with older women reporting more impaired social supports than the younger women.

> I think sometimes my friends with children dominate the conversation with talk about their lives and their children. They don't always ask about me and what I have been doing even though I have quite an interesting and busy life. So I guess this suggests a bit of a bias in how people view me and what is important. (ID 116; circumstantially childless; aged 52)

> My two close girlfriends cannot have children and think people who do not want children are selfish. It's negative for me as I cannot tell them my decision to not have children. (ID 124; voluntarily childless; aged 34)

Conclusions

The *Life as a woman with no children in Australian society: resources, opportunities and participation* study suggests women without children, aged 25–64 years, experience exclusion from social participation at the societal, community and individual level. The study has both strengths and limitations. The mixed-methods approach utilised facilitated a deeper understanding of social exclusion among women without children, however, the cross-sectional design precluded causal inferences being drawn and meant iterative data collection and analysis and participant validation were not possible. While this study included a large sample of women without children, the non-probability sampling approach limits the ability to generalise the findings. Despite these limitations, the empirical data presented are grounded in and supported by the relevant theoretical concepts.

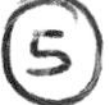

Women without children experience substantial social dislocation driven by prevailing and pervasive pronatalist ideologies. Pronatalism results in the negative stereotyping, stigmatisation and exclusion of women without children, rendering them as 'other' and having consequences for their social inclusion, connectedness and support. In order for women without children to experience full social participation, we need to challenge pronatalist discourses, narratives of the normative nuclear family and what constitutes 'family', and gender norm ideologies at all levels of society as these impact women at the micro, mesa and macro level. This does not mean women without children restricting themselves to social contexts and relationships favourable to their non-parenting status and thus 'normalising' their experiences, but rather addressing the social-cultural gender norms which define all women as mothers. Intersectional feminisms identify the importance of recognising the diversity of women's experience, influenced by many different factors, just two of which are whether they have children or not, and the reasons that this came about. Factors such as ethnicity, religion, dis/ability, are all important in the nuanced positioning of different individuals, at different times, in different contexts in relation to the challenges they face participating in the social domain of life, to the extent that they want, and in accessing support when they need it. A reorientation of social policy away from pronatalist ideologies is required to respect and respond to these multiple diversities and improve the social experiences and connectedness of women without children.

References

Albertini, M., & Kohli, M. (2009). What childless older people give: Is the generational link broken? *Ageing & Society*, *29*(8), 1261–1274.

Albertini, M., & Mencarini, L. (2011). *Childlessness and support networks in later life: A new public welfare demand? Evidence from Italy*. Italy: Collegio Carlo Alberto.

Anderson, M. J. (2007). Fertility futures: Implications of national, pronatalist policies for adolescent women in Australia. Paper presented at the International Women's Conference: Education, employment, and everything – the triple layers of a woman's life, Toowoomba, QLD, Australia.

Arendall, T. (2000). Conceiving and investigating motherhood: The decade's scholarship. *Journal of Marriage and the Family*, *62*, 1192–1207.

Australian Bureau of Statistics. (2012a). *2011 census community profiles: Time series profile* (Catalogue number 2003.0).

Australian Bureau of Statistics. (2012b). *2011 census community profiles: Time series profile* (Catalogue number 2003.0).

Bachrach, C. A. (1980). Childlessness & social isolation among the elderly. *Journal of Marriage and the Family*, *42*(3), 627–637.

Baron, A. (2009). *Social exclusion in later life. An exploration of risk factors*. London: Age Concern and Help the Aged.

Bays, A. (2017). Perceptions, emotions, and behaviors toward women based on parental status. *Sex Roles*, *76*(3/4), 138–155.

Berkman, L. F. (1984). Assessing the physical health effects of social networks and social support. *Annual Review of Public Health*, *5*, 413–432.

Berkman, L. F., & Glass, T. (2000). Social integration, social networks, social support and health. In L. F. Berkman & I. Kawachi (Eds.), *Social epidemiology*. New York, NY: Oxford University Press.

Breheny, M., & Stephens, C. (2009). 'I sort of pay back in my own little way': Managing independence and social connectedness through reciprocity. *Ageing & Society*, *29*(8), 1295–1313.

Burchardt, T., Le Grand, J., & Piachaud, D. (1999). Social exclusion in Britain 1991–1995. *Social Policy and Administration*, *33*(3), 227–244.

Campbell, R., & Wasco, S. M. (2000). Feminist approaches to social science: Epistemological and methodological tenets. *American Journal of Community Psychology*, *28*(6), 773–791.

Carey, G., Graham, M., & Shelley, J. (2009). Discourse, power and exclusion: The experiences of childless women. In A. Taket, B. Crisp, A. Nevill, G. Lamaro, M. Graham, & S. Barter-Godfrey (Eds.), *Theorising social exclusion*. London: Routledge.

Cohen, S. (2004). Social relationships and health. *American Psychologist*, *59*(8), 676–684.

Çopur, Z., & Koropeckyj-Cox, T. (2010). University students' perceptions of childless couples and parents in Ankara, Turkey. *Journal of Family Issues*, *31*(11), 1481–1506.

Culley, L., & Hudson, N. (2005). Diverse bodies and disrupted reproduction. *International Journal of Diversity in Organisations, Communities & Nations*, *5*(2), 117–125.

Dever, M. (2005). Baby talk: The Howard Government, families, and the politics of difference. *Hecate*, *31*(2), 45–61.

Doyle, J., Pooley, J. A., & Breen, L. (2013). A phenomenological exploration of the childfree choice in a sample of Australian women. *Journal of Health Psychology*, *18*(3), 397–407.

Dux, M., & Simic, Z. (2008). *The great feminist denial*. Melbourne: Melbourne University Press.

Dykstra, P. (2006). Off the beaten track: Childlessness and social integration in late life. *Research on Ageing*, *28*(6), 749–767.

Gillespie, R. (1999). Voluntary childlessness in the United Kingdom. *Reproductive Health Matters*, *7*(13), 43–53.

Gillespie, R. (2000). When no means no: Disbelief, disregard and deviance as discourses of voluntary childlessness. *Women's Studies International Forum*, *23*(2), 223–234.

Gillespie, R. (2003). Childfree and feminine: Understanding the gender identity of childless women. *Gender and Society*, *17*(1), 122–136.

Goffman, E. (1963). *Stigma notes on management of a spoiled identity*. Middlesex: Penguin Books.

Gotlib, A. (2016). 'But you would be the best mother': Unwomen, counterstories, and the motherhood mandate. *Journal of Bioethical Inquiry*, *13*(2), 327–347.

Graham, M., Hill, E., Shelley, J., & Taket, A. (2013). Why are childless women childless? Findings from an exploratory study of childless women in Victoria, Australia. *Journal of Social Inclusion*, *4*(1), 70–89.

Graham, M., McKenzie, H., & Lamaro, G. (2018). Exploring the Australian policy context relating to women's reproductive choices. *Policy Studies*, 39(2), 145–164.

Graham, M., McKenzie, H., Lamaro, G., & Klein, R. (2016). Women's reproductive choices in Australia: Mapping federal and state/territory policy instruments governing choice. *Gender Issues*, *33*(4), 335–349.

Graham, M., & Rich, S. (2012a). Representations of childless women in the Australian print media. *Feminist Media Studies, iFirst*, 1–16.

Graham, M., & Rich, S. (2012b). What's childless got to do with it? *Alfred Deakin Research Institute*, *2*(36), 16.

Heard, G. (2006). Pronatalism under Howard. *People and Place*, *14*(3), 12–25.

Heitlinger, A. (1991). Pronatalism and women's equality policies. *European Journal of Population/Revue européenne de Démographie*, *7*(4), 343–375.

Hinton, L., Kurinczuk, J. J., & Ziebland, S. (2010). Infertility; isolation and the Internet: A qualitative interview study. *Patient Education & Counseling*, *81*, 436–441.

Hird, M. J., & Abshoff, K. (2000). Women without children: A contradiction in terms? *Journal of Comparative Family Studies*, *31*(3), 347–366.

House, J. S. (1981). *Work stress and social support*. Philippines: Addison-Wesley Publishing Company Inc.

Hughes, C. (2002). *Key concepts in feminist theory and research*. London: Sage Publications.

Ireland, M. (1993). *Reconceiving women: Separating motherhood from female identity*. New York, NY: Guilford.

Ishii-Kuntz, M., & Seccombe, K. (1989). The impact of children upon social support networks throughout the life course. *Journal of Marriage and the Family*, *51*(3), 777–790.

Jackson, N., & Casey, A. (2009). Procreate and cherish: A note on Australia's abrupt shift to pro-natalism. *New Zealand Population Review*, *35*, 129–148.

Kohli, M., & Albertini, M. (2009). Childlessness and intergenerational transfers: What is at stake? *Ageing and Society*, *29*(8), 1171–1183.

Laakso, J. H., & Drevdahl, D. J. (2006). Women, abuse, and the welfare bureaucracy. *Affilia*, *21*, 84–96.

LaMastro, V. (2001). Childless by choice? Attributions and attitudes concerning family size. *Social Behaviour and Personality*, *29*(3), 231–244.

Lampman, C., & Dowling-Guyer, S. (1995). Attitudes towards voluntary and involuntary childlessness. *Basic and Applied Social Psychology*, *17*(1&2), 213–222.

Lang, F. R., Wagner, J., Wrzus, C., & Neyer, F. J. (2013). Personal effort in social relationships across adulthood. *Psychology and Aging*, *28*(2), 529–539.

Langford, C. P. H., Bowsher, J., Maloney, J. P., & Lillis, P. P. (1997). Social support: A conceptual analysis. *Journal of Advanced Nursing*, *25*(1), 95–100.

Larsson, K., & Silverstein, M. (2004). The effects of marital and parental status on informal support and service utilization: A study of older Swedes living alone. *Journal of Aging Studies*, *18*(2), 231–244.

Letherby, G. (1994). Mother or not, mother or what? Problems of definition and identity. *Women's Studies International Forum*, *17*(5), 525–532.

Letherby, G. (1999). Other than mother and mothers as others: The experience of motherhood and non-motherhood in relation to 'infertility' and 'involuntary childlessness'. *Women's Studies International Forum*, *22*(3), 359–372.

Letherby, G. (2000). Images and representations of non-motherhood. *Reproductive Health Matters*, *8*(16), 143.

Letherby, G. (2002a). Challenging dominant discourses: Identity and change and the experience of 'infertility' and 'involuntary childlessness'. *Journal of Gender Studies*, *11*(3), 277–288.

Letherby, G. (2002b). Childless and bereft?: Stereotypes and realities in relation to 'voluntary' and 'involuntary' childlessness and womanhood. *Sociological Inquiry*, *72*(1), 7–20.

Letherby, G., & Williams, C. (1999). Non-motherhood: Ambivalent autobiographies. *Feminist Studies*, *25*(3), 719–728.

Maher, J. M., & Saugeres, L. (2007). To be or not to be a mother?: Women negotiating cultural representations of mothering. *Journal of Sociology*, *43*(1), 5–20.

Major, B., & O'Brien, L. T. (2005). The social psychology of stigma. *Annual Review of Psychology*, *56*, 393–421.

McQuillan, J., Greil, A. L., Shreffler, K. M., Wonch-Hill, P. A., Gentzler, K. C., & Hathcoat, J. D. (2012). Does the reason matter? Variations in childlessness concerns among U.S. women. *Journal of Marriage and Family*, *74*(5), 1166–1181.

Miall, C. E. (1986). The stigma of involuntary childlessness. *Social Problems*, *33*(4), 268–282.

Miettinen, A., Rotkirch, A., Szalma, I., Donno, A., & Tanturri, M.-L. (2015). *Increasing childlessness in Europe: Time trends and country differences*. Families and Society Working Paper Series – Changing families and sustainable societies: Policy contexts and diversity over the life course and across generations, 33, pp. 1–66.

Moafi, F., Dolatian, M., & Alimoradi, Z. (2014). Impact of social support on infertile couples. *Iranian Journal of Reproductive Medicine*, *12*, 130–131.

Morell, C. (1994). *Unwomanly conduct: The challenges of intentional childlessness*. New York, NY: Routledge.

Morison, T., Macleod, C., Lynch, I., Mijas, M., & Shivakumar, S. T. (2016). Stigma resistance in online childfree communities. *Psychology of Women Quarterly*, *40*(2), 184–198.

Morrell, C. (2000). Saying no: Women's experiences with reproductive refusal. *Feminism & Psychology*, *10*(3), 313–322.

Mueller, K., & Yoder, J. (1997). Gendered norms for family size, employment, and occupation: Are there personal costs for violating them? *Sex Roles*, *36*(3/4), 207–220.

Mueller, K., & Yoder, J. (1999). Stigmatization of non-normative family size status. *Sex Roles*, *41*(11/12), 901–919.

Mumtaz, Z., Shahid, U., & Levay, A. (2013). Understanding the impact of gendered roles on the experiences of infertility amongst men and women in Punjab. *Reproductive Health*, *10*, 3.

Park, K. (2002). Stigma management among the voluntary childless. *Sociological Perspectives*, *45*(1), 21–45.

Park, K. (2005). Choosing childlessness: Weber's typology of action and motives of the voluntary childless. *Sociological Inquiry*, *75*(3), 372–402.

Pearson, J. E. (1986). The definition and measurement of social support. *Journal of Counseling & Development*, *64*(6), 390–395.

Penning, M. J., & Wu, Z. (2014). Marital status, childlessness, and social support among older Canadians. *Canadian Journal on Aging/La Revue Canadienne Du Vieillissement*, *33*(4), 426–447.

Popay, J., Escorel, S., Hernández, M., Johnston, H., Mathieson, J., & Rispel, L. (2008). *Understanding and tackling social exclusion*. Final Report to the WHO Commission on Social Determinants of Health From the Social Exclusion Knowledge Network.

Rich, S., Taket, A., Graham, M., & Shelley, J. (2011). 'Unnatural', 'unwomanly', 'uncreditable' and 'undervalued': The significance of being a childless woman in Australian society. *Gender Issues*, *28*(4), 226–247.

Riessman, L. (2000). Stigma and everyday resistance practices: Childless women in South India. *Gender & Society*, *14*(1), 111–135.

Schnettler, S., & Wöhler, T. (2016). No children in later life, but more and better friends? Substitution mechanisms in the personal and support networks of parents and the childless in Germany. *Ageing & Society*, *36*(7), 1339–1363.

Seccombe, K. (1991). Assessing the costs and benefits of children: Gender comparisons among childfree husbands and wives. *Journal of Marriage and the Family*, *53*(1), 191–202.

Shapiro, G. (2014). Voluntary childlessness: A critical review of the literature. *Studies in the Maternal*, *6*(1), 1–15.

Sherbourne, C. D., & Stewart, A. L. (1991). The MOS social support survey. *Social Science & Medicine*, *32*(6), 705–714.

Simpson, R. (2007). 'Defying nature'?: Contemporary discourse around delayed childbearing and childlessness in Britain. *GeNet seminar: Low fertility in industrialised countries: London School of Economics*. Edinburgh: Centre for Research on Families and Relationships.

Smith, D. E. (1987). *The everyday world as problematic: A feminist sociology*. Boston, MA: Northeastern University Press.

Somers, M. D. (1993). A comparison of voluntary childfree adults and parents. *Journal of Marriage and the Family*, *55*(3), 634–650.

Steuber, K. R., & High, A. (2015). Disclosure strategies, social support, and quality of life in infertile women. *Health Policy & Planning*, *30*(7), 1635–1642.

Taket, A. R. Crisp, B. R., Graham, M., Hanna, L., Goldingay, S., & Wilson, L. (2014). *Practicing social inclusion*. London: Routledge.

Taket, A., Crisp, B., Nevill, A., Lamaro, G., Graham, M., & Barter-Godfrey, S. (2009). *Theorising social exclusion*. London: Routledge.

Tietjens-Meyers, D. (2001). The rush to motherhood: Pronatalist discourse and women's autonomy. *Signs: Journal of Women in Culture & Society*, *26*(3), 735–773.

Turnbull, B., Graham, M., & Taket, A. (2016a). The nature and extent of social exclusion of Australian childless women in their reproductive years: An exploratory mixed-methods study. *Social Inclusion*, *4*(1), 102–115.

Turnbull, B., Graham, M., & Taket, A. (2016b). Pronatalism and social exclusion in Australian society: Experiences of women in their reproductive years with no children. *Gender Issues*, *34*, 333–354.

Turnbull, B., Graham, M., & Taket, A. (2016c). Social connection and exclusion of Australian women with no children during midlife. *Journal of Social Inclusion*, *7*(2), 65–85.

Veevers, J. E. (1974). Voluntary childlessness and social policy: An alternative view. *The Family Coordinator*, *23*(4), 397–406.

Vikström, J., Bladh, M., Hammar, M., Marcusson, J., Wressle, E., & Sydsjö, G. (2011). The influences of childlessness on the psychological well-being and social network of the oldest old. *BMC Geriatrics*, *11*(78), 1–11.

Wagner, J., Wrzus, C., Neyer, F. J., & Lang, F. R. (2015). Social network characteristics of early midlife voluntarily and involuntarily childless couples. *Journal of Family Issues*, *36*(1), 87–110.

Watson, S. (1995). Reclaiming social policy. In B. Caine & R. Pringle (Eds.), *Transitions: New Australian feminisms*. St. Leonards, NSW: Allen & Unwin.

Wenger, G. C., Dykstra, P. A., Melkas, T., & Knipscheer, K. C. P. M. (2007). Social embeddedness and late-life parenthood: Community activity, close ties and support networks. *Journal of Family Issues*, *28*(11), 1419–1456.

Wenger, G. C., Scott, A., & Patterson, N. (2000). How important is parenthood? Childlessness and support in old age in England. *Ageing and Society*, *20*(2), 161–182.

Chapter 6

'Join the Club' or 'Don't Have Kids'? Exploring Contradictory Experiences, Pressures and Encouragement to Have Children in Pronatalist Social Fields

Alyssa Mullins

Abstract

In childlessness literature, researchers often engage in a discussion of why some women (and men) intend or choose to remain childless, with an emphasis on macro-level or interpersonal experiences. However, further research is needed to identify the ways in which voluntarily childless (VC) adults actively negotiate the social world among structural influences that simultaneously value parenthood and place complex burdens on parents. Utilising the Bourdieuian concepts of habitus, capital and field, this chapter contributes to a shift in the conversation from 'why' individuals remain childless towards an understanding of 'how' childbearing preferences impact individuals' lives in practice.

This research compares experiences and characteristics of non-parents in relation to childbearing preferences. This study explores a sample of 972 participants' responses to two open-ended questions addressing particular social arenas or experiences where they feel pressured or encouraged to have children as well as those where they feel pressured or encouraged not to have children. Responses were coded using a general inductive approach to identify emerging themes regarding the social fields and the nature of the interactions relevant to childbearing preferences. A between group comparison of temporarily childless (TC) and VC participants indicated a number of similarities and differences that highlight the contradictions, hardships and benefits of actively deciding to delay or forgo having children.

Both groups frequently indicated family, friends, work or school, public spaces and other structural and cultural factors pressuring or encouraging them to have children, but also indicated pressures or encouragement within similar fields advising them not to have children. For both groups, many of the responses highlighted the contradictory nature of these messages. The similarities and differences between groups also highlight ways in which the current status of non-parent can lead to certain similar social experiences, regardless of personal preference for the future, while also showing a number of ways these encounters are experienced or perceived differently, based on this preference.

Keywords: Childfreedom; voluntary childlessness; Bourdieu; pronatalism; habitus; social fields

Introduction

Pronatalist ideologies, which encourage childbearing and consider parenthood the expected path towards adulthood, are deeply rooted within American culture (McQuillan et al., 2012; Newport & Wilke, 2013; Scott, 2009; Yaremko & Lawson, 2007). However, over time, macro- and micro-level factors have contributed to more active decision-making among individuals regarding when (or if) they plan to have children. Ideologies of individualism and rational choice (Cherlin, 2009), access to reliable reproductive technologies and women's educational and work pursuits (Cain, 2001) contribute to an overall trend of delaying marriage, having fewer children and having them later in life (Cherlin, 2005; Sassler & Miller, 2014). While more opportunities and identities become available for younger cohorts, increased demands and expectations may make these choices incompatible with each other (Cherlin, 2009). Contradictory climates and unmanageable expectations may contribute to the increased rates of delaying or forgoing childbearing as many adults feel as though 'they must either make a choice or compromise' (Scott, 2009, p. 37).

Actively deciding to become a parent or forgo childbearing is not consistent across all groups, due to socio-economic status, biological ability, etc. (McQuillan, Griel, & Shreffler, 2011; Morgan & King, 2001; Sassler & Miller, 2014; Shreffler, Griel, Mitchell, & McQuillan, 2015). However, academic and public discourses are paying increased attention to some adults' decisions remain childless, or 'childfree'.[1] Previous research often views voluntary childlessness as either an outcome of structural or personal factors (e.g. Christoffersen & Lausten, 2009; Hagestad & Call, 2007), or a contributing factor to a number of interpersonal or structural strains, such as stigma or care for an aging population (Lisle, 1996; Park, 2002, 2005; Wolf & Laditka, 2006). Yet, little research has explored how childfree adults actively negotiate the social world among pronatalist influences that simultaneously value parenthood and place complex burdens on parents (Coontz, 2005; Gerson, 2010; Hays, 1996).

I utilise a Bourdieusian (1990) theoretical model to conceptualise childbearing preferences as the *habitus* – individuals' deeply rooted dispositions which are shaped by the social world but also actively shape the social world around them. Framing childbearing preferences as a deeply rooted habitus contributes to an understanding of the complex interaction between individuals as active agents with deeply rooted ideologies as well as the interplay between personal preferences and external structures (*fields*). I aim to contribute to a shift in the conversation from 'why' men and women choose to remain childless towards an understanding of 'how' they act as social agents to simultaneously shape the social world while also being shaped by external social realities. This exploratory look into experiences in practice highlights one major theme related to the impact of the preference (not) to have children within structural fields. In particular, I explore similarities and differences in experiences of contradictory messages that non-parents receive about childbearing within various social arenas and interactions.

Literature Review

Contributions to Childbearing Intentions

Viewing childbearing as a distinct and active *choice* offers only a limited perspective on this complex reality. However, it is not uncommon for individuals to maintain an active and personal *intention* to have, or not

[1]Some believe that the term 'childless' implies a sense of absence or void, which does not accurately describe their preference not to have children. Others believe the term 'childfree' has its own implications, such as a dislike of children – which may also not be reflective of this identity. To avoid endorsing one term over the other, I intentionally use the terms interchangeably.

have, children (Houseknecht, 1979; Rovi, 1994). Many researchers consider how childbearing decisions involve an active cost/benefit analysis. For instance, adults intending to have children may believe the expressive, personal *rewards* of being a parent (i.e. happiness, pride and accomplishment) outweigh instrumental *costs*, including financial strain and responsibility (Senior, 2014; Yaremko & Lawson, 2007). On the other hand, childfree adults may associate these personal rewards with autonomy, travel, hobbies and relationships with other adults (Gillespie, 2003). Instrumental costs, such as an inability to balance work and family (Andrade & Bould, 2012), or a preference for economic stability and upward mobility (Xu, 2013), may deter others from having children.

However, factors that push or pull some adults towards childlessness are not exclusive to the childfree. Those that intend to become parents may delay childbearing to achieve financial stability, educational attainment or establish solid marital relationships (Sassler & Miller, 2014). Additionally, some who delay parenthood are taking time to become ready for a parenting lifestyle, which requires more selflessness, 'going out … less, and developing more patience'. (Sassler & Miller, 2014, p. 544). Among the childfree, education and financial explanations tend to vary by gender. Men are arguably more likely to cite financial concerns (Park, 2005) as a reason to forgo childbearing (Mahaffey & Ward, 2001; Waren & Pals, 2013), while increased education is linked with a higher likelihood of voluntary childlessness for women. Childfree women are also more likely to cite an inability to balance parenthood and careers or a lack of parental 'instinct' (Park, 2005; Waren & Pals, 2013).

Gendered differences in factors that push or pull men and women to remain childless (Gillespie, 2003) highlight broader cultural norms and contradictions. The United States is characterised by a culture of 'intensive mothering', a belief that mothers are responsible for the primary caretaking of children and, to be a *good* mother, this task should take priority over all other interests and desires (Hays, 1996; Senior, 2014). However, these ideologies contradict cultural and structural transformations which have made most families reliant on the economic contribution of wives and mothers and increasingly in favour of more egalitarian ideologies (Cowan & Cowan, 2009; Gerson, 2010; Hays, 1996; Kricheli-Katz, 2012). Women also experience a gendered 'double bind' that pits intensive mothering against cultural standards of the ideal worker (Hays, 1996; Sullivan, 2014). In the professional world, fathers tend to receive more financial and professional benefits than childless men (Bernard & Correll, 2010). In contrast, ideologies about mothers' competency and commitment to their careers paired with career interruptions due to pregnancy, childbirth and caretaking, negatively impact women's career paths and wages (Budig & England, 2001; Sullivan, 2014).

Contradictory pressures also pit working 'Super Moms' against traditional, stay-at-home mothers into an exaggerated, ideological 'mommy war' with 'no way for either type of mother to get it right' (Hays, 1996, p. 149). This no-win scenario, paired with technological advancements in reproductive health and increased autonomy for women, may make it easier for some women to 'decide' not to have children. However, women that opt to have no children in order to alleviate the tension between these conflicting identities are oftentimes viewed as 'cold, heartless, and unfulfilled …' (Hays, 1996, p. 133), further contributing to the no-win scenario that women must negotiate. Similarly, traditional gender ideologies disproportionately leave women with childcare and household duties, which may make it more appealing to forgo childbearing to focus on other priorities. On the other hand, 'the vast majority of all men, whether fathers or childless, believe that the rewards of being a parent are worth it despite … the work that goes into it' (Livingston & Parker, 2011, para. 4). Gendered gaps in earnings, workplace cultures and traditional family policies and norms continue to perpetuate expectations for fathers to have 'a greater responsibility for breadwinning and mothers for caregiving' (Wall & Arnold, 2007, p. 511). While fathers are becoming more involved parents and spending quality time with their children, this involvement frequently involves leisure or mentorship (Townsend, 2009; Wall & Arnold, 2007).

These explanations highlight the impact of cultural, social and economic resources on viewing childbearing as an active choice or intention. Working-class and poor adults tend to have less access to contraceptives, face higher rates of unplanned pregnancies early in life and are more likely to experience socialisation which elevates childbearing as one's most important life accomplishment (Edin & Kefalas, 2005; Edin & Nelson, 2013). Additionally, low-income women of colour may be less motivated to prevent unplanned pregnancies as economic prospects and alternate identities remain limited compared to white, middle-class Americans with whom voluntary childlessness is more commonly associated (Edin & Kefalas, 2005; Livingston, 2015). Low-income men and men of colour also experience distinct structural influences impacting meanings of parenthood compared to white and middle-class men. For many men, becoming a father alleviates the strain of racial prejudice, low-income neighbourhoods, poverty and limited education and opportunity (Edin & Nelson, 2013). In contrast, on average, middle-class

…ave more professional and educational opportunities and … to health care and reproductive control, granting them …omy to identify parenthood as *one of many* potential life …vements (Abma & Martinez, 2006; Gillespie, 2003; Senior, 2014).

However, those who become parents early in life and those who intentionally remain childless may also share similarities despite this major distinction (Christoffersen & Lausten, 2009). Unstable family background, including family discord or parental divorce (Cain, 2001), poverty and parental unemployment or disability (Christoffersen & Lausten, 2009) are also potential precursors for voluntary childlessness. Stable family backgrounds and higher education are more consistently associated with delayed, but eventual, childbearing (Christoffersen & Lausten, 2009). Thus, the childfree shares a number of similarities with non-parents who are actively delaying or planning parenthood as well as those who become parents earlier in life. Yet there are also several distinctions within and between each of these groups (Houseknecht, 1979). Even among those who have, or intend to have, children, parenthood can have substantially different meanings when paired with unequal access to economic, social, cultural and symbolic capital. Expectations about the timing or intention to have children, career or educational plans and other structural barriers or advantages provide insight into the complex interplay between an individual's personal decision about childbearing and factors that contribute to this decision.

Prevalence of Childlessness

Public and political discourses frequently attribute voluntary childlessness to structural and cultural changes, including feminism, women's increased autonomy, access to the workforce and higher education and greater access to quality contraceptives. However, despite the widespread impact of these social and structural changes, childfree adults tend to account for only a small portion of the population in the United States (Gillespie, 2003; Livingston & Cohn, 2010; Yaremko & Lawson, 2007). Arguably 'the transition to parenthood presents different and more confusing challenges for modern couples creating families than it did for parents in earlier times' (Cowan & Cowan, 2009, p. 257). As such, intentional childlessness is increasingly common among younger cohorts (Kelly, 2009; Livingston, 2015). However, on average, older women are currently more likely than younger women to express an intent to remain childless, suggesting that for some, the meaning of voluntary childlessness can arise through life experiences rather t static identity (Houseknecht, 1979; Kelly, 2009; Rovi, 1 childbearing intentions and experiences of childlessnes marital status. The experience of voluntary childlessness among ... or cohabitating adults is likely to be different from unmarried or unattached adults, whose perspectives may be more likely to shift if they feel their opportunities for childbearing are constrained by 'social norms and the absence of a partner' (Mosher & Bachrach, 1982, p. 521).

Experiences of Childlessness

Reasons for choosing childlessness and the meanings associated with this identity vary widely among individuals and over the course of a person's life. As a result, an emphasis on isolating reasons women (and men) remain childless provides an oversimplified and limited understanding of this identity. Pathways to childlessness 'may not necessarily represent clear choices or preferences; instead they reflect the changing influence of relationships, economic opportunities, and personal developments' (Koropeckyj-Cox, 2003, p. 263). Thus, childfreedom research would benefit from a shift from understanding '*why*' some men and women intentionally remain childless, towards '*how*' childfree men and women negotiate structural, interpersonal and individual factors in their everyday lives. Understanding voluntary childlessness as a complex and recurring interplay between structural forces and active agents may expose factors contributing to and resulting from the decision (not) to become a parent, and how these factors co-exist in a recurring and evolving manner.

Oftentimes, research addressing how childless adults negotiate the social world emphasises the distinct characteristics and experiences of childless adults in middle or old age, or consequences of childlessness on individuals or the broader society. These consequences highlight psychological well-being, social isolation or social support and the utilisation of health care services and assisted living services among childless adults (Koropeckyj-Cox & Call, 2007; Wolf & Laditka, 2006). Middle-aged, childless women experience anxieties related to stereotypes and stigma about aging without children, while also engaging in active efforts to establish emotional and social support systems that will aid them in the aging process (Koropeckyj-Cox, 2003). Commonly cited stigmas include perceptions of childfree adults as selfish, self-centred, materialistic, strange or taboo, cold, heartless and unfulfilled (Hays,

1996; Lisle, 1996; Park, 2002). Park (2002) identified how the management of these stigmas varied based on how central childlessness was to her participants' identities. For instance, some would hide this identity or mask their voluntary childlessness as involuntary, while others were more proactive in providing explanations about a lack of maternal instinct or condemning those that condemn childlessness (Park, 2002). While this research identified many experiences related to childbearing preferences, its focus is on *perceptions* of stigma and coping strategies in and the way *information* about childlessness is conveyed (Park, 2002). Thus, further research is needed to explore experiences and strategies in relation to pronatalist social or institutional interactions. Particularly, more research is needed on how these strategies or pressures vary based on the different audiences or contexts.

Some researchers argue that longitudinal analyses and studies of women beyond reproductive years offer the most valid measures of childlessness, as intentions may change over time (Christoffersen & Lausten, 2009). However, others acknowledge that while intentions and behaviours can shift, 'the response of "no [I do not want children]" ...' at any point during potential childbearing years '... *is of interest in and of itself*' (Rovi, 1994, p. 344). Regardless of whether individuals intending to remain childless will do so in practice, it is important to identify interactions or institutions contributing to the longevity of this decision, and the resources individuals use to negotiate this identity while the decision to avoid childbearing is most actively experienced by controlling procreation and negotiating pronatalist pressures and social norms (Gillespie, 2003).

This shift provides important insight into the experiences of childlessness and the social norms and expectations associated with this identity. Exploring experiences of voluntarily childless (VC) adults draws attention to informal social sanctions or punishments that arise from challenging pronatalism. As Scott (2009, p. 174) describes, '[i]t's non-normative to say "I don't have children, and I don't want any", and if you say that in several different environments, you will feel the sanctions'. Additionally, identifying ways childless adults negotiate informal and formal social norms and structures may highlight potential patterns in the process of becoming a parent or solidifying a childfree identity. This chapter contributes to this shift towards an understanding of how non-parents of childbearing age experience the complex interplay of active, individual (non-) childbearing intentions and the societal and familial pressures to conform to parenting norms.

Theoretical and Methodological Considerations

In this chapter, I propose a shift towards a Bourdieusian theoretical orientation to move beyond understanding childfreedom as an *outcome* of either structural or personal factors. Bourdieu (1990) emphasised the complex and recurring interplay between acting agents and external structures, arguing that an overemphasis on objectivist or subjectivist perspectives creates a false dichotomy in our understanding of the social world. Adopting this approach provides a perspective on 'the way ... individuals are able to exercise choices within the limits of ... social structure' regarding voluntary childlessness (Bourdieu, 1990, p. 53) as well as their experiences within various fields, or social arenas.

Childbearing preferences are conceptualised as the *habitus*, the subjective, deeply rooted and typically taken for granted ideologies or identities. Habitus are structured by the social world, yet also contain agentic perceptions of and actions towards that world. For instance, some VC adults cite a lack of a maternal or parental 'instinct' (Park, 2002; Waren & Pals, 2013) indicating ways in which this decision is perceived as a natural, deeply rooted identity. However, childbearing preferences may not necessarily remain static (in one direction or another) throughout the life course, highlighting structural or interpersonal influences as well as individuals' continued agency to modify the habitus when new ideas or experiences are interpreted in relation to these meanings and identities (Bourdieu, 1990).

Bourdieu also posed that preferences and practices are influenced by an interaction of habitus and capital. Capital includes the money and objects used to produce goods and services (economic capital); groupings and networking used to gain status or material goods (social capital); and interpersonal skills or knowledge associated with styles and practices valued by society (cultural capital). Capital is also symbolic, consisting of prestige, reputation and the ability to transform economic, social and/or cultural capital within social fields (Bourdieu, 1984, 1990).

Although the application of this theoretical approach is limited within childlessness literature, researchers have utilised a Bourdieusian perspective to theoretically and empirically address various topics in social science. For instance, Powell (2008) identified a complex interaction between structural gender norms and the creative acts of individual agency that correspond with the changing nature of young people's love/sex relationships, sexual pressures and consent. However, more broadly speaking, despite its usefulness to resolve gaps in explanatory research, a Bourdieusian conceptualisation of the interplay between macro- and micro-level forces typically remains latent in existing literature (Green, 2008).

Understanding negotiations between active agents and external structures can provide insight into broader social norms about the decision to become a parent. Exploring potential differences based on childbearing preferences provides insight into understanding (non-) parenthood as a consequence of an interplay between social sanctions/supports and personal accomplishments and identities (Edin & Kefalas, 2005; Edin & Nelson, 2013; Veevers, 1974). Since pronatalist ideologies permeate through most social arenas, including family life and intimate relationships (Cain, 2001), health care (Denbow, 2014), workplaces (Heitlinger, 1991) and social interactions/leisure activities (Parry, 2005), intentions to remain VC can impact access to capital and experiences within various fields. For example, increased economic capital in the form of quality and affordable health care may lead individuals to view childrearing as more of a personal choice. An individual's preference to have no children may also simultaneously shape their career path, which can result in greater economic resources.

Methodology and Sample

According to Bourdieu (1990), habitus (and capital) simultaneously shape and become shaped by the 'rules of the game' within various social fields. This chapter summarises open-ended responses from a larger, mixed method exploratory study (Mullins, 2016) contributing to an understanding of how childbearing habitus are experienced in social fields. Participants in the original study responded to a survey consisting of open- and closed-ended questions, distributed via online forums. Purposive and convenience sampling techniques were used to oversample VC adults. Eligibility requirements for the initial study limited the sample to childless men and women residing in the United States, between the ages of 25 and 40. Childlessness was defined as not having (or expecting) biological, adopted or step-children that they consider like their own. Participants were categorised as temporarily childless (TC) if they indicated wanting (or probably wanting) children in the future. Those that did not (or probably did not) want children were considered VC, or childfree. The initial sample included 972 respondents. Slightly more than half of the participants (59%) were childfree. On average, participants were middle-class (M = $61,479), white (89%), heterosexual (79%) and female (82%). The average age was 29.7. Approximately 75% had a bachelor's (four year) degree or higher. The sample disproportionately identified as Atheist (35% of TC and 51% of VC).

This chapter focuses on participants' responses to open-ended questions regarding pressures or encouragement to have children, as well pressures or encouragement not to have children. Approximately 76% of the total sample responded to the question regarding pressures or encouragement to have children and 66% participated in response to pressures or encouragement not to have children. I inductively coded responses for keywords with a focus on where, when and with whom these experiences arise. I also explored how participants describe these experiences. Findings suggest similarities among non-parents, as well as distinctions in perceptions and experiences based on preference (not) to have children.

Findings

Responses of temporarily and VC participants exposed a number of similar and distinct experiences, contradictions, hardships and benefits to actively delaying or forgoing having children. In particular, responses commonly revealed complex and contradictory pressures or encouragement (not) to have children. Childfree and TC participants identified pressures or encouragement to have children from family, friends, work, school, public spaces and other structural and cultural factors, but also felt pressured or encouraged not to have children within similar fields.

'Join the Club' versus 'Don't Have Kids'

For both groups, contradicting pressures or encouragement most commonly came from family members, especially during holidays. TC participants often indicated encouragement or support from family members while others felt pressured by a sense of urgency to have children. These respondents felt encouraged by observing or interacting with family members' children. For instance,

> Spending time with [my uncle's daughter] raised a fatherly instinct in me that I never knew I had. Would be interested in raising a child to hopefully right the wrongs of my upbringing and encourage them live a happy and fulfilling life … (TC Man, age 33)

Yet many TC participants' family members overtly asked them if they are expecting yet or when they are going to have children. These respondents were encouraged (and pressured) by their parents wanting grandchildren or grandparents 'wanting great-grandkids before they pass' (TC woman, age 25).

Similarly, VC respondents most frequently experienced overt pressures or encouragement to have children from family members. However, childfree participants more frequently expressed feeling pressure, guilt, agitation and devaluation. As one VC woman (age 32) notes, '... my step-mother gets all sobby about me not experiencing the joys of motherhood'. Another described the persistence and discomfort that arises at family get-togethers:

> ... They often joke about it at first, then try to explain the benefits, then state that everyone has kids (plus some reasons why I should too). If I am still firm, they will regress to 'what if you meet the right person?', 'what if your husband wants them?' After defending my position it ... ends with 'what if you get pregnant by accident?' ... to which I state my feelings on abortion. The conversation becomes very uncomfortable after that. (VC Woman, age 25)

Responses among the childfree are consistent with frequently cited stigmas (Park, 2005) attached to childfreedom in a pronatalist society. Family members of childfree respondents often called them selfish, persistently told them they will change their mind, pressured them to pass on the family name and engaged in other 'passive-aggressive remarks' (VC Man, age 30) like commenting on 'when' rather than 'if' he or she will have children.

For both groups, pressures and encouragement also came from friends or acquaintances that have children of their own. TC participants felt encouraged but also isolated from friends that are parents. As one respondent put it, 'I'm ... the last of my friends to not have a child. But I feel encouraged each time I spend time with them' (TC Woman, age 32). TC participants were also asked when they would 'join the [Parent] club' (Woman, age 40) so their children can play and grow up together. Childfree participants also received pressure/encouragement to 'join the club'. As one 29-year-old VC woman stated, '[e]very time ... I am with my family or my friends that have kids, they pressure me to have them. My sister and friends want me to have kids so we can "have kids together"'. A small number of VC participants also indicated that positive interactions with friends or family members' children occasionally made them 'question my childfree leanings' (VC Woman, age 29).

Interestingly, VC participants more frequently felt encouraged or pressured not to have children through overt discouragement from people that are parents, jokingly or otherwise. Others whom surrounded themselves with likeminded people or supportive friends and family members felt supported in their decision to remain childfree. For instance, one 40-year-old woman stated that '... friends with kids tell me don't have them'. Similarly, 'career focused acquaintances ... [whom] have expressed regret about their decision to have children ...' provided support for another respondent's childfreedom. '... To them, the alleged personal fulfilment/rewards of having children did not [offset] the costs'. (VC Man, age 25). Additionally, one 29-year-old woman's parents '... completely agree that children are too expensive and not a solid investment for the most part'. Another found support among a largely childfree, long-time friend group, stating '... [My friends with children] keep it real with us, saying that overall it's rewarding to them, but if you don't want children you definitely don't need to have them' (Woman, age 32).

TC respondents also felt pressured or encouraged not to have children by friends and family members, most frequently those with children of their own. Such as friends sharing stories of their child's latest troublemaking '[u]sually with the phrase, "don't have kids"' (TC Man, age 25) or their 'own mother saying that I would be a "terrible" parent' (TC Woman, age 31). Others noted pressures or encouragements through observations of others' experiences, such as

> ...I have a brother who has some mental health and personality disorders. After seeing his destructive nature cripple my parents emotionally, financially and sometimes physically I ... fear ... having a child like him. I would be afraid of living with the struggles my parents had ...[or] abandoning my child. (TC Woman, age 33)

In addition to direct interpersonal experiences with friends and family members, pressures/encouragement to have or not have children arise in public settings and broader societal arenas. For instance, TC participants highlighted various public settings, media representations and societal influences as pressures or encouragement to have children. Some participants felt pressure from social media, believing that '... everyone on Facebook has kids now' (Woman, age 25). Or,

> ...Society makes sure almost daily that I should have a child and they question why I don't. It gets questioned on Facebook and even in the supermarket by COMPLETE STRANGERS. ... I kid you not, I am asked a question about children at least once a week. (TC Woman, age 30, emphasis in original)

Similarly, childfree participants indicated pressure or encouragement to have children in 'most social interactions' or from media representations of families and the lack of media representation of childfree adults. For instance, one VC woman (age 28) feels encouraged to have children '[w]hen I see a close, happy family with adult children genuinely enjoying each other's company', while another noted that '...pressure ... sometimes comes from ... movies or shows where couples have their first kid and it's all sunshine and rainbows...' (VC Woman, age 25). TC and VC participants both expressed the influence of religion and cultural forces, including the importance of faith and its association with childbearing or the pressures of a particular ethnic culture. In addition to cultural and religious factors, childfree participants also indicated pressures based on their region of residence – particularly the 'Bible Belt' South. As one 25-year-old VC woman describes, in the South, '... people are expected to have children. If you're not married with kids by the time you're 30, they act like there's something wrong with you'.

Despite broad cultural pressures to have children, public arenas and other societal or structural factors also discouraged or pressured both groups not to have children. For instance, TC participants considered observing other people's children in public spaces as a type of discouragement. As a 25-year-old woman describes, '...anyplace I visit that has a disruptive child I'm glad that I don't have one of my own'. VC participants also frequently considered how the public world and other people's children encourage a life without children. For instance, '[w]henever I spend time with kids I know that it's not for me. Every story I hear about kids, and parents not being able to do anything because of their kids strengthens my decision' (VC Woman, age 31).

Childfree respondents frequently considered broad global, societal or structural factors as discouragement from having children. For example, 'news stories describing crime, terrorism, child molesters, murder, horrific accidents, ... diseases and ailments, abuse, alcoholism, usurious politicians' (Man, age 40) as well as environmental factors (i.e. overpopulation), and the belief that the 'US work ethic is extremely hostile to working parents' (Woman, age 29). Some TC participants also mentioned large scale factors such as overpopulation, maternity leave or the state of the world. For instance,

> Having children, while something that I very much want, is illogical. It's a major financial burden, there is massive overpopulation and I live in a high crime area. Really, any time that I have a discussion about the logic of procreation, I feel pressured to not have kids. (Woman, age 34).

Another TC woman (no age provided) feels discouraged from having children when she considers how the United States work environment makes childbearing

> impossible to afford… no paid [maternity] leave …[then] I suddenly have to be able to afford new day care experiences and the new cost of adding a child to my insurance plan!

Wait… But Do Not Wait Too Long

Both groups also experienced the contradictory nature of their age, lifestyle preferences or life course circumstances as contributors to the pressures to have and not to have children. TC participants in particular frequently expressed pressures/encouragements in favour of having children based on their stage of life. These experiences typically consist of internal and external pressures related to their age, milestones or their 'biological clock', and falling behind everyone they know. Some started feeling pressure once they entered their 30s, oftentimes because '…All adults are married with children. … it's like I haven't matured to true adulthood. Despite being educated and financially independent' (TC Woman, age 37). Another explicitly stated she felt pressure all the time, as '…a 32-year-old married woman and all my friends already have kids' (TC Woman, age 32).

VC participants were more likely to describe pressures or encouragement to have children based on life course milestones or age in relation to others' expectations for them. For instance,

> … people just seemed to think babies were the next step [after getting married] and they weren't shy about saying so. … especially whenever someone else in the family is pregnant/just had a baby, the pressure is on for me to do

> so too. …'X's baby is so cute, when are you going to start a family?' 'You would have the most adorable babies; don't you want that?' (Woman, age 37).

A few childfree participants mentioned internal pressures, like a concern about being cared for into old age, biological clocks or comparing their lives to peers. Unlike those in the TC group, childfree respondents citing the influence of a 'biological clock' or a fear of regret for not having children mentioned those feelings go away pretty quickly or included justifications, such as 'Hopefully I'll be an awesome aunt and my niece will help out if I'm, like, fully senile' (VC Woman, age 35) or, 'I feel motivated to have kids when I am dissatisfied with some major factor in my life … [but] the feeling goes away when I make a change in another area of my life…' (VC Woman, age 26).

Participants who felt pressured or encouraged not to have children were more likely to feel they should *delay* having children, but not to avoid having kids all together. For instance, a TC woman's (age 25) mother-in-law 'blatantly states "you really shouldn't have any kids until you've finished some sort of upper-level degree"'. Another TC woman (age 33) felt pressured to wait until she and her husband (both with PhDs) were established in their careers. On the other hand, some TC respondents felt pressured or encouraged not to have children due to lifestyle preferences or circumstances, such as prioritising leisure and hobbies or managing difficult health and financial barriers. For instance, one woman (age 35) considered her life full of leisure, hobbies, personal quiet time and a number of material belongings that are not child proof. However, as she explains, 'We do have a lovely life… I know children are going to ruin all of this, but I can't think my way out of wanting them…' Similarly, another TC man (age 27) expressed how a child could introduce additional emotional and financial strain to his current way of life.

> For example, putting money toward new flooring in a home and the child does something to damage it beyond repair… adds a great deal of financial stress and I'd hate to lose my temper at my child over something so silly … possibly instilling in them that they aren't as important as carpet. Also, I suffer from chronic major depression. I'd feel horrible for my children to see their father in such a pathetic state. (TC Man, age 27)

A small portion of childfree participants felt pressure or encouragement not to have children due to lifestyle preferences or circumstances, including hobbies, relationships or other responsibilities and hardships (such as financial strain). For example:

> ...Thinking about how little time I have already to work on my books, music, and drawings while working a full-time job ... and how much ... they're what really keeps me alive; and knowing that art can leave a far greater and longer legacy than a child (who may or may not do anything for society). (Non-binary, age 28)

Work Hard, but Have a Family Too

Workplaces and school settings frequently contributed to contradicting experiences in favour and in opposition to having children. For both groups, work or school responsibilities and the perceived inability to balance work and family life highlighted reasons not to have children. For instance, many TC respondents acknowledge the predicament that family leave policies have on their ability to maintain a career and a family. As one 26-year-old TC woman explains,

> ...I find myself discouraged by the possibility of being a working mom, and so much of my identity is about being a programmer that if I couldn't have both I would pick work over motherhood...

The type of work that people engage in can also be a barrier to childbearing. As one 25-year-old mental health therapist who wants children notes,

> ... I see children with severe behavioural difficulties or developmental delays on a daily basis. After an especially hard day it is difficult to imagine having a child ... like the children with whom I do therapy.

VC respondents also expressed the nature of their work or the difficulties balancing work and family life correlating with their preference to remain childfree:

> I'm a lecturer in academia (physical sciences). My job and its demands are incredibly incompatible with childcare. ...

> Pre-tenure women faculty are rare and usually super human beings when you find one. Of course, by the time you get tenure, your fertility would be shit. … (VC Woman, age 34)

On the other hand, the nature of work can also be a source of pressure in favour of having children. For instance, one 25-year-old TC school teacher noted that '[p]arents don't take professional advice as seriously from a teacher who doesn't have kids because "What do they know about parenting?"' Similarly, a 31-year-old childfree school teacher noted that '[p]eople …outright assume that [elementary] teachers … should be married with a family'. Casual conversations with classmates or co-workers also correlate with pressures or encouragement to have children. Some respondents felt isolated from co-workers with children, as '[parenting is] part of almost everyone's daily conversation in the workplace' (TC Woman, age 28). Descriptions of isolation from co-workers varied among the TC. Those who expressed isolation and pressure from co-workers were more likely to cite struggles with fertility, while those actively delaying childbearing were more encouraged or excited when hearing about other people's parenting experiences. Childfree participants were more likely to express feelings of frustration or harassment from co-workers who '… sometimes make insensitive comments about how I have "no responsibilities" or that I don't have a "real family" without kids' (VC Woman, age 30) or 'always talk as though it is inevitable I am going to have kids …' (VC Woman, age 28).

Discussion

Childbearing Preferences in Social Fields

In short, participants' responses indicate a number of ways a shared status of non-parent can lead to similar social experiences, regardless of personal preference to have children in the future. Yet, there are also a number of ways these encounters are experienced or perceived differently, based on childbearing preference. Generally speaking, both groups experienced pressures or encouragement to have children consistent with pronatalist ideologies. However, both groups were also pressured or discouraged from having children based on others' experiences with their children, difficulty balancing work and family life or the financial or instrumental costs of prolonged education, professional development and interpersonal and societal considerations. Many pressures or encouragement to have children came from the same groups or fields as the pressures or encouragement not to have children.

For instance, participants frequently mentioned family as a major source of pressure or encouragement to have children. However, many respondents also claimed their families were a major source of pressure not to have children – or to delay having children to pursue other goals. Similarly, respondents noted that their close friends and acquaintances consistently urge them to have children (with the exception of likeminded companions among the childfree). Family and friends often express to non-parents that they should 'join the [parent] club' so their children can play and grow up together. On the other hand, participants were also discouraged from having children by friends and family members that are parents themselves. Some had friends with children overtly say things like 'don't have kids' or 'don't do it yourself', particularly when describing a hardship that their children have caused for them.

Additionally, while the responses in the current sample support the belief that the workplace is often considered a 'greedy institution' (Sullivan, 2014), there is also evidence that fields of work and school have not escaped pronatalist ideologies. In fact, in many cases it seems that participants' contradictory experiences in the workplace can assist in identifying the interplay between various ideologies, as well as how individuals' habitus can shape and be shaped by various fields. In this case, it appears that, *structurally*, childlessness serves the workplace as a 'greedy institution' in that non-parents can be viewed as committed, ideal workers, contributing to the constant demands of the workforce. However, *interpersonally*, childfree and childless members are viewed as deviant to pronatalist ideologies that workers carry in to this field, thus making it difficult for childless members to interact, relate and prove their credibility among their colleagues, clients and superiors.

While these experiences and pressures were similar, participants typically articulated or rationalised their experiences consistent with their distinct habitus differences. TC participants were more likely to report pressure to have kids before they were ready or able to – either due to financial, lifestyle or fertility-based circumstances – while VC respondents were more likely to feel pressured to 'change their minds'. Similarly, TC participants who experienced pressures or encouragement counter to their initial perspective ultimately reverted back to a perspective of either 'I can't think my way out of wanting them, as much as that would simplify everything' (TC) or 'every story I hear … strengthens my decision' (VC). Experiences and interpretations of contradicting social messages about parenthood highlight informal and formal social pressures, sanctions and support systems available as well as the *perceived* impact of structural forces on childbearing decisions and deeply rooted differences in preferences among non-parents.

Limitations/Future Research

In short, this chapter considers a shift towards an underutilised theoretical paradigm that may assist researchers in resolving complexities of structural and subjective forces seemingly at odds in existing childlessness literature (Gillespie, 2003). An emphasis on the interplay of habitus, capital and fields also contributes to a shift towards an understanding of how childfree experience the social world, rather than simply why some individuals choose childlessness. This approach views childbearing habitus as simultaneously shaping and shaped by the various fields in which individuals interact. While a more complex measurement of this interplay is beyond the scope of this discussion, similarities and differences in non-parents' experiences provide preliminary support for a shift towards a Bourdieusian theoretical understanding of childfreedom. This analysis includes a risk for coding bias due to limited intercoder reliability. Findings should be interpreted with caution and researchers should continue exploring various methods and patterns to represent the complex interplay of habitus, capital and fields in greater detail.

Future studies should also explore narrative differences between and among groups based on childbearing preference, biological ability to reproduce, gender, sexual orientation and so forth to identify additional themes in the interplay among habitus, capital and fields. For instance, my TC participants included both planners and those struggling with fertility. While the purpose of this discussion was to assess experiences based on *preference* to have children rather than ability, it is important to note that experiences in the social world among the involuntarily childless are likely to be distinct from those intentionally postponing or actively trying to have children. Future examinations would benefit from deeper explorations into differences among the group homogenously categorised here. Similar distinctions are needed among the childfree to explore how this identity and experiences vary based on access to capital not explored here.

This discussion is also limited in exploring experiences of marginalised groups, as the sample was largely white, middle-class, heterosexual and female. For example, future research should continue exploring experiences and intentions of LGBT+ non-parents, including the distinct stigmas, barriers or support experienced in relation to public and political discourses about same sex relationships and parenthood (Cain, 2001; Harris, 2005; Mezey, 2010). Similarly, there are substantial gaps in literature exploring non-parenthood among different class positions and racial and ethnic groups regarding the intersection between race, class and meanings of parenthood (Kelly, 2009).

References

Abma, J. C., & Martinez, G. M. (2006). Childlessness among older women in the United States: Trends and profiles. *Journal of Marriage and Family*, *68*, 1045–1056.

Andrade, C., & Bould, S. (2012). Child-care burden and intentions to have a second child: Effects of perceived justice in the division of child-care. *International Review of Sociology: Revue Internationale de Sociologie*, *22*, 25–37.

Bernard, S., & Correll, S. J. (2010). Normative discrimination and the motherhood penalty. *Gender & Society*, *24*, 616–646.

Bourdieu, P. (1984). *Distinction: A social critique of the judgment of taste*. Cambridge, MA: Harvard University Press.

Bourdieu, P. (1990). *The logic of practice*. Stanford, CA: Stanford University Press.

Budig, M. J., & England, P. (2001). The wage penalty for motherhood. *American Sociological Review*, *66*, 204–225.

Cain, M. (2001). *The childless revolution: What it means to be childless today*. Cambridge, MA: Perseus Publishing.

Cherlin, A. J. (2005). American marriage in the early twenty-first century. *The Future of Children*, *15*, 33–55.

Cherlin, A. J. (2009). *The marriage-go-round: The state of marriage and the family in America today*. New York, NY: Vintage Books.

Christoffersen, M. N., & Lausten, N. (2009). Early and late motherhood: Economic, family background and social conditions. *Finnish Yearbook of Population Research 2009*. Retrieved from https://journal.fi/fypr/article/download/45046/11324.

Coontz, S. (2005). *Marriage, a history: How love conquered marriage*. New York, NY: Penguin Books.

Cowan, P., & Cowan, C. P. (2009). New families: Modern couples as new pioneers. In A. S. Skolnick & J. H. Skolnick (Eds.), *Family in transition* (15th ed., pp. 255–275). New York, NY: Pearson Education, Inc.

Denbow, J. (2014). Sterilization as cyborg performance: Reproductive freedom and the regulation of sterilization. *Frontiers*, *35*, 107–131.

Edin, K., & Kefalas, M. (2005). *Promises I can keep: Why poor women put motherhood before marriage*. Berkley and Los Angeles, CA: University of California Press.

Edin, K., & Nelson, T. J. (2013). *Doing the best I can: Fatherhood in the inner city*. Berkley and Los Angeles, CA: University of California Press.

Gerson, K. (2010). *The unfinished revolution: Coming of age in a new era of gender, work, and family*. New York, NY: Oxford University Press.

Gillespie, R. (2003). Childfree and feminine: Understanding the gender identity of voluntarily childless women. *Gender & Society*, *17*, 122–136.

Green, A. I. (2008). Erotic habitus: Toward a sociology of desire. *Theory and Society*, *37*, 597–626.

Hagestad, G. O., & Call, V. R. A. (2007). Pathways to childlessness: A life course perspective. *Journal of Family Issues*, *28*, 1338–1361.

Harris, J. (2005). Lesbian motherhood and access to reproductive technology. *Canadian Woman Studies*, *24*, 43–49.

Hays, S. (1996). *The cultural contradictions of motherhood*. New Haven, CT: Yale University Press.

Heitlinger, A. (1991). Pronatalism and women's equality policies. *European Journal of Population*, *7*, 343–375.

Houseknecht, S. K. (1979). Timing of decision to remain voluntarily childless: Evidence for continuous socialization. *Psychology of Women Quarterly*, *4*, 81–96.

Kelly, M. (2009). Women's voluntary childlessness: A radical rejection of motherhood? *WSQ: Women's Studies Quarterly*, *37*, 157–172.

Koropeckyj-Cox, T. (2003). Review of women without children: Nurturing lives. *Journal of Marriage and Family*, *65*, 263–264.

Koropeckyj-Cox, T., & Call, V. R. A. (2007). Characteristics of older childless persons and parents. *Journal of Family Issues*, *28*, 1362–1414.

Kricheli-Katz, T. (2012). Choice, discrimination, and the motherhood penalty. *Law & Society Review*, *46*, 557–587.

Lisle, L. (1996). *Without child: Challenging the stigma of childlessness*. Routledge: New York.

Livingston, G. (2015). *Childlessness*. Pew Research Center, May 7. Retrieved from http://www.pewsocialtrends.org/2015/05/07/childlessness-falls-family-size-grows-among-highly-educated-women/. Accessed on July 10, 2015.

Livingston, G., & Cohn, D. (2010). *Childlessness up among all women; down among women with advanced degrees*. Pew Research Center, June 25. Retrieved from http://www.pewsocialtrends.org/2010/06/25/childlessness-up-among-all-women-down-among-women-with-advanced-degrees/. Accessed on June 5, 2015.

Livingston, G., & Parker, K. (2011). *Chapter 2. Attitudes about fatherhood*. Pew Research Center, June 15. Retrieved from http://www.pewsocialtrends.org/2011/06/15/chapter-2-attitudes-about-fatherhood/. Accessed on June 5, 2015.

Mahaffey, K. A., & Ward, S. K. (2001). The gendering of adolescents' childbearing and educational plans: Reciprocal effects and the influence of social context. *Sex Roles*, *46*, 403–417.

McQuillan, J., Griel, A. L., & Shreffler, K. M. (2011). Pregnancy intentions among women who do not try: Focusing on women who are okay either way. *Matern Child Health J*, *15*, 178–187.

McQuillan, J., Greil, A. L., Shreffler, K. M., Wonch-Hill, P. A., Gentzler, K. C., & Hathcoat, J. D. (2012). Does the reason matter? Variations in childlessness concerns among U.S. women. *Journal of Marriage and Family*, *74*, 1161–1181.

Mezey, N. J. (2010). *New choices new families: How lesbians decide about motherhood.* Baltimore, MD: John Hopkins University Press.

Morgan, S. P., & King, R. B. (2001). Why have children in the 21st century? Biological predisposition, social coercion, rational choice. *European Journal of Population, 17*, 3–20.

Mosher, W. D., & Bachrach, C. A. (1982). Childlessness in the United States: Estimates from the national survey of family growth. *Journal of Family Issues, 3*, 517–543.

Mullins, A. R. (2016). *'I kid you not, I am asked a question about children at least once a week': Exploring differences in childbearing habitus in pronatalist fields.* Unpublished doctoral dissertation. University of Central Florida, Orlando, FL.

Newport, F., & Wilke, J. (2013). Desire for children still norm in U.S. *Gallup* September, 25. Retrieved from http://www.gallup.com/poll/164618/desire-children-norm.aspx. Accessed on June 4, 2015.

Park, K. (2002). Stigma management among the voluntary childless. *Sociological Perspectives, 45*, 21–45.

Park, K. (2005). Choosing childlessness: Weber's typology of action and motives of the voluntarily childless. *Sociological Inquiry, 75*, 372–402.

Parry, D. C. (2005). Women's leisure as resistance to pronatalist ideology. Abstract of the Paper presented at the Eleventh Canadian Congress on Leisure Research, May 17–20, 2005.

Powell, A. (2008). Amor fati? Gender habitus and young people's negotiation of (hetero)sexual consent. *Journal of Sociology, 44*, 167–184.

Rovi, S. (1994). Taking 'no' for an answer: Using negative reproductive intentions to study the childless/childfree. *Population Research and Policy Review, 13*, 343–365.

Sassler, S., & Miller, A. J. (2014). 'We're very careful...': The fertility desires and contraceptive behaviors of cohabitating couples. *Family Relations, 63*, 538–553.

Scott, L. S. (2009). *Two is enough: A couple's guide to living childless by choice.* Berkeley, CA: Seal Press.

Senior, J. (2014). *All joy and no fun: The paradox of modern parenthood.* New York, NY: HarperCollins Publishers.

Shreffler, K. M., Griel, A. L., Mitchell, K. S., & McQuillan, J. (2015). Variation in pregnancy intendedness across U.S. women's pregnancies. *Maternal and Child Health Journal, 19*, 932–938.

Sullivan, T. A. (2014). Greedy institutions, overwork, and work-life balance. *Sociological Inquiry, 84*, 1–15.

Townsend, N. (2009). The four facets of fatherhood. In A. S. Skolnick & J. H. Skolnick (Eds.), *Family in transition* (15th ed., pp. 283–293). New York: Pearson Education, Inc.

Veevers, J. E. (1974). Voluntary childlessness and social policy: An alternative view. *The Family Coordinator, 23*, 397–406.

Wall, G., & Arnold, S. (2007). How involved is involved fathering? An exploration of the contemporary culture of fatherhood. *Gender & Society, 21*, 508–527.

Waren, W., & Pals, H. (2013). Comparing characteristics of voluntarily childless men and women. *Jounal of Population Research, 30*, 151–170.

Wolf, D. A., & Laditka, J. N. (2006). *Childless elderly beneficiaries' use and costs of Medicare services.* Final report. U.S. Department of Health and Human Services.

Xu, Q. (2013). Absent or ambivalent mothers and avoidant children – An evolutionary reading of Zhang Kangkang's motherhood stories. *Finnish Yearbook of Population Research, XLVIII*, 147–168.

Yaremko, S. K., & Lawson, K. L. (2007). Gender internalization of expressive traits, and expectations of parenting. *Sex Roles*, *57*, 675–687.

SECTION III
INTERSECTIONAL PERSPECTIVES ON CHILDLESSNESS

Chapter 7

Are Loneliness and Regret the Inevitable Outcomes of Ageing and Childlessness?

Rose O'Driscoll and Jenny Mercer

Abstract

Discourses on ageing and childlessness coalesce around the notion that childless women will experience regret and loneliness in old age. In the United Kingdom, the idea that children (mostly women) will provide care in old age tends to be normalised and underpins social care provision. In recent times, media coverage of childless women has also tended to sustain and promote this. This discourse occurs within a context where childlessness is on the rise and where there is little academic interest in the topic.

Our chapter will report on a constructivist grounded theory study with women who choose not to have children. A key aim of the study was to explore the consequences of participants' choices on their lives. Twenty-one women aged between 45 and 75, from across England, Scotland and Wales participated. The age criteria were chosen to reflect the category that is used by the Office of National Statistics to denote that women's reproduction ends at 45. This also helps to construct a social norm that women aged 45 and over are seen as older women. Findings reveal that most participants experience no regrets following their choice not to have children. Some express 'half regrets' while all challenge the societal expectation that without children there will be no one to care for them when they are older.

This supports the limited, mainly autobiographical literature, on loss and regret. It also refutes the unquestioned and widely believed assumption that women who choose not have children will live to regret it. For participants, the choice for motherhood was but one choice from a menu of many others. Their choice was for something more meaningful for them rather than a choice against motherhood. Consequently, participants had no reason to experience loss or regret. These findings also question the discourse, which implies that children will ensure care in older age. It presents a challenge to the myth that the family is a haven of happiness and support in an ever-changing world. Crucially, it supports calls for more inclusive policy making to address the care needs of all older people.

Keywords: Women's experiences; choice; childlessness; ageing; regret; grounded theory

Introduction

An increasing number of women in the UK are childless by the age of 45 (ONS, 2013). Despite this, childless women are still perceived as somehow in deficit and are positioned negatively within society. This was illustrated by Gillespie (2000) who revealed that there are no positive words to describe women without children. Instead they are, *'perceived as maladjusted selfish and immature'* (p. 142). Additionally, the language used to describe 'childless' women denote loss or absence. As Wager (2000) argued, 'The problem for childless women, then, is that as "real women" something is missing; there is a flaw in our identity and lifestyle' (p. 3). Such negativity portrays them as marginalised and renders them as the 'other', a term Letherby (2002, 1999) noted to be in direct opposition to 'mother'. We stated in a previous chapter that both mainstream and feminist writers have largely overlooked childless women (O'Driscoll & Mercer, 2015). The more popular focus has been on childbirth, infertility, motherhood and reproduction. Where they do appear in literature, such women are typically seen as problematic.

This negative image of childless women resonates with discourses surrounding ageing. In contemporary societies, older people are often portrayed as a passive and dependent group. The language used to describe older women is often negative, patronising and insulting; for example: 'little old ladies', 'bats', 'witches' and 'hags' (Bearon, 2002). We constantly hear the refrain from politicians and media commentators about the 'problems of old age' and 'the burden of an ageing population' (Branfield & Berersford, 2010). Such language helps perpetuate the notion of a 'deficit' model of ageing and promotes the idea that all older people will need care. A common assumption is that childless women will experience significant loneliness, isolation and regret as they age (Gillespie, 2000; O'Driscoll & Mercer, 2015; Wager, 2000).

Traditionally older people have received informal care from families, typically from daughters/women. In the UK, women are more likely to be carers than men (Carers UK, 2017). The idea that children (mostly women) will care for their parents tends to be normalised and appears to underpin current and future social care provision. Such discourses occur at a time when the numbers and proportions of older people have grown and continue to grow significantly. In addition, birth rates are declining (ONS, 2014). There are increasing cuts to health and social care budgets and calls from political leaders to do more to look after ourselves. This raises important questions such as where does this leave ageing women who have no children (and may also be in caring roles for their own parents)? Do discourses about ageing which focus on the 'crisis' in social care offer another means to marginalise this group of women? Will they be seen as an additional 'drain' on a system, which is already struggling to cope with care in later life?

The aim of this chapter is to report on findings from a constructivist grounded theory study. Drawing on the voices of women who chose not to have children, the findings challenge the prevailing belief that loneliness and regret are inevitable outcomes of ageing and childlessness. First, we will outline the methodological approach and fieldwork. Second, we present the findings on regret giving primacy to the voices of participants. Finally, we relate and discuss the findings to previous substantive research, relevant literature and to the current public policy debate.

Terminology Adopted

Initial literature searches revealed that the most common terms used were 'voluntary' and 'involuntary childlessness'. 'Voluntary childlessness' tends to be defined as making a choice not to have children and 'involuntary childlessness' as not able to have children. However, in our study, we elected not to use the word voluntary childlessness since we did not feel it accurately reflected the complexity of choice these women made. Instead, we chose to use the phrase, 'women who choose not to have children'.

Methodology

For reasons such as those highlighted thus far, we felt that it was essential for the topic of women who chose not to have children to be viewed through a feminist lens. Feminist research remains rooted in a desire to address prejudice and social inequalities (Hesse-Biber, 2014; Letherby, 2003; Oerton, 2014) associated with women's lives. It is about recognising the need for social change for women, which makes it avowedly political (hooks, 1989; Wikinson, 1998). Thus, we did not approach our research from a 'neutral' or 'objective' stance and we wanted our findings to challenge the status quo. For this reason, we needed to contextualise our research within current political thinking.

Embracing this also entailed selecting a methodological approach, which placed the narratives of childless women centre stage. Writers such as Chodorow (1989, 1998) and Letherby (2003) argued that hearing female voices are a key goal of feminist scholarship; yet childless women's voices have been largely silent and marginal within feminist discourse. From a research perspective, Chodorow suggests that both qualitative and reflexive methodologies are apposite tools to facilitate this approach. We selected Kathy Charmaz's constructivist grounded theory for this purpose. What follows is an account of why and how we embraced it.

Charmaz (2016) summarised the ways in which her approach to grounded theory was different from earlier versions by:

- assuming a relativist epistemology;
- acknowledging researchers' and research participants', multiple standpoints, roles and realities;
- adopting a reflexive stance towards backgrounds, values, actions, situations, relationships with research participants and representations of them; and
- situating research in the historical, social and situational conditions of its production (p. 1).

Parallels can be clearly drawn between ideas outlined above relating to feminist approaches to research, and constructivist grounded theory.

Intersectionality

Our approach was further enhanced by acknowledging the principle of intersectionality. Collins (2000) defines intersectionality as the ways in which gender, race, sexuality, class, different biographies and locations situate our individual experiences and life chances. Thus as Cho, Williams-Crenshaw and McCall (2013) argue, 'the dynamics of intersectionality' serve as 'both as an academic frame and as a practical intervention in a world characterized by inequalities' (p. 807). In adhering to this principle, we were conscious of how women's lived experiences differs based on geographical, structural and ideological factors (Collins, 2000; hooks, 1981).

Reflexivity

An integral part of this approach is reflexivity. Feminist scholars have spearheaded a substantial body of literature on the significance and importance of reflexivity in the research process (e.g. Charmaz, 1996, 2006, 2014, 2016; Chodorow, 1998; Delamont, 2003; Letherby, 2003, 2015; Moch & Gates, 2000; Roberts, 2007; Wikinson, 1998). As researchers, our ideas and theories are in constant interaction with the data and permeate the research from start to finish (Crotty, 2003; Grix, 2004); we need to be aware how our own lives and values may affect research. In doing this, it is not necessary to reveal intimate details of our lives. However, we need to be aware of them and how they can influence our own preconceptions on data and concepts.

Our account would therefore be incomplete without some information about the authors to provide a reflexive frame of reference for the reader. This chapter takes a category from the first author's doctoral study about women who choose not to have children (O'Driscoll, 2017). The second author supervised the work. It has been further developed here by discussing it in the context of the implications it has for ageing. Both writers are female, and have no children. They are within the same age bracket set as the inclusion criteria for participants who took place in the study. For them, the choice came at different stages of adulthood: for Rose, her choice not to have children was made during her mid-20s, while for Jenny it became clear in her mid to late thirties, based on a long-term relationship with a partner who already had children and did not want any more. Both work in higher education and have social science backgrounds; Rose in sociology, Jenny in social psychology. While there is some overlap between these disciplines, the analysis was largely produced from a sociological stance. Rose conducted the interviews and participants were informed when she introduced herself that she has chosen not to have children.

Data Collection

The inclusion criteria comprised women aged 45 and over who had chosen not to have children. This age range was chosen to reflect the category that is used by the Office of National Statistics (ONS) to denote that women's reproduction ends at 45 (ONS, 2013). We elected to use this because it also plays a role in constructing a social norm that women aged 45 and over are seen as 'older' women. Twenty-one women aged between 47 and 75, from different social class backgrounds, across England, Scotland and Wales participated.

Six out of the twenty-one participants were recruited from the older women's feminist network in London. These women shared a largely feminist view of the world. Their feminist consciousness was a key liberatory factor in their personal journey towards choosing not to have children. It could be argued that this data may have had undue influence on the findings. On the one hand, we can see this as a reasonable critique. However, on the other hand, this critique is balanced to some extent in that many of the other participants did not share a feminist analysis. Moreover, and as importantly, these women wanted to be involved and had distinct and varied experiences.

The demographics of the participants can be found in Table 1 below.

Semi-structured interviews were guided by questions covering key areas in relation to the research aim. Initially, the women were asked to share their biographies and family backgrounds. This was followed by more focused questions exploring relationships, marriage, choices not to have children and how and why they made their choices. The later questions referred to participants' experiences arising from their choices.

The research comprised two phases, a preliminary and a main study. The purpose of the preliminary study was to collect a corpus of data from which tentative categories were drawn and further explored in the second phase of data collection. This process allows one to check the feasibility of the findings while ensuring that the knowledge construction is grounded in the data and words of the participants. Four women with ages ranging from 47 to 52 years were recruited via convenience sampling. Four tentative categories were constructed from the data from these interviews. In a grounded theory study, initial categories are always provisional, tentative and hazy, or as Charmaz (2014) states, 'analytically thin… insufficiently supported' (p. 212). All were explored further in the main study, but it is the preliminary category of 'Loss and

Table 1. Profile of Participants for Preliminary and Main Study.

Participant Number	Age	Parental Social Class as Defined by Participants	Self-defined Social Class	Location
1	52	W/C	M/C	Wales
2	48	M/C	M/C	Wales
3	51	W/C	M/C	Wales
4	47	M/C	M/C	Wales
5	58	M/C	M/C	Wales
6	57	M/C	M/C	London
7	47	W/C	W/C	London
8	65	W/C	M/C	Watford
9	75	W/C	M/C	Watford
10	59	M/C	Poor	London
11	55	W/C	M/C	Kent
12	67	W/C	M/C	Yorkshire
13	60	W/C	M/C	Wiltshire
14	48	M/C	M/C	Wales
15	65	M/C	M/C	Kent
16	67	M/C	M/C	London
17	67	W/C	M/C	Scotland
18	67	W/C	M/C	Essex
19	70	Upper M/C	M/C	Essex
20	67	M/C	M/C	Wales
21	48	M/C	M/C	Sussex

Note: Middle class: **M/C,** Working class: **W/C**

regret as normal elements of everyday life', which is of relevance to this chapter.

For the main study, a UK-wide recruitment of participants was undertaken. In keeping with the principles of theoretical sampling required in grounded theory, a non-probability sampling approach, purposive sampling was employed. A list of UK-wide women only organisations were contacted requesting the inclusion of an advertisement in their publications or on their websites. A poster was also displayed in local hairdressers, slimming clubs, charity shops and leisure clubs. One of the women's organisations (Women's History Group) placed the advertisement on their website. The Older Feminist Network based in London also placed details in their magazine. Over a period of 12 months, 26 women expressed an interest in participating. Most responded to the magazine advert. One participant responded to the website advertisement. None responded to the poster. This generated a second sample of 17 women, aged between 47 and 75 years of age. These came from London, Yorkshire, Wiltshire, Sussex, Scotland and Wales.

During the preliminary study, only one of the women had expressed loss and regret at her choice not to have children. The other three participants, while acknowledging regret as a potential element of such a life-changing choice, did not report experiencing any loss or regret. When contact was made with prospective participants for the main study, they were sent the provisional categories identified in the preliminary study. Most felt they could identify with certain elements of the first three; yet what stood out was that they reported feeling least identification with the category around loss and regret. In the sixth interview, the participant opened her interview by saying, 'you said some of them were sad about it, having made that choice … and I think having made that choice, why would you be sad?' (P6). This validated the decision to include loss and regret as an area of exploration in the main study. It also opened up a very insightful dialogue on regret, which led to the construction of a category around this concept, to which attention is now turned.

Findings: Regret

Analysis of the data revealed that most participants ($N = 16$) experienced no regrets following their choice not to have children. Only one participant (who took part in the preliminary study) expressed a deep sense of loss at her choice. Others ($N = 4$) were more ambivalent, which was coded as half regrets. These participants acknowledged and accepted an element of regret from their choices. Landman, Vandewater, Stewart, and Malley (1995) referred to this as 'counterfactual thinking', which she defined as, 'the process of imagining alternatives to reality, what might have been' (p. 87). All pondered the potential for regret when older and in need of care.

No Regrets

The majority of participants felt no regrets for choosing not to have children as revealed in some of their comments:

> I don't regret not having kids, no. (P7)
>
> Never really thought about loss or regret. (P5)
>
> No loss or regret, no, not at all, always happy with my choice. (P13)
>
> Absolutely no regrets and I don't feel I have missed out on anything. (P14)
>
> I have no regrets about not having children, definitely no regrets. (P17)

Several different, but related, reasons were cited as to why they did not express regret. An important reason for some was that the desire to have children was never part of their life plans. The plan was always to live lives of their own making outside motherhood. For this participant, not having children meant that she could be, 'incredibly productive, so not having children means I can fulfil more desires and I don't have to worry about a child or children' (P12). From this perspective, it was about wanting more autonomy and personal freedom. As another stated, 'I never wanted one [child], I wanted to have a really good life, I wanted to have a life of freedom without responsibilities. No loss, no regret, personal choice' (P11).

In the same vein, others wanted to pursue education, find rewarding work and have a home of their own. Moreover, in pursuing personal goals, they did not feel guilty as this participant asserted:

> I don't feel guilty for my lifestyle either; I enjoy it. I don't think there is anything wrong with it and I'm glad I never had children. No regret and no loss, no, because I have lived my life, so I feel relief. I have a life, I have an education, I have work, I have my own place. (P20)

Another reason offered centred on the commitment involved with not having and rearing children. For instance, as a young woman, one participant experienced a mothering role with siblings. She did not enjoy this role and it made her aware of the demands of motherhood. She asserted:

> I have no reason to regret. What I thought about the bringing up of children and the commitment is as true today as it was when I was 14. I can see what it means; I think it is a fairly mature decision and recognition of myself. Did I want that sort of responsibility; no, I did not. (P8)

For another, it appeared to be more about the loss of self often associated with motherhood. She expressed the view that some mothers appeared to live their lives through their children. Thus, they had little or no identity other than being a mother. She argued that this could lead to a resulting merging of identities – woman and motherhood. She accepted that some women are happy to accept that role. However, she realised early on that, had she chosen to have children she, 'would not have had a life; your life would have been like all women before you, your children' (P9).

Others had a more political and feminist view of life and felt such ideals were more important for them. As one participant stated, 'politics, environment … we can't have children, we are too busy saving the world' (P1). This stance reflects a view that 'saving the world' is also an important project and maybe has equal or even greater social value than being a mother.

Half Regrets

However, this challenge could be somewhat addressed by what we theorised as, 'half-regrets'. A small number of participants ($N=4$) acknowledged the inevitably of regret from making a major life choice. For these, regret was not having the *experience* of motherhood or rearing a child to adulthood. There was a sense of inevitability expressed about having at least some element of regret following any major life choice. As this participant observed:

> I think I hold contradictory views like most people do, which is I do have regrets; there is a lack of something I could have done [having children] that would have been creative and would have been satisfying. (P15)

The fourth participant agreed and stated that it is unrealistic not to experience some regret from choosing not to have children:

> I knew I would regret not having children, because to imagine you can go through life and never have that feeling is unrealistic. I thought lots of time, will I regret it, but wouldn't it be worse if you regretted having them. (P4)

Another concurred with the view that intrinsic to choice are elements of regret. She said that her choice meant she rejected motherhood because it is not something she desired for her own life. Nevertheless, she accepted that because of her choice there was regret, 'yes there will always be regret but not enough to do anything about it, so I guess they are not big regrets' (P1). She acknowledged that being a mother might have been an interesting experience. However, at the same time she believed motherhood is only one experience in life and not the only way to find fulfilment, stating 'the desire to have a child could not have been that strong, otherwise I would have pursued it' (P1). Instead, she pursued activities for her that were interesting, satisfying and creative. For example, she was involved in politics and women's groups with people who shared her views on life and with whom she built rewarding and lasting connections, 'it [having a child] was only one experience in life; there were also other as important things to do … politics, environment' (P1).

One participant shared a deep sense of loss and personal failure at her choice. This participant enjoyed a very successful life. Yet, despite enormous professional achievements, not having a child created an acute sense of failure:

> It's probably something in me that I feel a sense of failure to take up the challenge, was weak, was some sort of reject … If you've got the mother tag, it rolls off the tongue, it's a description that fills out a whole life history very easily, you've obviously spent your time wisely, because you have been a mother … you could have buried people in the back garden, but you've been a mother so you're covered. (P2)

She was also regularly reminded by negative societal perceptions of women without children, 'being a wife has solved quite a few societal conventions, God forbid if I hadn't been married, having been married takes the heat off' (P2).

It should be stressed that making the choice not to have children was a complex process involving considerable introspection and the working through of competing influences. As noted earlier participants' social class had a significant influence on their capacity to choose not to have children. Despite their social class and age differences, there was no noticeable difference in how participants responded to the question on regret. For some, the best way to deal with this tension was to take responsibility for their choices. As this participant stated:

> You know, life is full of half regrets and ponderings over what it would have been like … it's about taking responsibility for your choices. I mean God help me if I was dogged by regrets of not having children, what a waste of emotion. (P4)

Regret and Ageing

A number of participants referred to ways in which they were often reminded both privately and publicly that their choice not to have children meant there would be no one to care for them in old age. However, they did not accept the correlation between not having children and the lack of care when older. Challenging what she believed was a misconception, this participant asserted that, 'I don't look to my old age thinking, "God, there is no one to look after me", I don't, I just don't' (P21). Another supported this view and thought the idea that, 'oh your children will look after you in your old age, is a load of rubbish' (P5).

Others were less certain and more circumspect, 'you know there will come a time when the clichéd fear of being old with nobody around hits you', (P4). This sentiment was also reflected in other responses. This woman had fears that she would be vulnerable and isolated when older:

> Until ten years ago, I would have said 100% no regrets. But now sometimes I regret it partly because I am an outsider and a loner and that is hard sometimes. I am also 64, my body is disintegrating, I think of having a nice daughter to look after me in my ailing years …, and I guess love. I'm not in a relationship at the moment, there is not enough love in my life, and I would like that ordinary love some friends have with their daughters, that profound connection with someone. But 60% [of her regret] is about

> lifestyle, 25% is about not having blood relations and 15% is about not having a child. (P12)

A participant who lived in a rural area with poor transport links shared her caring experiences of a friend, 'who will care for me, crossed my mind last year when a friend of mine died; like running people to hospital and, you know, that kind of thing' (P17). However, she went on to say there is no guarantee that even if one had children that they would care for their parents:

> I look around other friends with children and by the time they have got to this stage, the children have got lives of their own; they are married with their own families. (P17)

Some felt that even if children are in a position to help they might not want to do so. One person recalled her neighbour, who was over 90 years old. She went on to say, 'she had a son who she absolutely doted on, and you know he wouldn't even send her a birthday card, and it was just sad because she had somebody who just wasn't there for her' (P14).

Participants whose parents live abroad pointed out that it was not possible to provide care in such circumstances. Any care they were able to offer was remote,

> My Mum lives in X, I live here, so does my brother. She sees us once a year. I speak to her almost every day, that is my choice, so having children does not guarantee care. I am not there looking after them physically and everything I do is remote, but if they were relying on me in old age, it is not going to happen. (P22)

> Look at my parents, I am not able to offer care and attention to them, I live on the other side of the world. (P2)

Discussion

The evidence from this study suggests that most women who chose not to have children do not experience regret, as they age. In fact, participants wondered why others would assume that their choices would lead to regret and loneliness in old age. Indeed, many recalled being told by others that their lives would be inadequate and meaningless without a child. These assumptions are consistent with other studies. Nunez (2015), herself a childless woman, in her autobiographical work stated that people would say to her, 'but you love children … Meaning, surely I must have regrets' (p. 116).

Reflecting on our findings, it appears that participants' disclosures around regret were linked to prejudicial attitudes about ageing and childlessness. In contrast, for participants, regret was framed in more feminist terms. This echoes Houston (2015) who citing a friend, wrote, 'I will never regret not having children. What I regret is that I live in a world where in spite of everything, that decision is still not quite okay' (p. 171). The important insight here is that feelings of regret are to be expected where gendered expectations are deeply embedded within society and where motherhood has been the measure by which we define women (Ireland, 1993; Rich, 1977). In such a context, women who do not have children go against tradition and deeply ingrained biological, cultural and societal practices (de Beauvoir, 1972; Woolf, 2004). Childless women can find themselves on the outside, isolated and subject to derision. Consequently, regret and loss may be inevitable and a woman can feel like, 'a zero, a nothing … a gap … a blank … a space' (P2).

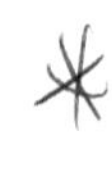

Our findings also reveal that having children does not mitigate against isolation or a guarantee of care from family members in later life, 'I don't look to my old age thinking god there is no one to look after me, I don't, I just don't' (P21). 'oh your children will look after you in old age, is a load of rubbish' (P5). This finding concurs with evidence from the field of gerontology, which reveals a more complex story. While these theorists do not specifically deal with regret, they refer to related concepts of isolation and loneliness as correlates of ageing. Wenger, Davies, Shahtahmasebi, and Scott (1996) review of research in this area found that isolation and loneliness are only widespread among the very old. This suggests that their prevalence as a natural and inevitable part of the general ageing process may have been overestimated. Reporting specifically on a sample of over 85-year-old childless people who took part in a longitudinal study, Wenger (2009) found that adaptation had taken place by this stage of the lifespan. Individuals typically had established closer relationships with collateral kin (e.g. siblings, nephews and nieces), friends and neighbours than their counterparts who had children. Wenger's work (2001, 2009) also revealed that, generally, childless women demonstrate more positive adaptations in later life than men do.

It is noteworthy that childless people are more likely to enter residential care earlier, due to having fewer formal networks of care (Wenger,

2009). However, this is, once again towards the end of their life when health is likely to have deteriorated. The message we can take from such research is that social isolation and loneliness are dependent on a range of interacting factors such as gender, class, marital status and social networks (Wenger, Scott, & Patterson, 2000). Being a childless woman does not necessarily equate to an unfulfilling and lonely life as one ages.

Reynolds (2009) study with childless women and men found that they referred to 'family' in a much wider context, one that did not necessarily mean having their own children and grandchildren to care for them. 'Family' included connections with friends, community, neighbours' children and grandchildren. Instead of expecting children to care for older parents, there is a need to rethink current provision and government policies on care for older people without children, 'I sometimes think of the future and wonder about what it will be like, we need to rethink provision we need for [all] older people' (P13). This echoes the sentiments in relation to the concept of 'generation strain' identified in the Institute of Public Policy Research report by McNeil and Hunter (2014). They provided evidence for a growing 'family care gap' where the number of ageing individuals requiring support and care is set to outnumber the adult children who can do this. The authors predicted that this will occur by 2017. Pickard (2013) estimates a further 60% increase in England by 2030 among the number of people who are ageing without adult children. Current demographics reveal that the number of people who will be able to care for older people will have increased by only 20% in this period. The idea that families are the solution for the crisis in social care is not a viable option.

Despite acknowledgement of the 'generation strain', media reports of calls by politicians for children to be responsible for their ageing parents suggests that this message still needs to be embraced by government. For example, in 2013, Jeremy Hunt (the then newly appointed Health Minister) talked of a 'social contract' where grandchildren could observe their parents caring for grandparents and recognise that this will eventually be their responsibility (Butler, 2013). Again, in 2017, David Mowat the Social Care Minister in England placed responsibility on adult children to look after their parents to tackle the crisis in social care (Ashtana, 2017). The finding from this study challenges such assertions; we would argue that ageist and family-centric discourses only transpire to feed insecurities.

The fact that childless women will have had less interrupted employment histories than those with children means that they are likely to have paid taxes more consistently. Similarly, they are not going to have made demands on the healthcare system for paediatric care or on the public education system (Wenger, 2009). The likelihood that they *may* need more state support in later life should not be seen as another reason to view such women as a drain and in deficit. Yet, such ideas continue to reinforce the message previously highlighted by sociologists such as Letherby, that having children is the preferred societal option and promises security and care in old age (Letherby, 2002). A consistent discourse is that the family is the place of love, warmth, comfort and care in old age (Bauman & May, 2001; Finch, 1989; Parsons, 1956; Young & Wilmott, 1957). Our findings reveal that such ideas are often too simplistic, drawn on outdated social norms, and are based on rhetoric, rather than facts. In a world of increasing individualisation, commodification and change, the rhetoric that stresses the value and sanctity of family life offers very little comfort for support in old age.

Conclusion

The findings from this study suggest that most women who choose not to have children do not experience regret as they age. Children do not mitigate against loneliness and isolation and neither are they a guarantee of care in later life. This evidence runs counter to ageist discourses about childlessness, and the assumption that women without children will inevitably experience significant loss and regret. They challenge ageist discourses, which conflates the notion that having children guarantees care when older. Participants' experiences of choice and regret reveal a more realistic picture that reflects the changing nature of families and communities. Crucially, the findings call for more inclusive social policies, which consider the diversity of *all* older people.

References

Ashtana, A. (2017). Take care of your elderly mothers and fathers, says Tory minister. *The Guardian*, January 31. Retrieved from https://www.theguardian.com/society/2017/jan/31/take-care-of-your-elderly-mothers-and-fathers-says-tory-minister. Accessed on April 24, 2017.

Bauman, Z., & May, T. (2001). *Thinking sociologically*. Oxford: Blackwell.

Bearon, L. B. (2002). *Little old ladies & grumpy old men: How language shapes our views about aging*. Retrieved from https://learn.gold.ac.uk/pluginfile.php/72839/mod_resource/content/0/Little_Old_Ladies.pdf Accessed on May 20, 2017.

Branfield, F., & Berersford, P. (2010). *A better life: Alternative approaches from a service user perspective*. York: Joseph Rowntree Foundation.

Butler, P. (2013). Jeremy Hunt: UK should adopt Asian culture of caring for the elderly. *The Guardian*, October 18. Retrieved from https://www.theguardian.com/politics/2013/oct/18/jeremy-hunt-uk-families-asia-elderly. Accessed on February 21, 2017.

Carers UK. (2017). *Facts about carers*. Retrieved from http://www.carersuk.org/for-professionals/policy/policy-library/facts-about-carers-2015. Accessed on April 21, 2017.

Charmaz, K. (1996). The search for meanings – Grounded theory. In J. A. Smith, R. Harre, & L. Van Lagenhove (Eds.), *Rethinking methods in psychology* (pp. 27–49). London: Sage.

Charmaz, K. (2006). *Constructing grounded theory. A practical guide through qualitative analysis*. Los Angeles, CA: Sage.

Charmaz, K. (2014). *Constructing grounded theory* (2nd ed.). Los Angeles, CA: Sage.

Charmaz, K. (2016). Constructivist grounded theory. *The Journal of Positive Psychology*, doi:10.1080/17439760.2016.1262612

Cho, S., Williams-Crenshaw, K., & McCall, L. (2013). Toward a field of intersectionality studies: Theory, applications, and praxis. *Signs: Journal of Women in Culture and Society*, *38*(4), 785–810.

Chodorow, N. J. (1989). *Feminism and psychoanalytic theory*. Cambridge, MA: Polity Press.

Chodorow, N. J. (1998). Seventies questions for thirties women: Some nineties reflections. In S. Wilkinson (Ed.), *Feminist social psychologies: International perspectives* (pp. 21–50). Buckingham: Open University Press.

Collins, P. H. (2000). *Black feminist thought: Knowledge, consciousness and the politics of empowerment*. London: Routledge.

Crotty, M. (2003). *The Foundations of social research. Meaning and perspective in the research process* (2nd ed.). London: Sage.

de Beauvoir, S. (1972). *The second sex*. Harmondsworth: Penguin.

Delamont, S. (2003). *Feminist sociology*. London: Sage.

Finch, J. (1989). *Family obligations and social change*. Cambridge: Polity Press.

Gillespie, R. (2000). When no means no: Disbelief, disregard and deviance as discourses of voluntary childlessness. *Women's Studies International Forum*, *2*(2), 223–234. *Ingentaconnect*. Retrieved from: http://www.sciencedirect.com/science/article/pii/S0277539500000765. Accessed on June 14, 2015.

Grix, J. (2004). *The foundations of research*. Basingstoke: Palgrave Macmillan.

Hesse-Biber, S. N. (2014). *Feminist research practice: A primer* (2nd ed.). London: Sage.

hooks, b. (1981). *Ain't I a woman: Black women and feminism*. Boston: South End Press.

hooks, b. (1989). *Talking back: Thinking feminist, thinking black*. Toronto: Between the Lines.

Houston, P. (2015). The trouble with having it all. In M. Daum (Ed.), *Sixteen writers on the decision not to have kids* (pp. 163–185). New York, NY: Picador.

Ireland, M. S. (1993). *Reconceiving women: Separating motherhood from female identity*. New York, NY: Guilford Press.

Landman, J., Vandewater, E. A., Stewart, A. J., & Malley, J. E. (1995). Missed opportunities: Psychological ramifications of counterfactual thought in midlife women. *Journal of Adult Development*, *2*(2), 87–97. Retrieved from http://link.springer.com/article/10.1007/BF02251257. Accessed on April 18, 2014.

Letherby, G. (1999). Other than mother and mothers as others: The experience of motherhood and non-motherhood in relation to 'infertility' and 'involuntary childlessness. *Women's Studies International Forum*, *22*(3), 359–372. Retrieved from: http://www.sciencedirect.com/science/article/pii/S027753959900028X. Accessed on March 4, 2013.

Letherby, G. (2002). Childless and bereft? Stereotypes and realities in relation to 'Voluntary' and 'Involuntary' childlessness and womanhood. *Sociological Inquiry*, *72*(1), 7–20. Retrieved from http://onlinelibrary.wiley.com/doi/10.1111/1475-682X.00003/abstract. Accessed on September 28, 2012.

Letherby, G. (2003). *Feminist research in theory and practice*. UK: Open University Press.

Letherby, G. (2015). Gender-sensitive method/ologies. In V. Robinson & D. Richardson (Eds.), *Gender & women's studies* (4th ed., pp. 76–92). London: Palgrave.

McNeil, C., & Hunter, J. (2014). *The generation strain: Collective solutions to care in an ageing society*. London: Institute for Public Policy Research.

Moch, S. D., & Gates, M. F. (Eds.). (2000). *The researcher experience in qualitative research*. London: Sage.

Nunez, S. (2015). The most important thing. In M. Daum (Ed.), *Sixteen writers on the decision not to have kids* (pp. 97–119). New York, NY: Picador.

O'Driscoll, R. (2017). *'I was looking for something different and I found it'. A constructivist grounded theory study with women who choose not to have children*. Unpublished PhD, Cardiff Metropolitan University, Cardiff, Wales.

O'Driscoll, R., & Mercer, J. (2015). Women who choose not to have children: A preliminary study. *Psychology of Women Section Review*, *17*, 21–30. Retrieved from https://repository.cardiffmet.ac.uk/dspace/bitstream/10369/7801/3/Women%20who%20choose%20not%20to%20have%20children-Mercer%20J.pdf

Oerton, H. (2014). Emerging feminists. *Psychology of Women Section Review*, *16*, 2–4.

ONS. (2013). Office for National Statistics. *1 in 5 women are childless at 45*. Retrieved from http://www.ons.gov.uk/ons/rel/fertility-analysis/cohort-fertility–england-and-wales/2011/sty-1-in-5-women-are-childless-at-45.html. Accessed on March 8, 2013.

ONS. (2014). Office for National Statistics, *Birth summary tables, England and Wales*. Retrieved from https://www.ons.gov.uk/peoplepopulationandcommunity/birthsdeathsandmarriages/livebirths/bulletins/birthsummarytablesenglandandwales/2015-07-15/previous/v1#main-points. Accessed on May 6, 2017.

Parsons, T. (1956). *Family: Socialisation and interaction process*. London: Routledge and Kegan Paul.

Pickard, L. (2013). A growing care gap? The supply of unpaid care for older people by their adult children in England to 2032. *Ageing and Society*, *35*(1), 96–123. Retrieved from https://www.researchgate.net/publication/272008784_

A_growing_care_gap_The_supply_of_unpaid_care_for_older_people_by_their_adult_children_in_England_to_2032. Accessed on February 4, 2017.

Reynolds, J. (2009). Older people without children. *Solo Living*, 26 October, Edinburgh, UK. Retrieved from http://oro.open.ac.uk/24436/. Accessed on May 16, 2017.

Rich, A. (1977). *Of woman born – Motherhood as experience and institution*. CA: Bantam Books.

Roberts, B. (2007). *Getting the most out of the research experience. What every researcher needs to know*. London: Sage.

Wager, M. (2000). Childless by choice? Ambivalence and the female identity. *Feminism and Psychology*, *10*(3), 389–395. *Sage Journals*. Retrieved from http://fap.sagepub.com/. Accessed on April 25, 2012.

Wenger, G. C. (2001). Myths and realities of ageing in rural Britain. *Ageing and Society*, *21*, 117–130.

Wenger, G. C. (2009). Childlessness at the end of life: Evidence from rural Wales. *Ageing and Society*, *29*(8), 1243–1259. Retrieved from https://www.cambridge.org/core/journals/ageing-and-society/article/childlessness-at-the-end-of-life-evidence-from-rural-wales/DA012D72A391978D3B98CF658492B412. Accessed on October 22, 2015.

Wenger, G. C., Davies, R., Shahtahmasebi, S., & Scott, A. (1996). Social isolation and loneliness in old age: Review and model refinement. *Ageing and Society*, *16*, 333–358.

Wenger, G. C., Scott, A., & Patterson, N. (2000). How important is parenthood? Childlessness and support in old age in England. *Ageing and Society*, *20*(2), 161–182.

Wikinson, S. (Ed.). (1998). *Feminist social psychologies: International perspectives*. Buckingham: Open University Press.

Woolf, V. (2004). *A room of one's own*. London: Penguin.

Young, M., & Wilmott, P. (1957). *Family and kinship in East London*. London: Routledge and Keegan Paul.

Chapter 8

Age Identity and Never-married Childless Older Women

Kate de Medeiros and Robert L. Rubinstein

Abstract

Although childless women comprise around 17% of women aged 65 and over in the US (Census Bureau, US, 2016) and up to 20% in other places in the world (Dykstra, 2009), the intersection of childlessness, female gender and old age has not been as widely explored as is necessary; older women have historically been and continue to be overlooked in feminist research compared to other groups of women (Browne, 1998; Ray, 1996; Twigg, 2004). Therefore, how childlessness affects identity and identity, childlessness in later life is not well understood. Our analysis considered: How do never-married, childless women identify themselves in terms of age? What are the key features of such an age identity? And, do these identities align with progress narratives or narratives of decline? For this chapter, interviews with 53 older women (22 African American, 31 White) aged 60 and over, who described themselves as never married and without biological children, were analysed. Questions were semi-structured and open-ended and covered background health information, a life story interview, questions about social networks, various forms of generativity and the sample's views about the future. Overall, these women negotiated their age identity not necessarily in relation to others (e.g. child, spouse) but in relation to themselves as social actors with an orientation towards the future – what will tomorrow bring? These forward-thinking narratives point to a new and important way to consider progress narratives and to rethink trajectories of the experience of aging.

Keywords: Age identity; childless; older women; never-married; progress narratives; feminist gerontology

Introduction

While there have been decades of feminist work addressing the unique aspects of childlessness and its effect on women's identity constructions and power relations, most of this work, with a few exceptions, has focused on girls or women in early or mid-life (Chodorow, 1978; Gilligan, 1982; Ruddick, 1980; Sorell & Montgomery, 2001). The focus of this chapter is therefore on how age identity can be understood in a group of never-married, childless older women. In 2016, 17% of women aged 45–50 were childless in the US and around 3 million women aged 65 and over were without children (Census Bureau, US, 2016). Yet, there is limited feminist work on childless older women – or on older women in general (Browne, 1998; Calasanti, Slevin, & King, 2006; Garner, 1999). This oversight has lead feminist gerontologists to equate the absence of aging women (and men) in current feminist scholarship to the absence of class, colour and other overlooked inequalities in second-wave feminism (Browne, 1998; Calasanti, 2004; Calasanti & Slevin, 2006; Macdonald & Rich, 1983; Ray, 1996; Twigg, 2004). For example, Davis (2008), in her work on the importance of intersectionality in feminist theory, writes, 'feminist journals are likely to reject articles that have not given sufficient attention to "race", class, and heteronormativity, along with gender' (p. 68). Age, however, is not included in this 'must-have' list. Rosenthal (2014) argues that '[i]t is time to round out the feminist agenda with issues of deep concern to women at midlife and beyond' and that 'research stops short of recognizing that these same core feminist issues continue to be concerns in the last third of women's lives' (pp. 1–2). To overlook age and the unique ways it affects power structures for women and men in various social categories is to overlook phenomena that affect a growing percentage of the population and another essential piece of inequity.

From the gerontology side, feminist perspectives are given little voice, especially in gerontology research journals. Although there was a spurt of interest in the late 1990s/early 2000s, truly feminist perspectives are rare in gerontology (Garner, 1999, 2014; Ray, 2003), save for the occasional book chapter in large edited volumes on gerontological theory. As ethicist Holstein (2015) notes, 'For a variety of reasons, old women, understood through feminist lenses, have not been well attended in gerontology or women's or gender studies' (p. 17). In reality, not only have feminist perspectives been missing, gender itself – regardless of perspective – is often either ignored entirely or controlled for statistically in gerontology research; there is little 'thick description' and also little 'thin description'. Consequently, gendered experiences and their implications for later life are not well addressed and many questions remain.

We note that there is a small literature on childlessness and aging. In addition, aside from Rubinstein's work in the late 1980s to early 1990s (Rubinstein, 1987; Rubinstein, Alexander, Goodman, & Luborsky, 1991), there have been few studies looking at childless older persons from non-deficit models (Black, Hannum, Rubinstein, & de Medeiros, 2014; de Medeiros, Rubinstein, Doyle, Rowles, & Bernard, 2013). Most papers that do address childlessness focus on negative aspects such as depression, loneliness and social isolation (Albertini & Mencarini, 2014; Aykan, 2003; Hansen, Slagsvold, & Moum, 2009; Rowland, 1998) rather than trying to understand the breadth of experiences – good or bad – and intergenerational relations of this group. Overall, this points to several levels or types of marginalisation: childless status, female, over age 65; and, for some, poor and/or minority status.

Older Age, Gender and Feminist Lenses

Older age and gender are critical points for consideration of childlessness for several reasons. Later life is greatly influenced by earlier experiences, expectations, opportunities and oppressions (Calasanti & Kiecolt, 2012). The culmination of women's unequal access to education, type of job and paid work across their life course, for example, means that many women, especially never-married women, have limited resources in retirement despite women's overall longevity compared to men (Calasanti & Slevin, 2001; Dannefer, 2003; Ferraro & Shippee, 2009). Also, adoption aside, most women know they will be childless years before they reach age 65, although this may not be true for men, who may believe they may have more time to become a parent. Further, a disparity in retirement is especially true for women from ethnic and racial minority groups (Dannefer, 2003; Ferraro & Shippee, 2009). With regard to longevity, life expectancy at birth for all women in the US in 2015 was 81.2 years compared to 76.4 years for men (He, Goodkind & Kowal, 2016). Euro-American women's (and men's) life expectancy was higher than for African American/Black women and men: 81.4 years for Euro-American women compared to 78.4 for African American women; 76.7 years for White men compared to 72.5 years for African American men (He et al., 2016). In the US, women, regardless of child status, comprise the majority of residents in nursing homes and assisted living facilities (around 75%), have higher poverty levels in people 65 and over (25.6%) than do men, 16.5%; (Aykan, 2003; OECD, 2015) and have much higher rates of living alone than men. Of the 12.5 million non-institutionalised persons over age 65 in the US living alone, 8.8 million were women; 46% of women aged 75 and over live alone (Aging, 2014). Although women live longer on average, they do so in poorer health and with fewer resources and supports.

Other oppressions include the caregiving roles that older women are assigned – as carers for their spouses and other family members, including grandchildren. The 'grandmother hypothesis', a theory from evolutionary biology, even suggests that the reason why women survive past their reproductive years is so that they can function as caregivers to younger children and thereby propagate the species (Alvarez, 2000; Hawkes, 2004; Von Hentig, 1946). Finally, ageism, or the systematic devaluation of people and their abilities (Butler, 1969; Jönson, 2013; Laws, 1995), has a potentially profound effect on older women in particular. Because, culturally, women's worth is linked to beauty while men's worth is linked to power, women suffer from ageist attitudes at a much younger chronological age than men (Laws, 1995; McHugh, 2003; Twigg, 2004; Woodward, 1999). These are all issues relevant to comparative gender identities and feminist lenses.

Intersectionality

Just as old age has been largely absent from feminist scholarship and, conversely, feminist scholarship from gerontology, so has intersectionality been missing from gerontological research. In addressing the lack of work on intersectionality within the social sciences – to include gerontology, Calasanti and King (2015) point to the willingness of researchers to discuss differences in demographic characteristics (e.g. age, gender, race and sexuality) but not to the interactions among systems of inequality. Calasanti and Kiecolt (2012) define systems of inequality as 'a relationship of privilege and oppression based on group membership' (p. 265). These often invisible systems are embedded within institutions such that enactments of oppression and privilege seem 'natural'. An example is women's informal care work, which has been viewed as 'natural' and has also been primarily examined through heterosexual, married women's experiences (Zajicek, Calasanti, Ginther, & Summers, 2006). It is therefore important to carefully consider how complex systems and multiple oppressions and privileges operate in the context of age identity to include assumptions about 'motherhood status'; lifetime access to opportunities to include marriage and paid labour; ageism; and others.

Age Identity

As mentioned earlier, the focus of this chapter is on how age identity can be understood in a group of never married, childless older women. We focus on the never married since most identity work in aging has looked to age identity relative to one's position to children and/or spouses and through one's role (e.g. grandparent.) Graham, Sorell, and Montgomery (2004) define identity as 'the conscious awareness of knowing who one is' (p. 253) through components of identity that may include ego identity, social identity and personal identity. Age identity has been described as the subjective experience of the age one feels, regardless of chronological age. An underlying component of age identity is that the meaning of age itself is a cultural construction whereby one internalises and activates the performance of age based on cultural expectations (e.g. What should a 65-year-old woman wear?), which bears many similarities to gender performance (Butler, 1986; Calasanti & Slevin, 2001; Hazan & Raz, 1997; Twigg, 2004).

Several researchers have linked 'role' identity with age identity. For example Kaufman and Elder (2002) suggest that

> people feel old at different ages, and this difference stems from the idea that individuals' perceptions of themselves are based not only on what age society defines as 'old' but also on what is happening in their life course. (p. 170)

Kaufman and Elder (2003) also explored age identity in grandparents specifically. They write,

> Being a grandmother has been found to be an important factor in age identity. While being a parent and grandparent are important in themselves, the number and ages of children and grandchildren have also been found to have an effect on age identity. (Kaufman & Elder, 2003, p. 271)

They also cite other researchers who suggest that having older children and grandchildren is associated with an older age identity since people gauge their own age in relation to others in their immediate family. Age identity has therefore been described as 'relational' as people tend to understand their own age in comparison to others (e.g. children, spouses). We were interested in moving beyond pronatalist assumptions.

Many informants in the study discussed here said they never felt old until they got a chronic illness in old age. For many of these informants, 'traditional' life course transitions such as 'age at first marriage' or 'age when first child was born' were deeply rooted in pronatalist and heteronormative assumptions, in which they lacked children or spouses. Rubinstein et al. (1991) did explore key relationships in a sample of never-married childless older women with an interest in how these women identified themselves within social and familial networks. Although the focus of their work was not on age identity specifically, their findings do suggest that relationships play a role in how people derive a sense of self and identity, albeit more from a social perspective in this case (e.g. what is my place in the larger societal structure?) than in an age identity one (e.g. how do I define my age roles based on my perceptions of my friends' and family members' age roles?).

In our discussion of age identity, we argue that what is missing, besides a focus on childless older persons, is the idea that identity is not singular or unified or simply the sum of the three parts (i.e. ego, social relationships with others, social roles). Instead, people experience multiple identities, some of which may be actively managed by the individual and some which are externally imposed on the person by the larger socio-cultural context (de Medeiros, 2005; Ewing, 1990). For example, in the case of age, a 70-year-old woman might assume the identity of someone who has a lot to offer. She may be identified, however, as someone who is no longer of value (de Medeiros, 2005). Similar arguments could be made for other cultural categorisations such as race, ethnicity, gender, sexual orientation, socio-economic status and so on. Recognising the multiple ways that identity can be experienced and conferred is therefore important.

Cultural Narratives and Ageing

If identities are created through complex layering of internal and external expectations and judgements, it is important to consider how age identities are grounded in larger external cultural narratives as well as internally established life histories. Gullette (2004) introduced the idea of the progress narrative in resistance to scripts of decline in older age, arguing that interpreting the events in one's life as part of a continuum rather than as a decline after 'peaking' in middle age, can be a source of strength and continued growth in later life. In addition, narratives of progress and decline can be found in age autobiographies, stories which compose part of one's age identity. Gullette asks:

> How do the subjects of a particular culture come up with narratives of aging – comprehensible stories, prospective and retrospective, about moving through all the given ages of life? These supply meanings of what other people normally call aging, which age critics investigate as being aged by culture. These stories have intensely personal aspects, but the narratives are comprehensible because they are tied to shared, dominant models of 'the way aging really goes'. (p. 102)

She goes on to argue that it is the cultural value that a given society places on how various life stages are experienced that contribute to the age autobiography. The master culture narrative for most, internally and externally, is one of decline, especially one's own decline in relation to those of another. In opposition to the narrative of decline, of aging as a downward trajectory, is the *progress narrative* whereby old age presents new opportunities for growth; a new door that has opened.

We therefore consider: How do never-married, childless women identify themselves in terms of age? What are the key features of age identity for them? And do these identities align with progress narratives or narratives of decline? The importance of these questions to feminist perspectives lies in the lack of knowledge due to the omission of work on childless older women. As Dykstra (2009) writes, 'By focusing on individuals who do not make the transition to parenthood, one gains insight into mechanisms that produce social inequality and social cohesion, insofar they are linked with parenthood' (p. 681). This is certainly true for age identity as well.

Methods

Our current sample was drawn from a larger, four-year qualitative study of 180 women (90 African American/Black women and 90 Euro-

American/White women aged 65 and over, living in the mid-Atlantic region of the US, who described themselves as 'childless'[1] (see Rubinstein, Girling, de Medeiros, Brazda, and Hannum (2015)[2] for a description of the original study and methods). Women were asked to participate in three one-on-one oral interviews at a place of their choice, usually in their homes. The same interviewer conducted all three interviewers, once a week for three consecutive weeks. Each interview lasted from 1 to 2 hours giving us around 3–6 hours' worth of interview data for each participant. All interviewers were female to facilitate discussions about and sensitivity towards sexuality and reproduction that might otherwise be uncomfortable for some women to discuss with male interviewers or that men may not be aware enough of to ask (e.g. the emotional meaning of menstruation and questions about pregnancy).

The interviews were semi-structured. Rather than ask each woman the same questions, the goal of the interviews was to guide discussion around some key concepts: the life story, types of generativity, views towards childlessness and views towards the future. Therefore, specific questions were omitted if the interviewer felt that, in the course of the interview, the subject was sufficiently addressed. While the interviewer asked follow-up questions for clarity, she gave primary control of the interview to participant, allowing participants to talk at length on topics that were salient to them. Interviews were transcribed verbatim and checked for accuracy by the interviewer against the original recording. ATLAS.ti was used to manage the data and facilitate analysis.

From the larger sample, we focused on the women who described themselves as never married to explore age identity. We selected never married women to better understand whether comparison to others was common relative to discussions on how one 'knew' her age. Since same-sex marriage was not legal at the time the women were interviewed, we recognise that some women in our study may have been in long-term partnered relationships. We did not provide any definitions for what 'never married' meant and allowed women to identity their own marital status. We did not ask about sexual orientation for several reasons that include lack of relevance to our original research questions and the fact that due to long-held societal biases and dangerous discrimination tactics against lesbian/bisexual/gay/transgender/queer women, women of

[1]A few women either had biological children who had died or had step-children. If a woman considered herself childless, she was enrolled in the study.

[2]Sponsored by a grant from the National Institute of Aging, 1-R01-AG03061-01A1.

this cohort who identified themselves as other than heterosexual female might be unlikely to talk with us about their experiences.

Data Analysis

Analytic Strategy for the Master Study

Thematic coding for transcripts was accomplished in three basic stages. In Stage 1, initial codes were constructed using theoretical concepts (e.g. biological generativity, relational generativity) and anticipated themes addressed in the project's funding proposal. The codebook was tested using a team coding process in which all members of the research team used the codebook to code the same set of transcripts. Performance of existing codes was discussed at subsequent team meetings and modifications made to the codebook (additions, deletions, changes to definitions) based on team consensus. This method was repeated until the team reached consensus that the codebook had been sufficiently refined into the largest blocks of thematic units possible. In Stage 2, the codebook was further tested by splitting the team into pairs of coders who independently coded and reconciled sets of transcripts. This allowed the codes to be tested on a much larger selection of transcripts and to potentially reveal any omissions or discrepancies. As in Stage 1, codebook performance was discussed at team meetings and changes decided by group consensus. Reliability was established when pairs were able to independently code transcripts with close agreement, determined during code reconciliation. In Stage 3, individual coders used the final codebook to code 80% of the remaining interviews. Every fifth interview (20% of the total sample) was team coded to ensure uniformity of coding throughout the study.

Analytic Strategy for the Subsample

All in all, 53 women (22 African American women, 23 White women) were in our subsample for this chapter. The mean age in years for the subsample was 75.8 years (standard deviation of $\pm$8.4). The mean age for the African American/Black participants was 77 years and 75 years for White participants. To make sense of the subsample interviews in light of our current focus on age identity, categories were developed by examining data for answers to several questions: What do the data say about informants' ideas on self-identity? What do the data say about decline versus progress? Through the use of the ATLAS.ti software, excerpts for the codes 'accomplishments', 'age', and 'self-statements' were pulled for all women in the subsample and read for any reference to age as a type of referential marker beyond chronology. These include statements such as 'I don't know how I got to be this age' or 'I don't feel as old as I am'. In addition, ATLAS.ti allows the researcher to view the coded excerpt within the larger transcript. Therefore, if the excerpt seemed particularly rich, we were able to return to the transcript and reread it to see if any additional linkages to age identity appeared. We note that since we included large chunks of text in our initial coding strategy versus short excerpts, we were able to reread the extracted codes within the larger context of the interview.

Results

In rereading the 53 transcripts for the purpose of writing this chapter, the first author was able to develop analytical categories in relation to the notion of age self-identity that successfully categorised the informants as well offered a new way of looking at their narrative content in relationship to decline versus progress narratives. Based on the method described in the previous section, we came up with three categories about these topics. (1) ways of knowing age; (2) accomplishments; and (3) current and future roles through work. Rather than existing as discrete categories *per se*, these three connect to a type of flow within person's perceived place within her larger life course trajectory (the present, upward trajectory, downward trajectory). Each is discussed below.

Ways of Knowing Age

This category includes talk by the participants that specifically discussed how they *externally* confirmed their age through things such as the actions of others, or comparisons to others (or themselves in age stages over time). For example, Ms. Adams, a Euro-American woman, told the interviewer during the first of three interviews:

> I know physically because my body tells me that I'm 66 years old but I don't think of myself as that age. You know, like I look at that gathering we had on the Fourth

> of July and think, 'How did we get this old?' Which realistically, I know we are and I feel it and I see it in my friends, sometimes it's a little disconcerting. My friend and I will go someplace together and, like maybe to the movies or something, and the movie person doesn't even ask us if we're seniors or not and I think to myself, you know, it shows. I feel it.

Ms. Adams is reminded of her age by what she sees in her friends and how others treat her. Having the person at the movie assume she meets the criteria for a 'senior' discount reinforces age. She is externally identified as 'older' although she also mentions that internally, she feels '66'. She said in a later interview, 'So, that's been a realization, probably within the last five years I think, that I have to remind myself of my age and my physical limitations with some things'. Unlike the earlier interview, she suggests here that she has to remind herself of her age, which also suggests that she is trying to maintain an age identity that corresponds with how others are treating her. This further suggests the notions of an age identity *balance*, when identity inside and outside in most ways match. This, then also suggests that a focus on the present day includes both narratives of decline and progress (or a continuum.)

Another participant, Ms. Smith, a 78-year-old woman who described herself as 'black', spoke about looking at pictures of herself over time to gauge her age. She said:

> I got pictures in albums but I don't think anybody would look at the albums. They're just pictures of, mostly, mostly pictures of me (chuckle) … It's pictures of me when I was in my 20s, pictures of me when I was in my 40s, 50s, 60s, and 70s … And the pictures of my parents.

Here she suggests that part of her age identity is rooted in her own appearance of age, that to know her age is to look at her age through photos over time, even comparing her own aging to her parents. Her focus on the present involves a constant comparison of different pasts. It is unclear whether she views these pasts as decline or progress.

In a slightly different way, Ms. Phillips, a 71-year-old Euro-American woman, explained her own disconnect from time. She said,

> We had a resident [at her retirement community] who died a few months ago, age 96, and somebody said her daughter was coming to see her. And it took me a while to

> register that I shouldn't be looking for a young person. When I saw her daughter in the front lobby, I thought, 'If you're 96, your daughter is not 30'.

Although this observation doesn't apply to her own aging, it does suggest that generationally, she was looking for someone within a certain age category who would have the role of 'daughter', even though that age category (i.e. 30) was not correct. Her 'way of knowing' was therefore linked to her realisation that she was not immediately aware of the passage of time in terms of family structure. The term 'daughter', for example, initially brought up an image of 'younger person' in her mind until, through further thought, she was able to realise that the daughter in this case would likely be in her 60s. Ms. Phillips came to know age relationally through another member of her community.

A 79-year-old African American woman, Ms. Johnson, told the interviewer, 'See, I don't go by chronological age. I say chronological age has nothing to do with how old you are. It's what you do and how you think of yourself'. She then went on to describe some trips she was going to be taking and compared herself to another woman at her retirement community. She said, 'This little old lady, she's two years younger than me. People thought she was my mother'. Like the previous participant, Ms. Johnson uses a familial, relational comparison (mother–daughter). However, as Ms. Phillips points out, she is actually two years older than the person people thought was her mother. Given that there is generally an age difference of around a 20 years or so between mothers and daughters, Ms. Phillips' observation suggests that she positions her own experienced age as being much younger than the younger person in her retirement community. Hers is a progress narrative in that she describes herself in terms of a positive progression especially when compared to others, who she uses a decline narrative in contrast to her own aging.

Finally, Ms. Roberts, a 73-year-old African American was asked what she thought her life would be like in five years. She said:

> I hope I make it. Let's see, I'm 73 now. I'll be 77 years old. I hope I make it and I just thank the Lord above that I'm still here. It's the only thing I can say.

When the interviewer asked about 10 years in the future, she responded:

> I haven't thought that far ahead (chuckle). I haven't thought that far – really I was thinking just the other day,

> one of the friends here, we're just talking in general, and I said when I was young, like my 20s and 30s, I never thought I'd live to be the age I am now, 73 years old. And they say the same thing. And now that I am, I'm proud. I'm very proud to be my age. And if I do live ten years from now I'll be prouder than what I am now, you know, because thank God, like I say, my dad lived to be 91 and that was beautiful. I didn't know I was going to have him that long, you know? So I haven't thought ten years [ahead], though. [Laughter] Not yet. But if I live five years from now, I think that would be beautiful. I'll be proud and happy to be the age I am.

From this passage, age identity doesn't seem to play a salient part in her life. However, the interviewer asked her to comment on her present and her future. In this case, Ms. Roberts uses her father as a reference point. Her way of knowing age is related to her father's experience of living until 91 years, which she describes as beautiful. Like Ms. Phillips, Ms. Roberts' narrative is also one of progress.

Accomplishments

In response to the question, 'What would you say were your biggest accomplishments?', Ms. Conrad, an 80-year-old Euro-American woman, laughed and responded:

> Well, first the move [into the retirement community where she lived] which actually was, it will be five years ago this July. Just, uh, the ability to find [the community], to make, as a single woman, to make all the arrangements, to sell the apartments, to downsize, to move, to call on friends, two of whom were marvellous .... So, um, you know, just pulling it together to do that kind of thing.

This informant is clearly able to identify some activities as accomplishments and appears quite proud of her demonstrated competence in pulling it all together. Her reference to the period five years earlier, when she was around 75, does not suggest any type of decline but instead stresses her abilities.

Ms. Jenkins, a 78-year-old African American woman, in talking about her biggest accomplishments, said, 'It was important that

I finished high school, that I advanced in my workplace because I started out being a maid and a kitchen worker and then I advanced to being a dental assistant and then a dental office manager. So I think that was a great accomplishment and I'm very proud of that'. She had been retired for 10 years at the time of her interview, but said that she used the time to travel and read, which she enjoyed. For her, retirement was a time of exploring parts of her interests that she was unable to do at earlier points in life because of time and money constraints.

Ms. Mandley, a 64-year-old African American woman, was asked to describe her biggest accomplishments in the last five years. She said:

> In my lifetime, oh, Hell, oh, excuse me. Uh, (pause) last five years. Well, I guess, nothing big, just being able to continue to work and to enjoy life I guess, I mean. Nothing super-duper, you know, and being able to continue being physically active I guess, that's a major accomplishment, you know.

The word 'continue' is aligned with Gullette's notion of 'progress'. When asked about accomplishments in her life as a whole, she said:

> Hum, my life has not been that exciting (chuckle). Well, I guess, you know, finishing college. I did end up getting a Master's, that was a struggle, a Master's Degree, and, um, hum, and I guess just having the ability to work and to get out and meet folks, you know, and staying as healthy as I can these days, you know, it's a challenge. So and then dealing with, you know, maybe financial challenges or, you know, unemployed or being laid off, just coming through all those things and I guess keeping the faith and knowing that I'll get through it and pick up something else and keep going, you know what I mean? Moving forward. But nothing spectacular, you know what I mean?

In answering this question, this informant traces the entire history of her work and school life, seeming to indicate that her entire life was a struggle of sorts, in which she overcame, bringing her to the present day. The idea of 'moving forward' is a strong theme in her interview, which again speaks to the idea of progressing through life rather than peaking at middle age and experiencing decline thereafter.

Current and Future Roles in through Work

Unlike the previous category, 'accomplishments', current and future roles speak directly to identities that women claimed with regards to work. For example, Ms. Lind, a childless, never-married woman, is an Episcopal priest who retired from her congregation, but continues to work for a local funeral home, officiating funeral services for people who request a religious service but are not affiliated with any particular church or denomination. Her overarching narrative is one of progress: of overcoming challenges in the 1970s with ordination of women in the Episcopal Church. She talked at length about how the struggle to change women's roles in the church from 'nun' to 'priest' was difficult, costing her many friendships and associations. However, she eventually persevered, was ordained a priest, and found a congregation willing to have her. Through this experience, she developed a strong awareness of labels and their power. She therefore talked about the importance of laying claim to labels and experiences as a way of destigmatising them.

For example, she described her experience with a group of lesbian parents that called themselves 'Tykes and Dykes'. She said:

> I knew a couple of people who belonged. They said, 'our children are going to hear people call us dykes and if they associate it with a nice group that goes to the park and has ice cream, we're Okay'. I think the same thing about age. I hate the thought of 'golden years' vocabulary. I've got my own fight with the administration around here who have gone all squishy about the term 'assisted living'. The assisted living unit is now known as Fountain View. Which is, I'm sorry, it sounds like the name of a burial plot. I'm not supposed to say, 'Oh, you're looking for Betty?' She's in assisted living. I'm supposed to say, 'Betty is in Fountain View'... as if it were shameful.

Her resistance to labels, including labels associated with aging, suggests a resistance to the scripts of decline or living out one's life in later life without an opportunity for purpose or to contribute. Instead, she uses words of empowerment such as 'fight', which suggests forward moving action rather than acceptance.

Another woman, Ms. Taylor (an 80-year-old Euro-American woman) said:

> I'm still teaching. Now it's part-time, but I mean now they are 14, you know 14-week courses. But they're non-credit, no tests in my class, just the test is for me to put it together. And this summer is a new *course*.

In a similar way, Ms. Fields, a 64-year-old African American woman also talked about the importance of working. She said, 'People ask me now, when are you going to retire? When are you going to retire? And, I say, "I don't know. Retire for what?"' She adds:

> I like what I do still and it gives me an opportunity to travel so I can go and see different parts of the country. And I like meeting people and interacting with people and, you know, and laughing with people and having fun, so why retire?

In this example, Ms. Fields equates retirement with a type of decline. She suggests that retirement means withdrawing from people and opportunities, or a type of giving up. Instead, she intends to move forward, to continue her work and pursue her interests. Like the other two women, her trajectory isn't downward but rather upward as she continues to seek out new opportunities.

Discussion

Earlier, we posed the questions: How do never-married, childless women identify themselves in terms of age? What are the key features of age identity for them? And do these identities align with progress narratives or narratives of decline? As our findings suggest, age is dictated, relational, and fluid as well as external and internal to the self. As such, it is a master symbol in society, thick with meaning. It reflects and refracts other social and cultural concerns while enrobing the person with meanings, all derived from culture, which surround the person, are internalised by her, and are externally projected. Age identity is both solid (one cannot get away from how old others think you are) and fluid (most people don't feel their age and it is not germane to that much). While a large body of work has suggested that people generally report being chronologically older than they feel (Keyes & Westerhof, 2012; Westerhof, Whitbourne, & Freeman, 2012), much of that work linked subjective age to health status or to a role within the heteronormative family (Kaufman & Elder, 2002, 2003).

For the women in our sample, age identity did not appear to be that important to how they identified themselves. In other words, they might recognise that they are of a certain age category when certain social situations arose, such as the woman who said she had to remind herself of her age from time to time, but they did not appear to make age a central characteristic. That age was not central to the everyday self is an important insight since much of the literature on age identity does assume certain role transitions nested in parenting and the heteronormative family. Challenging what is 'normative' with regards to older age and reconsidering how age identity is negotiated and experienced in groups such as childless older people could provide new perspectives on how people experience age.

The other categories, 'accomplishments' and 'current and future roles through work', suggested that these older women were forward-thinking (using an overarching progress narrative, not a narrative of decline). Most resisted or never entertained narratives of decline. This is related to age-identity negotiation. Although societally, negative age identities might be placed on certain women (e.g. childless and never-married equates to lonely and depressed), these women suggested they had power and control over their lives and were less burdened by demoing relationships. Further, while none had children, many were engaged in generative relationships with younger people in their lives. In keeping with the idea of progress narratives and narratives of decline, this shows resistance to the stereotypical image of older women who are either functioning in the role of grandmother, debilitated due to illness or otherwise declining.

This idea of strength and forward progression relates to an observation of Browne (1998), that:

> unknowingly, the strengths of older women are neglected if conceptualization of power and empowerment is one of domination and control, as opposed to capacity and relatedness … feminist conceptualizations of empowerment often begin with social relatedness, energy, capacity, and an emphasis on community good. (p. 216)

Lacking children of their own, we found that the women in our sample did not look back that often, did not dwell on the past, had engaged lives, looked forward to the next day, and supplemented whatever sense of loss they might have had in being childless with relationships of significance with peers, nieces and nephews, younger students and younger people they mentored.

As gerontology and feminist scholarship move forward, both would benefit from understanding age as a critical site for knowledge. By omitting older women from many inquiries from the meaning of later life to skewed and oppressive power structures, both areas of studies are missing out on potentially rich perspectives. As the women in our sample have strongly suggested, advancing age can be a source of great power and ability if there can be a shift away from how old age 'looks' to how old age 'feels'. Several women mentioned comparing images of their younger selves to the present to try to discern in a way what age they were supposed to be. It was as if they were figuratively studying a script to better understand what they *should* do and feel, which was often in contrast to how they viewed themselves. Overall, by exploring the possibility of the progress narrative as a counter narrative to cultural stories of decline, both gerontology and feminist studies can have much to offer women and men in later life.

Acknowledgements

We would like to thank the National Institute on Aging for supporting this research (1-R01-AG03061-01A1). We would also like to thank all of the women who shared their stories and experiences with us.

References

Administration on Aging. (2014). *Aging statistics*. Washington, DC. Retrieved from http://www.aoa.gov/Aging_Statistics/

Albertini, M., & Mencarini, L. (2014). Childlessness and support networks in later life: New pressures on familistic welfare states? *Journal of Family Issues*, *35*(3), 331–357.

Alvarez, H. P. (2000). Grandmother hypothesis and primate life histories. *American Journal of Physical Anthropology*, *113*(3), 435–450.

Aykan, H. (2003). Effect of childlessness on nursing home and home health care use. *Journal of Aging & Social Policy*, *15*(1), 33–53.

Black, H. K., Hannum, S. M., Rubinstein, R. L., & de Medeiros, K. (2014). Generativity in elderly oblate sisters of providence. *The Gerontologist*, doi:10.1093/geront/gnu091

Browne, C. (1998). *Women, feminism, and aging*. New York, NY: Springer.

Butler, J. (1986). Sex and gender in Simone de Beauvoir's second sex. *Yale French Studies*, (72), 35–49.

Butler, R. N. (1969). Age-ism: Another form of bigotry. *The Gerontologist, 9*(4 Part1), 243–246. doi:10.1093/geront/9.4_Part_1.243

Calasanti, T. (2004). Feminist gerontology and old men. *The Journals of Gerontology Series B: Psychological Sciences and Social Sciences, 59*(6), S305–S314. Retrieved from http://psychsocgerontology.oxfordjournals.org/content/59/6/S305.full.pdf

Calasanti, T., & Kiecolt, K. J. (2012). Intersectionality and aging families. *Handbook of families and aging*, (2nd ed., pp. 263–286). Santa Barbara, CA: Praeger.

Calasanti, T., & King, N. (2015). Intersectionality and age. *Routledge handbook of cultural gerontology* (pp. 193–200). London: Routledge.

Calasanti, T. M., & Slevin, K. F. (2001). *Gender, social inequalites, and aging.* Lanham, MD: Alta Mira Press.

Calasanti, T. M., & Slevin, K. F. (Eds.). (2006). *Age matters: Realigning feminist thinking*. Abingdon: Taylor & Francis.

Calasanti, T. M., Slevin, K. F., & King, N. (2006). Ageism and feminism: From 'et cetera' to center. *NWSA Journal, 18*(1), 13–30.

Census Bureau, US. (2016). Fertility of women in the United States: 2016. Retrieved from https://www.census.gov/data/tables/2016/demo/fertility/women-fertility.html

Chodorow, N. (1978). *The reproduction of mothering*. Berkeley, CA: University of California Press.

Dannefer, D. (2003). Cumulative advantage/disadvantage and the life course: Cross-fertilizing age and social science theory. *The Journals of Gerontology Series B: Psychological Sciences and Social Sciences, 58*(6), S327–S337.

Davis, K. (2008). Intersectionality as buzzword: A sociology of science perspective on what makes a feminist theory successful. *Feminist Theory, 9*(1), 67–85.

de Medeiros, K. (2005). The complementary self: Multiple perspectives on the aging person. *Journal of Aging Studies, 19*(1), 1–13. doi:10.1016/j.jaging.2004.02.001

de Medeiros, K., Rubinstein, R. L., Doyle, P., Rowles, G., & Bernard, M. (2013). 'A place of one's own': Reinterpreting the meaning of home among childless older women. In G. Rowles & M. Bernard (Eds.), *Environmental gerontology: Making meaning places in old age* (pp. 79–104). New York, NY: Springer.

Dykstra, P. A. (2009). Childless old age. In P. Uhlenberg (Ed.), *International handbook of population aging* (pp. 671–690). New York, NY: Springer.

Ewing, K. P. (1990). The illusion of wholeness: Culture, self and the experience of inconsistency. *Ethos, 18*(3), 251–278.

Ferraro, K. F., & Shippee, T. P. (2009). Aging and cumulative inequality: How does inequality get under the skin? *The Gerontologist, 49*(3), 333–343.

Garner, J. D. (1999). Feminism and feminist gerontology. *Journal of Women & Aging, 11*(2–3), 3–12.

Garner, J. D. (2014). *Fundamentals of feminist gerontology*. New York, NY: Routledge.

Gilligan, C. (1982). *In a different voice*. Cambridge, MA: Harvard University Press.

Graham, C. W., Sorell, G. T., & Montgomery, M. J. (2004). Role-related identity structure in adult women. *Identity, 4*(3), 251–271.

Gullette, M. M. (2004). *Aged by culture*. Chicago, IL: University of Chicago Press.

Hansen, T., Slagsvold, B., & Moum, T. (2009). Childlessness and psychological well-being in midlife and old age: An examination of parental status effects across a range of outcomes. *Social Indicators Research*, *94*(2), 343–362.

Hawkes, K. (2004). Human longevity: The grandmother effect. *Nature*, *428*(6979), 128–129.

Hazan, H., & Raz, A. E. (1997). The authorized self: How middle age defines old age in the postmodern. *Semiotica*, *113*(3–4), 257–276.

He, W., Goodkind, D., & Kowal, P. (2016). *US Census Bureau, international population reports*. P95/16-1, An Aging World: 2015.

Holstein, M. (2015). *Women in late life: Critical perspectives on gender and age*. New York, NY: Rowman & Littlefield.

Jönson, H. (2013). We will be different! Ageism and the temporal construction of old age. *The Gerontologist*, *53*(2), 198–204. doi:10.1093/geront/gns066

Kaufman, G., & Elder, G. H. (2002). Revisiting age identity: A research note. *Journal of Aging Studies*, *16*(2), 169–176.

Kaufman, G., & Elder, G. H. Jr (2003). Grandparenting and age identity. *Journal of Aging Studies*, *17*(3), 269–282. doi:10.1016/S0890-4065(03)00030-6

Keyes, C. L. M., & Westerhof, G. J. (2012). Chronological and subjective age differences in flourishing mental health and major depressive episode. *Aging & Mental Health*, *16*(1), 67–74.

Laws, G. (1995). Understanding ageism: Lessons from feminism and postmodernism. *The Gerontologist*, *35*(1), 112–118. doi:10.1093/geront/35.1.112

Macdonald, B., & Rich, C. (1983). *Look me in the eye: Old women, aging and ageism*. Tallahasee, FL: Spinsters Ink.

McHugh, K. E. (2003). Three faces of ageism: Society, image and place. *Ageing and Society*, *23*(02), 165–185.

OECD. (2015). *Pensions at a glance 2015*. OECD Publishing.

Ray, R. E. (1996). A postmodern perspective on feminist gerontology. *The Gerontologist*, *36*(5), 674–680.

Ray, R. E. (2003). The uninvited guest: Mother/daughter conflict in feminist gerontology. *Journal of Aging Studies*, *17*(1), 113–128.

Rosenthal, E. R. (2014). *Women, aging, and ageism*. London: Routledge.

Rowland, D. (1998). Consequences of childlessness in later life. *Australian Journal on Ageing*, *17*(1), 24–28.

Rubinstein, R. L. (1987). Childless elderly: Theoretical perspectives and practical concerns. *Journal of Cross-Cultural Gerontology*, *2*(1), 1–14.

Rubinstein, R. L., Alexander, B. B., Goodman, M., & Luborsky, M. (1991). Key relationships of never married, childless older women: A cultural analysis. *Journal of Gerontology*, *46*(5), S270–S277.

Rubinstein, R. L., Girling, L. M., de Medeiros, K., Brazda, M., & Hannum, S. (2015). Extending the framework of generativity theory through research: A qualitative study. *The Gerontologist*, *55*(4), 548–558. doi:10.1093/geront/gnu009

Ruddick, S. (1980). Maternal thinking. *Feminist Studies*, *6*(2), 342–367.

Sorell, G. T., & Montgomery, M. J. (2001). Feminist perspectives on Erikson's theory: Their relevance for contemporary identity development research. *Identity: An International Journal of Theory and Research*, *1*(2), 97–128.

Twigg, J. (2004). The body, gender, and age: Feminist insights in social gerontology. *Journal of Aging Studies*, *18*(1), 59–73.

Von Hentig, H. (1946). The sociological function of the grandmother. *Social Forces*, *24*(4), 389–392.

Westerhof, G. J., Whitbourne, S. K., & Freeman, G. P. (2012). The aging self in a cultural context: The relation of conceptions of aging to identity processes and self-esteem in the United States and the Netherlands. *The Journals of Gerontology Series B: Psychological Sciences and Social Sciences*, *67B*(1), 52–60. doi:10.1093/geronb/gbr075

Woodward, K. M. (1999). *Figuring age: Women, bodies, generations* (Vol. 23). Bloomington, IN: Indiana University Press.

Zajicek, A., Calasanti, T., Ginther, C., & Summers, J. (2006). Intersectionality and age relations. Unpaid care work and Chicanas. In: T. M. Calasanti & K. F. Slevin (Eds.), *Age matters: Re-aligning feminist thinking* (pp. 175–198). New York, NY: Routledge.

SECTION IV
LIVED EXPERIENCES OF CHILDLESSNESS

Chapter 9

The Intentionally Childless Marriage

Laura Carroll

Abstract

This essay examines the lives of opposite-gender, cisgender, heterosexual married couples who have no children by choice, why the intentionally childless marriage lacks acceptance in society, and what is necessary for full societal acceptance. It discusses how intentionally childless married couples make the decision to have no children; the nature of their married lives and what a fulfilling marriage means to these couples; how these married couples are misperceived, stereotyped and why; the social and cultural pressures these couples face as well as ways they can address this issue in their personal and professional relationships; the research debate on whether marriages with children or without are happier; and the lives of these married couples in their elder years. In addition to relevant feminist theory, it discusses pronatalism as a powerful influence on why intentionally childless marriages remain judged and criticised. It looks at the societal progress that has been made to accept this kind of marriage, makes recommendations on what it will take for it to be accepted in society, and what today's men and women can do to further promote its acceptance. The essay draws on: (1) research for *Families of Two: Interviews with Happily Married Couples Without Children by Choice* (2000) which included interviews with 100 happily married opposite-gender, cisgender, heterosexual couples across the United States and in-depth interviews with 40 of them who span a wide range of ages and lifestyles; (2) relevant research discussed in *The Baby Matrix: Why Freeing Our Minds From Outmoded Thinking About Parenthood & Reproduction Will Create a Better World* (2012); (3) grounded theory qualitative data collection since the year 2000; and (4) recent research literature in this area of study.

Keywords: Marriage; couples; pronatalism; childfree; relationships; childless

The Intentionally Childless Marriage

In the late 1990s, I searched for a book on happily married couples who did not have children by choice. At the time, I had been happily married for 10 years, had no children by choice and wanted to learn more about opposite-gender, cisgender, heterosexual couples who had been married a long time and had made the same choice. Not finding such a book inspired the interview research for and publication of *Families of Two: Interviews with Happily Married Couples Without Children by Choice* (2000). For it, I interviewed 100 intentionally childless married couples in the United States and conducted in-depth interviews with 40 of them. Interviews and photos of 15 couples who best represented all of the interviews were selected for publication. Subsequent study led to the development of *The Baby Matrix: Why Freeing Our Minds From Outmoded Thinking About Parenthood & Reproduction Will Create a Better World* (2012), which in part examines why society finds the choice not to have children difficult to accept, and discusses research on intentionally childless marriages. Since the year 2000, I have also utilised grounded theory qualitative methodology to continue researching opposite-gender, cisgender, heterosexual married couples, primarily in the United States, who have no children by choice. Data collection has included online surveys and, as of this writing, over 5,000 electronic interviews and communications with married men and women with no children by choice. Findings discussed in this chapter draw from these sources of research.

The literature has historically termed those who choose not to have children as the 'voluntary childless'. This chapter instead uses the alternative term 'intentionally childless' to describe married couples. As Morell describes in *Unwomanly Conduct: The Challenges of Intentional Childlessness* (1994), the word 'intentional' more clearly denotes intent of action. In intentionally childless marriages, the choice not to bring parenthood into the marital relationship is a deliberate and purposeful act.

In the course of history, intentionally childless marriages are a recent phenomenon. For generations, childbearing came with marriage. In the United States, important social and legal events of the twentieth century influenced a shift in the historical connection between marriage and having children. Key court rulings related to contraception played a central role. In 1936, *United States v. One Package* opened the door for the medical community to begin distributing contraceptives. In 1965, the landmark Supreme Court case, *Griswold v. Connecticut*, ruled that a state's ban on the use of contraceptives violated the right to marital privacy. With regard to intercourse and reproduction, rulings like these put individual reproductive rights first and made it legally legitimate for marriage not to be inextricably connected to having children (Carroll, 2012a).

With the rise of feminism and the women's rights agenda in the 1960s, Betty Friedan's groundbreaking book, *The Feminist Mystique* (1963), spurred society to question the ingrained belief that becoming wives and mothers formed women's identities and gave them true fulfilment in life. These times inspired women to explore their fuller selves, including looking beyond the idea that marriage and having children must go hand in hand. With the advent of the pill in particular, couples could control childbearing. More women worked outside the home and began to realise there was more to marriage than motherhood. As women's identities expanded, many women saw how parenthood did not need to be the core of their marital union. They began to realise that it was possible for parenthood not be a part of their union at all. In this time of empowerment, men and women were marrying first and foremost for love.

With social and cultural developments like these, one might predict that decades later society would see more marriages with no children by choice. One might also expect that we would see societal acceptance of this kind of marriage. There are many reasons why this has not been the case.

Why Intentionally Childless Marriages Lack Societal Acceptance

Intentionally childless marriages continue to live outside the norm. According to the US Census Bureau, in 2014, 10% of ever-married women ages 40–44 had no children, and 11% of ever-married women ages 45–50 had no children. The 2014 census numbers do not differentiate between ever-married women with no children by choice and ever-married women who want(ed) children but do not have them. The 2014 census numbers and those before it do not track these kinds of statistics for men. Yet, since intentionally childless women are a subset of the ever-married numbers the census does track, it is clear that the numbers of intentionally childless married couples fall into the minority as well.

Long-held social and cultural reasons have prevented society's acceptance of intentionally childless marriages. The reasons relate to a set of beliefs that goes back many generations called pronatalism. The trailblazing book on the topic, *Pronatalism: The Myth of Mom & Apple*

Pie, defines pronatalism as '… an attitude or policy that is pro-birth, that encourages reproduction, that exalts the role of parenthood' (Peck & Senderowitz, 1974, p. 2).

From as far back as the time of Augustus' Laws, parenthood was promoted to ensure a country's survival and increase its power (Carroll, 2012a). During times of rural settlements, having many children was also important to family survival. However, in times past, for women in particular, having children came with physical risks. According to sociologist E. E. Le Masters, when a social role carries risk or is difficult, a romantic myth needs to surround it (Peck & Granzig, 1978). In her 1913 paper, 'Social Devices for Impelling Women to Bear and Raise Children', early feminist Leta Hollingworth discusses social devices or forms of social control that promoted myths about motherhood and parenthood (Peck & Senderowitz, 1974). Social devices include prominent pronatalist assumptions about intentionally childless marriages that have existed in society for many years and remain today.

One such pronatalist assumption I call the 'Destiny Assumption' (Carroll, 2012a). It reflects the belief that we are all biologically wired to want children. Despite society fostering this belief for many generations, there is no evidence to support the notion that everyone innately wants to have children. As Peck and Senderowitz (1974) write, 'Conception is biological; pregnancy is biological. Birth is biological. Parenthood is psychological in its application' (p. 137). Couples in a marital relationship have the biological ability to conceive and bear children, but this does not mean they have an instinctive desire to become parents or even have the ability to parent.

Even though this is the case, the pronatalist Destiny Assumption has been in society's social and cultural hardware for so long that the masses see it as a truth about ourselves and our adult lives. Society brings this mindset to marriage – that all married couples should want to have and raise children. Seeing this as a truth about life and marriage makes it difficult to understand, much less accept without judgement, couples who don't bring parenthood into their marriage experience.

Another pronatalist belief, I describe as the 'Normality Assumption' (Carroll, 2012a). It speaks to the belief that there is something wrong with people if they don't want children and includes three components of normality. For men and women, pronatalism tells us that wanting children is a sign of psychological health. It promotes the belief that having children marks the attainment of adult maturity. It also fosters the idea that wanting children reflects having a normal sense of identity.

For many years, society has tied identity to gender, and for women, womanhood has been viewed as synonymous with motherhood. Third-wave feminism challenged this idea. As Ireland (1993) writes in *Reconceiving Women*, motherhood is 'only one facet of female identity, and not central to the development of a woman's sense of her adult self' (p. 6). When it comes to defining one's sense of identity, third-wave feminism ultimately says to women, 'It's yours to create' (Carroll, 2012a, p. 43). This third-wave ideology holds for men as well. In the third-wave spirit, men can create and live out a sense of identity based on characteristics, traits and roles they feel are true expressions of themselves and who they want to be in the world. Despite this expanded thinking, society still has a hard time accepting that motherhood does not have to be part of a woman's sense of identity at all. While not as powerful as the historically synonymous description of womanhood and motherhood, society also views fatherhood as an important part of a man's identity.

The pronatalist Normality Assumption extends to married couples as well. Many years of pronatalist influence have instilled a mindset that an intentionally childless marriage is not a normal marriage, and that something is wrong with the partners such that they do not want to raise children. Although the reality is that marriage and parenthood no longer need to be experienced together, people have believed the Normality Assumption for so long they deeply believe that the normal course of life after one marries is to have children.

A third pronatalist assumption I call the 'Fulfilment Assumption', which reflects the strongly held belief that the ultimate path to fulfilment in life is parenthood (Carroll, 2012a). This pronatalist belief tells people they may have careers that mean a great deal to them, and do many other things in life that are important to them, but life is really about becoming mothers and fathers. Many married couples do find great meaning in life together from raising children. However, it is also true that couples have fulfilling lives together without this experience. Hundreds of years of being told that the ticket to fulfilment is parenthood and that everything else lags as a distant second makes it hard for people to believe that marriages that include parenthood reflect only one way to experience marital fulfilment. In a pronatalist world, a marriage that does not include the parenthood experience simply can't be as fulfilling, or even more fulfilling, than one in which the partners become parents.

The continued perpetuation of pronatalist assumptions like these stand in the way of seeing how they are either outmoded or have never been true at all. As long as pronatalist beliefs remain a dominant social and cultural force, marriages that don't put parenthood first stay in the tributaries of society. Ultimately, a pronatalist society makes reproduction a focal point in a marital union, not just one potential aspect of the union. It keeps intentionally childless marriages as outlier unions – life partners that could never match a union with the raising of children as its purpose.

How Intentionally Childless Couples Make the Decision to Not Have Children

Despite being in the minority, many couples go against pronatalist norms and decide not to have children. How married couples jointly make this decision varies. As Scott (2009), author of *Two Is Enough*, writes, '... how do couples come to this agreement – on the first date, or after five years together? Both, as it turns out' (p. 112). Qualitative analysis of interviews for *Families of Two* (2000) shows many couples did not jointly make the decision before they got married; they let it evolve over time once they were married. Qualitative analysis of interviews with 21 women and 10 men conducted by Blackstone and Stewart (2016) has similar findings; women and men reported that they made their decision consciously and experienced it as a process.

However, for other couples, the decision can come quickly. As this study by Edina Kurdi of Middlesex University found:

> Many are agreeing not to have children in one conversation, or in an unspoken way. One possible reason that couples did not need to talk about the issue much is that they could accurately sense their partner did not want children from their beliefs and lifestyle. (Wood, 2014, April)

Qualitative analyses for *Families of Two* (2000) and subsequent qualitative data collection have revealed that when couples discussed whether they wanted to become parents, the female spouse did not solely drive the decision. Many of the male spouses felt strongly about not wanting children. Interview analyses and subsequent data gathering have also revealed that many couples had concerns about how having children would impact the freedom and independence they had in their lives, which was important to them. Both have additionally identified that many couples have concerns about how having children would affect their marital relationship. They want to keep their marriage as their number one priority and do not think having children would impact their marriage in a positive way. As sociologist Blackstone notes, for these couples, 'it's all about intimacy and focussing their love on their partner' (Pawlowski, 2016).

Qualitative analyses for *Families of Two* (2000) and subsequent data collection have also indicated that couples have concerns regarding financial costs of raising a child, and about bringing a child into today's world and the environmental consequences of bringing another person into such a world. While they may have rational concerns like these, ultimately the couple's decision has rested in their lack of emotional desire to have and raise a child.

The Nature of Intentionally Childless Couples' Lives

How society commonly perceives intentionally childless couples' lives and the realities of their lives often differ. For example, the 12 August 2013 cover of *TIME* magazine which shows a beautiful couple happily lounging on the beach reflects common myths about intentionally childless married people: they are of upper-middle socio-economic level or higher, they have a good amount of disposable income, and have ample free time for vacations and travel (Carroll, 2013).

When research for *Families of Two* (2000) began, I received hundreds of calls and emails from couples from a range of socio-economic backgrounds. Of the 100 couples interviewed, 40% described their socio-economic status as middle class. Thirty per cent described themselves as upper-middle class and 30% third-lower middle class. Subsequent qualitative data collection on intentionally childless couples since its publication has shown that these married couples exist in every socio-economic stratum. It has additionally shown that they have a wide range of lifestyles and can't be described as a homogenous group.

Qualitative analysis of interviews for *Families of Two* (2000) also reveals that intentionally childless couples' roles and the way they set up their day-to-day lives exemplify liberal feminism in the marital relationship. Couples often have egalitarian roles; they do not follow traditional gender roles in their marital relationship. For example, most of the couples interviewed described how they equally share household domestics. It was not uncommon for women to have typical 'male' roles, from being the main breadwinner to taking the lead on house repair projects or yard work.

Interview and subsequent qualitative data collection have indicated that intentionally childless couples have a range of friends, some who are parents and some who are not. Couples have a variety of experiences with friends who have children. Some of them find, it difficult to maintain friendships with couples who became parents because they did not have children in common. Many others feel they have a more difficult time finding friends because they do not have children. This feeling was actually a popular reason for wanting to participate in the interviews for *Families of Two* (2000); a good number of participants requested that couples be offered the chance to give their names and contact information for possible communication with each other once the book was published.

The interviews and subsequent data collection have also revealed how intentionally childless couples place their relationship as the central priority in their lives and hold a very high value on making time to nurture it. However, unlike the portrayal on the cover of *TIME*, taking vacations and time off is not always easy for them. Many couples have reported how, like other families, job demands, avocations and other life responsibilities often make it challenging to spend as much time as they want together.

Misperceptions and Stereotypes

The influence of pronatalism plays a powerful role in why intentionally childless marriages remain judged and criticised. In addition to being in the higher socio-economic echelons, having a good deal of free time and disposable income, there are a number of other ways these couples are misperceived and stereotyped.

During 2010–2012, I conducted monthly online surveys with intentionally childless adults. One survey asked what stereotype they felt they had been subjected to the most in their lives (Carroll, 2011). Of the 642 respondents, 9 of the most common stereotypes or ways in which they felt they were misperceived included: they must have had bad childhoods; they are odd, eccentric types of people; they are career-driven types; they are cold-hearted; they suffer from a lack of meaning in their lives; they are not 'real' adults – they lack adult maturity; they are materialists; they hate children; and they are selfish people. The most common response to this online survey had more to do with how others seemingly understood those who claim they don't want children. It relates to this common comment they receive: 'You will change your mind'. To the online survey respondents, this kind of comment meant that others seem think those who say they don't want children don't know themselves well enough to know what they truly and will eventually want – children.

Qualitative analyses of interviews for *Families of Two* (2000) and subsequent qualitative data collection have shown how these stereotypes and misperceptions apply to intentionally childless couples as well. The most common misperception that they'll change their minds takes a sub-form with these couples. Many of them have reported being told by others that when they meet that 'right' person, and marry him or her, they will want a baby with that person. Qualitative analyses conducted since the year 2000 have not shown this to be the case.

In addition to these misperceptions and stereotypes, others pertain to intentionally childless couples in their elder years. Most common misperceptions relate the idea that because they will not have adult children in their lives at this time, partners in these marriages will have less emotional well-being, be isolated and lack social support. However, research (Hagestad & Call, 2007) has found that above having children, being married was a better predictor of well-being and satisfaction in one's later years. Research has also shown (Zhang & Hayward, 2001) that not being with one's spouse, or never having had one, particularly for men, has an impact on well-being. For example, divorced men with no children, widowed men with no children and men who had never married and had no children have been shown to have higher rates of loneliness compared to women with the same background. Divorced and widowed men with no children also had higher levels of depression than divorced and widowed women with no children.

Other research has identified another predictor of depressive symptoms in later life: net worth. For example, a study by Plotnick (2009) at the University of Washington looked at older married and unmarried men and women and found not children, but sufficient wealth contributed most to one's well-being in later years. Taken together, when it comes to married couples, having one's spouse there and having financial security can better predict well-being later in life than the existence of adult children.

With regards to being isolated and having lack of support, research tells us otherwise as well. Studies that focus on the social lives of the older intentionally childless have found that those with children and without children tend to be equally socially active. For example, a study by Wenger, Dykstra, Melkas, and Knipscheer (2007) that looked at older people in the United States, UK, Australia, Finland, Germany, Israel,

Netherlands and Spain indicated that those with no children were just as likely to be active in their communities and volunteer organisations as older persons who were parents. In this study, in some countries, it was found that being married and not being parents made the difference in terms of the strength of support networks. Those with no children can have smaller social networks but be equally strong and active as the social networks of those with adult children (Dykstra, 2006).

Qualitative analyses of interviews for *Families of Two* (2000) and subsequent data collection have supported this finding. While typically not large, long-time married intentionally childless couples have tended to have strong social and support networks. They have self-described themselves as more socially active than many of their neighbours in senior and assisted-living communities who have adult children and families. Like the misperception that older intentionally childless couples have less well-being than elderly people with adult children, they are no more likely to be isolated or lacking in social support solely due to the fact that they do not have children.

The Pressures to Have Children

The pressure to have children that intentionally childless couples receive comes from choosing a life that does not conform to reproductive norms. Collecting qualitative data since the year 2000 has revealed four kinds of pressures these couples commonly face (Carroll, 2012a).

Relational Pressure

One type of pressure I call 'relational pressure'. It comes from intentionally childless couples' friends, families and loved ones. Relational pressure involves comments designed to influence intentionally childless couples to decide to have children so that their relationship with them can grow ever closer. For example, this is when close friends who are parents comment on how great it would be if they could experience the raising of children together as a way to deepen their friendship bond. It is also when parents remark how wonderful it would be to have grandchildren as a way to make the extended family even closer. The intent behind the pressure is wanting to share and experience together what others believe will deepen already existing bonds.

This kind of pressure can often be negative, however. It can include comments that make intentionally childless couples feel judged. Often it can directly or indirectly insinuate others think the couples are selfish and self-involved for not wanting to become parents. Rather than closeness, judgement about them as people can create distance with close relations. Instead of trying to understand couples and what is right for them, this kind of pressure stems from loved ones believing couples will eventually do what they did – what all people are supposed to want to do. When this does not happen, intentionally childless couples can experience a loss of a sense of belonging in their friendship networks and families.

Shame-driven Pressure

Another kind of pressure I term 'shame-driven pressure'. It deepens the judgements and is designed to make intentionally childless couples feel like something is wrong with them for not wanting parenthood to be part of their marriage experience. Comments from others make them feel that not only is the choice wrong, but their lack of desire points to how they are abnormal to not want to become parents. Intentionally childless couples can easily feel shame when they internalise from others the idea that something is wrong with them. Often wanting to appear and feel 'normal' can be a powerful influence on couples to rethink their decision, which is exactly what others want them to do.

Guilt-driven Pressure

Intentionally childless couples can receive what I describe as 'guilt-driven pressure'. The purpose of this kind of pressure is to make intentionally childless couples feel badly about not doing what others want them to do. It can include comments about how their choice to not have children disappoints other family members and prevents their parents from having fulfilling elder years. Very often with this kind of pressure, gossip can operate as a back door to guilt. This happens when couples learn about others' disappointment and disapproval through someone else. It is designed to make them feel that their decision negatively affects others they love.

Invasive Pressure

Intentionally childless couples can also experience what I call 'invasive pressure'. This occurs when intentionally childless couples are asked intrusively personal questions related to why they don't have kids or don't want to have them. The questions can include asking directly about potential physical, emotional and psychological problems or personal decisions such as birth control use. Invasive pressure does not only come from people couples know well; it can come from complete strangers. This occurrence reflects the pronatalist norm that it is acceptable to ask others, even those one does not know, personal questions about their parental status.

How Intentionally Childless Couples Can Address the Pressures

Studying intentionally childless marriages since the year 2000 and having communicated with hundreds of intentionally childless couples during this time have led me to develop strategies on how to deal with these different types of pressures (Carroll, 2012a). A common response strategy that ultimately does not serve intentionally childless couples is lying. In generations past, intentionally childless couples lied as a common way of dealing with the pressures. Unfortunately, in present pronatalist times, couples still choose to lie over telling the truth. One lie entails creating the impression that the couple 'is trying' – that they do want a child and are trying to conceive – when this is far from the case. Another lie involves telling those who are pressuring them to have children that they can't have children, or an explanation that creates the impression of fertility issues. This kind of explanation often results in more concealment, such as the need to act sad and grief-stricken. Instead of deception, having the courage to communicate honestly and doing so with the following four-part strategy proves to be far more effective (Carroll, 2012a).

Clarity of Mind

First, it is very important that intentionally childless partners be very clear in their own minds why they do not want children. Not only do they need to know this for themselves, but they need to know it so they can clearly articulate it to others. In talking with those who are pressuring them, this can include being willing to explain myths and inaccurate stereotypes about those who don't have children by choice. For example, the female spouse can explain that the idea of the biological clock is not true for her, and that there is no real evidence that the clock exists at all. They can choose to explain how there is nothing wrong with them just because they choose not to have the experience of parenthood. Or they can explain that while parenthood brings fulfilment to many people, it is not the way for everyone and not the way for them. This can be followed by talking about what fulfilment in life means to them individually and as a couple.

A United Front

If both partners in the marriage clearly vocalise their position, it is harder for others to blame one or the other person in the relationship for their decision not to have children. Both partners need to talk without one or the other dominating. When one partner dominates, this can be perceived as one partner having made the decision while the other may not feel the same but is 'going along with it', or a related kind of misinterpretation. A united front also relates to responding to judgements or pressures from others. Both partners need to be willing to talk about where they stand.

Speak Up Sooner Rather than Later

Most often, tolerating direct or indirect pressures ultimately does not work. Negative feelings can fester, which will not serve intentionally childless couples when they do decide to speak up. When couples 'sit on' the pressures they feel from others, the conversation can easily end up being a heated one when it finally takes place. Speaking up sooner rather than later can fend off quarrels that could have been avoided.

Seek Mutual Understanding

A crucial step in alleviating pressure is to seek mutual understanding with others. After communicating honestly and clearly about why they do not want to have children, intentionally childless couples need to probe into why those who are pressuring them are pressuring them. They need to have the courage to ask others, 'Why is it that you want us to have children?'

Intentionally childless couples need to get others to see what is motivating them to pressure or judge. It can include asking parents why they want grandchildren, or if they have concerns about how they will be perceived; for example, that something was wrong with how they parented such that their adult children do not want to do the same. Seeking mutual understanding means talking with others until they can understand and acknowledge the motivations behind their pressures or judgements. Having a discussion that creates this kind of mutual understanding greatly increases the odds that the pressures from others will stop.

Are Intentionally Childless Marriages Happier than Marriages with Children?

Quite a history of marital happiness research exists, and in recent years, a good number of studies have compared happiness in marriages with and without children. Some of the most extensive studies have shown that intentionally childless marriages are happier. For example, an analysis of almost 100 marital satisfaction studies from the 1970s (Twenge, Campbell, Keith, & Foster, 2003) found that couples' overall marital satisfaction went down if they had children, and that parents' marital satisfaction has declined with every successive generation. Another study looked at data collected from 13,000 Americans by the National Survey of Families and Households, and found 'no group of parents – married, single, step or even empty-nest – reported significantly greater emotional well-being than people who never had children' (Ali, 2008, June).

Other studies show cycles in marital happiness when couples have children. In the book, *Stumbling on Happiness*, Gilbert (2007) discusses how several studies have found that marital satisfaction decreases dramatically after the birth of the first child and increases when the last child leaves home. Other studies have found that marital happiness increases over time as the child grows up, and still others have indicated that marital happiness moves in cycles, decreasing, for example, when a child is born, increasing when children are 6–13 years old, and decreasing again when the children reach their teens.

Whether the study shows parent or non-parent couples as happier, across studies, research flaws exist (Carroll, 2014). All too commonly, the studies do not differentiate between non-parents who want children and don't have them, those who want children but don't want them yet, and those who have no children by choice. They also do not operationally define 'happiness'. For these kinds of studies to better differentiate between different sample groups, happiness needs to be defined and measured. Without being operationally defined, respondents use what it means to them, which can be many things; it is unique to each person and each couple. Because of these issues, when it comes to which kind of marriage is happier, as the adage goes, 'the jury is out'. Rather than continuing to attempt to determine which kind of marriage is happier, there is greater research value in studying how married couples themselves define what a happy marriage means to them, and how having children or not fits into the picture.

The Road to Societal Acceptance

While it continues to remain outside the norm, from studying intentionally childless marriages since the year 2000, I have found that it gains more acceptance with every generation. In the 1950s, as an intentionally childless woman in *Families of Two* (2000) named Carol recalled, being married and choosing not to have children was 'a very unusual thing'. At that time, it was much more unusual to be intentionally childless than in today's times. When she and her husband were in their 60s, she described how others had long seen them as two 'exotic birds' (Carroll, 2000, p. 79).

Since the year 2000, views have shifted. The evolution of the digital world has fuelled awareness and education of the intentionally childless marriage and those who choose it (Carroll, 2016). However, society still has a long way to go to reach full societal acceptance. Since the publication of *Families of Two* (2000), subsequent qualitative analyses have revealed what can be characterised as 'temporary acceptance'. This commonly occurs when friends, loved ones or family members who are parents (or who want to be) accept the couple's intentionally childless status but believe they will ultimately change their minds and eventually will want to have children. Since the year 2014, qualitative data from electronic communications have revealed another common attitude that can be called 'nimby acceptance' – nimby standing for 'not in my backyard' (Carroll, 2012b). This is when parents of adult married children say they are fine with people opting out of parenthood until their own adult sons or daughters and their spouses decide not to have children.

From a Pronatalist to Post-pronatal Mindset

'Nimby' and 'temporary acceptance' types of attitudes point to what is necessary to attain full societal acceptance of the intentionally childless marriage. The long-held pronatalist assumption that people marry to have children now reflects outmoded thinking. It is time for society to begin living from a 'post-pronatal' mindset that speaks to what is true about marriage today. This post-pronatal mindset is: people marry as a way to bring them happiness and fulfilment in life. Marital happiness and fulfilment can take many forms. How Carole and Rich express it in *Families of Two* (2000) rings true for many intentionally childless couples; they see their intentionally childless marriage as 'more about a connection with someone on an intimate level they choose not to have with anyone else, and the institution of marriage is the ultimate commitment to that connection' (p. 142). One could call this form of marriage a 'connection marriage'.

In *The New I Do* (2014), Pease Gadoua and Larson expand forms of marriage outside the 'parenting marriage', including the companionship marriage, the distant marriage, the covenant marriage, the safety marriage and open marriage. All of these and the intentionally childless marriage show by example how a fulfilling marriage does not need to be defined solely by whether children are part of it. The marriage is defined by each couple and what they determine a successful marriage means to them. Each couple holds the keys to creating a relationship that is all their own and what makes theirs the most fulfilling for them individually and together in the marital relationship.

Adopting other post-pronatal mindsets will support the social and cultural acceptance of the intentionally childless marriage (Carroll, 2012a). This includes moving away from the notion that humans are biologically supposed to want children to the fact that our very biological capacities allow us to make parenthood a choice. It also means rejecting the idea that the only path to fulfilment in life is parenthood and adopting the true mindset that it can be one path to fulfilment. It includes rejecting the idea that something is wrong with people when they don't want to have children and embracing the truth that it is just as normal to not want children as it is to want them.

Fostering Post-pronatal Mindsets

In addition to exemplifying a post-pronatal mindset about marriage, intentionally childless married couples can more directly expose and educate others on outmoded or untrue pronatalist beliefs and post-pronatal mindsets surrounding marriage and children. For example, if a friend brings up how her biological clock is going off, the couple can talk about how, beyond the biological, powerful pronatalist social and cultural influences drive this thinking. When others say they want children, intentionally childless couples can enquire into why they think they want children and broach the lack of evidence to support the idea that all people are wired to desire children. Intentionally childless couples can help others see the truths about marriage and why it's time to move to post-pronatal mindsets that support those truths (Carroll, 2012a).

Intentionally childless married couples can also exemplify post-pronatal mindsets by how they plan for and live their later years. The old pronatalist assumption has been that a couple's children will be there for them when they are old (Carroll, 2012a). Because this will not be the case for the intentionally childless couple, they can embody and model an alternative assumption that planning for their later years is their responsibility. Couples who have adult children can benefit from this mindset as well. While one's children may be there for them when they are old, this is no longer a time in history when couples who are parents can unquestionably assume this will be the case. With or without children, to prepare for their later years, couples need to answer questions like: How do we envision our elder years? What kind of living environment do we want? What do our financial goals need to be in order to have this living environment when we will need it? What do we envision our support network to look like, and what can we do now to cultivate that support structure? Answering these questions and taking action well in advance to make intentionally childless couples' answers a reality will greatly help them fulfil their vision for their elder years. It can also show those with children ways in which they can do the same.

The Intentionally Childless Marriage as a Feminist Act

For the intentionally childless marriage, an important part of shifting from outmoded pronatalist beliefs to post-pronatal mindsets that reflect realities involve the expansion of marital identity. Just as third-wave feminism has allowed for the expansion of female identities beyond motherhood, the intentionally childless marriage broadens the ways in which married couples can identify with what their marriage means and represents to them as well as how the partners see themselves within that marriage. Choosing not to reproduce, which strongly represents their reproductive rights as a couple, is a central characteristic of this marital identity.

As feminism seeks equal personal and social rights for women, the acceptance of the intentionally childless marriage will mark the advancement of personal and social rights for couples who choose this form of marriage. Societal acceptance will mean the intentionally childless marriage is equally valued, respected and seen to be just as valid as marriage with children. More broadly, whether in marriage or not, when the choice not to reproduce is equally valued, respected and recognised to be just as legitimate as the choice to reproduce, it will mark a significant pinnacle in reaching full reproductive freedom in our society.

References

Ali, L. (2008, June 28). Does having kids make you happy? *Newsweek*. Retrieved from http://www.newsweek.com/2008/06/28/having-kids-makes-you-happy.html

Blackstone, A., & Stewart, M. D. (2016). There's more thinking to decide: How the childfree decide not to parent. *Family Journal, 24*(3), 296–303. Retrieved from http://journals.sagepub.com/doi/abs/10.1177/1066480716648676

Carroll, L. (2000). *Families of two: Interviews with happily married couples without children by choice*. Bloomington: Xlibris/Random House.

Carroll, L. (2011, September 1). *Reporting Back: The August 2011 on-the-ground question*. Retrieved from https://www.lauracarroll.com/reporting-back-the-august-childfree-on-the-ground-question/

Carroll, L. (2012a). *The baby matrix: Why freeing our minds from outmoded thinking about parenthood & reproduction will create a better world*. San Francisco: LiveTrue Books.

Carroll, L. (2012b, September 26). *Why not wanting kids is hard for society to accept*. Retrieved from https://www.lauracarroll.com/not-want-kids-hard-for-society-to-accept/

Carroll, L. (2013, August 6). *The childfree making the cover of TIME*. Retrieved from https://www.lauracarroll.com/childfree-making-cover-of-time/

Carroll, L. (2014, January 17). *Weighing in on kids-no kids happiness research*. Retrieved from http://www.lauracarroll.com/happiness-research/

Carroll, L. (2016, January 15). *Where are we, after 40+ years of talking about the childfree choice?* Retrieved from https://www.lauracarroll.com/where-are-we-after-40-years-of-talking-about-the-childfree-choice/

Dykstra, P. (2006). Off the beaten track: Childlessness & social integration in late life. *Research on Aging*, *28* (6), 749–767. doi:10.1177/0164027506291745

Gilbert, D. (2007). *Stumbling on happiness*. New York, NY: Vintage.

Hagestad, G., & Call, V. R. A. (2007). Pathways to childlessness: A life course perspective. *Journal of Family Issues*, *28* (10), 1338–1361. doi:10.1177/0192513X07303836

Ireland, M. (1993). *Reconceiving women: Separating motherhood from female identity*. New York, NY: Guildford Press.

Morell, C. (1994). *Unwomanly conduct: The challenges of intentional childlessness*. New York, NY: Routledge.

Pawlowski, A. (2016, August). I don't think this is for me: 7 reasons why people choose to be childfree. *TODAY*. Retrieved from http://www.today.com/health/i-don-t-think-me-7-reasons-why-people-choose-t102160

Pease Gadoua, S., & Larson, V. (2014). *The new I do: Reshaping marriage for skeptics, realists and rebels*. Berkeley, CA: Seal Press.

Peck, E., & Granzig, W. (1978). *The parent test: How to measure and develop your talent for parenthood*. New York, NY: GP Putman's Sons.

Peck, E., & Senderowitz, J. (1974). *Pronatalism: The myth of mom & apple pie*. New York, NY: Thomas Y. Cromwell Company.

Plotnick, R. (2009). Childlessness and economic well-being of older Americans. *The Journal of Gerontology Series B: Psychological Sciences and Social Sciences*, *64B*(6), 767–776. doi:10.1093/geronb/gbp023

Scott, L. (2009). *Two is enough: A couple's guide to living childless by choice*. Berkeley, CA: Seal Press.

Twenge, J., Campbell, W. K., & Foster, C. (2003). Parenthood and marital satisfaction: A meta-analytic review. *Journal of Marriage and Family*, *65* (3), 574–583. doi:10.1111/j.1741-3737.2003.00574.x

US Census Bureau. (2014, June). *Children ever born and percent childless by age and marital status: June 2014*. Washington, DC: U.S. Government Printing Office. Retrieved from https://www.census.gov/data/tables/2014/demo/fertility/women-fertility.html#par_list_57

Wenger, C., Dykstra, P., Melkas, T., & Knipscheer, K. (2007). Social embeddedness and late-life parenthood: Community activity, close ties, and support networks. *Journal of Family Issues*, *28*(11), 1419–1456. doi:10.1177/0192513X07303895

Wood, J. (2014, April). Remaining childless requires little conversation. *Psych Central*. Retrieved from https://psychcentral.com/news/2014/04/26/remaining-childless-requires-little-conversation/69037.html

Zhang, Z., & Hayward, M. D. (2001, September). Childlessness and psychological well-being of older persons. *The Journal of Gerontology Series B: Psychological Sciences and Social Sciences*, *56* (5), S311–S320. Retrieved from http://www.ncbi.nlm.nih.gov/pubmed/11522813

Chapter 10

Finding 'Mr Right'? Childfree Women's Partner Preferences

Helen Peterson

Abstract

This chapter explores an aspect of voluntary childlessness that has been neglected in previous research; how voluntarily childless (i.e. childfree) women engage in partnership formation processes and how they perceive that these processes become influenced by their voluntarily childless status. Drawing on interviews with 21 voluntarily childless, heterosexual, Swedish women, this chapter highlights how their childfree decision(s) impacted their partnering behaviour, their chances to form an intimate relationship and their preferences concerning partners and partnerships. The results show some of the challenges these women faced as they engaged in partnership formation processes concerning; for example, constraints in partner availability and potentially conflicting preferences regards autonomy, reproduction and intimacy. In addition, partnership formation was complicated due to a lack of communication, misunderstandings and disbelief in their childfree choices. The analysis illustrates that it was of utmost importance to these women that their intimacy goals were respected and protected during these processes but that some of them were also willing to negotiate their partner ideal. Nevertheless, this chapter ends with a discussion of relationship dissolution due to ambivalence concerning childfree choices and intimacy goals both on behalf of the childfree woman and her partner.

Keywords: Childlessness; Voluntary; Women; Relationships; Partnership; Intimacy

Introduction

This chapter explores how heterosexual voluntarily childless women in Sweden engage in partnership formation processes and how these processes are guided by their partner preferences and intimacy goals. How individuals form and sustain personal, informal and intimate relationships is one of the key issues, not only in sociology (Allan, 2001), but also in evolutionary psychology (Koyama, McGain, & Hill, 2004; Thomas & Stewart-Williams, 2018). Partnership formation processes, in a society where a majority still follows the expected life course, usually involve finding a partner with whom to form a monogamous and exclusive relationship and eventually have children (Frisén, Carlsson, & Wängqvist, 2014). This means that most women and men are expected to go through a series of status transitions – from living a single life to entering into an intimate couple relationship and to go from childless to becoming a parent (Mullins, 2016).

Partnership formation processes for voluntarily childless women deviate from this expected route, not only because they remain childless. Previous research has revealed that these women also are more likely to reject marriage and prefer to remain single, thereby achieving social and economic independence (see e.g. Dykstra & Hagestad, 2007; Houseknecht, 1987; Peterson, 2015). However, we know little about voluntarily childless women's partnership formation processes and their partner preferences. Deviating from the expected status transitions and having preferences that deviates from the great majority potentially poses some challenges for voluntarily childless women. Partner preferences constitute the foundation of partnership formation processes and are usually associated with similarities in attitudes, beliefs and interests (Bredow, 2015). The expected status transitions described above presuppose shared intimacy goals, including childbearing intentions (Sanderson, Keiter, Miles, & Yopuk, 2007). However, sex differences in mate preferences have also been established, with men giving precedence to fertility and physical attractiveness, and women placing greater importance on a potential mate's ability to acquire resources and good earning potential (Koyama et al., 2004). If a majority of men can be expected to have intimacy goals that include becoming a father (see Hakim, 2000), this is likely to influence 'mate availability' for voluntarily childless women and their chances to meet a 'well-matched partner' (Bredow, 2015; Thomas & Stewart-Williams, 2018). Even if women usually are expected to aspire to motherhood to a higher degree than men are expected to desire fatherhood (Bartholomaeus & Riggs, 2017), partnership formation processes could potentially prove challenging for voluntarily childless women. So, how do childfree women define 'Mr Right' and which search strategies, if any, do they adopt in order to find him?

This study adds to previous research by shifting the focus from investigating why some women have preferences for a childfree lifestyle, to investigating how these preferences influence their partnering behaviour, their chances to form an intimate relationship and their standards for a partner (see Bredow, 2015; Mullins, 2016). The analysis in this chapter investigates, firstly, voluntarily childless women's preferences concerning partnership formation and partner characteristics. Second, it investigates how these preferences influenced how these women navigated the dating scene, adopting different relationship initiation strategies. Third, the chapter explores challenges concerning partnership formation these women experienced.

Interpretative Framework

Previous Research

Previous research has investigated women's lifestyle preferences and childbearing intentions in order to understand and predict changes in fertility and employment patterns in modern, industrialised societies (Hakim, 2000; Nilsson, Hammarström, & Strandh, 2017). Previous research on voluntary childlessness has often centred on understanding the underlying values and attitudes that, together with a specific historical context, shapes individuals' preferences for a childfree lifestyle (Heaton, Jacobson, & Holland, 1999; Park, 2005). Voluntarily childless women have been depicted as having strong preferences for greater opportunities for self-fulfilment; career satisfaction; improved financial position; and decreased domestic responsibilities (Dykstra & Hagestad, 2007; Tanturri & Mencarini, 2008). Freedom to pursue professional possibilities has been named as one of the main reasons for women's decision to live without children (see e.g. Kemkes-Grottenthaler, 2003; Koropeckyj-Cox & Pendell, 2007; Veevers, 1979). These preferences set voluntarily childless women apart from the majority of women (Hakim, 2003a).

Previous research has also pointed out some patterns concerning voluntarily childless women's lifestyle preferences and preferences concerning intimate relationships (Abma & Martinez, 2006; Avison & Furnham, 2015). Voluntarily childless women are, for example, associated with a preference to cohabit without ever entering into marriage

(Mulder, 2003). Previous research shows that being unmarried is one of the strongest predicators of childlessness (Heaton et al., 1999; Park, 2005). Many of the women who reject motherhood also reject marriage and continue to stay single, which is a pattern that already Houseknecht (1987) has identified. She described how these women forgo 'not only one, but two of society's major role expectations' (Houseknecht, 1987, p. 376). Relationship status (single, cohabitation and married) is therefore intimately linked with having children or not (Keizer, Dykstra, & Jansen, 2007; Tanturri & Mencarini, 2008).

This study investigates voluntarily childless women's preferences in Sweden. Childlessness, both voluntary and involuntary, is relatively common in Sweden, over 20% for men and around 14% for women (Persson, 2010). Sweden also belongs to the group of Nordic countries with the highest concentration of single-person households in the EU (Eurostat, 2015). Moreover, Sweden is one of the most gender-equal societies in the world. Previous research has highlighted that voluntary childlessness is less disapproved of in more gender-equal countries, among them Sweden (Rijken & Merz, 2014). In countries such as these, women's choice to pursue a professional career is better understood and supported. Similarly, according to Tanaka and Johnson (2016), Sweden is a nation characterised by a low proportion of people believing motherhood is necessary for a woman – something that often correlates with childless people being happier and more satisfied than in other countries. However, women's decision to forgo motherhood has been associated with their unwillingness to give up a more gender-equal lifestyle as non-mothers – in the labour market and in the private sphere – also in Sweden (Peterson, 2015, 2017; Peterson & Engwall, 2013, 2015).

Theoretical Framework

The main interpretative tool used in the analysis in this chapter is the concept '*preference*', which in sociology is associated with the theoretical framework developed by Hakim (2003a, 2006). In her research, she investigates variation in women's career and employment patterns and explains them with reference to variation in women's preferences for how they want to live their life, focusing on work-family preferences. She highlights the dissonance between women's and men's preferences due to enduring sex differences in life goals (Hakim, 2006), and how men generally have a higher degree of uncertainty about having children compared to women (Hakim, 2003a). Hakim's proposed theory has received criticism because it underplays the importance of constraints and structural factors (Kan, 2007; McRae, 2003). McRae (2003) has therefore emphasised the importance of not only researching personal lifestyle preferences but also the constraints that affect women differently.

The analysis in this chapter acknowledges this criticism. Using 'preferences' as a theoretical concept, therefore, does not imply that the aim is to elaborate on the extent to which preferences are actually predicators of behaviour (Vitali, Billari, Prskawetz, & Testa, 2009) or that the aim is to explain gender inequality using preferences (Nilsson et al., 2017). It does not suggest that unconstrained choices determine how people live their lives (McRae, 2003). Instead, investigating preferences implies that the analysis is person-centred, focused on personal values and decision-making on a micro-level and recognises that people have agency and choices. The analysis also acknowledges differences and variations within groups (Hakim, 2003b). The aim of investigating individuals' preferences in this sense is to increase our understanding of their attitudes, motivations, values and life goals, while also taking contextual cultural and social constraints into account and how individuals interpret and respond to them (Hakim, 2000; Kan, 2007; McRae, 2003).

The concept 'partner preference' is used here to refer to people's beliefs about which characteristics are important in a potential partner (see Koyama et al., 2004). The analysis thus explores voluntarily childless women's partner preferences with a focus on what they considered as realistic preferences (see Bredow, 2015) in relation to constraints such as partner availability (see Thomas & Stewart-Williams, 2018) and in relation to potentially conflicting preferences concerning autonomy, reproduction and intimacy (see Koyama et al., 2004).

Methodological Framework

The chapter empirically draws on qualitative, in-depth interviews with 21 Swedish women, who defined themselves as voluntarily childless. All women presented themselves as heterosexual in the interviews and were between 29 and 54 years old (mean age: 39.6). Nine of the women were single and only one of them was married at the time of the interview. However, three more had been married before but were now divorced. Seven of the interviewees were cohabiting with a man. Four of them lived in long-term relationships with a man without sharing household with them, so called LAT-relationships (Living Apart Together). Table 1 below gives an overview of the respondents and the pseudonyms they are

Table 1. Summary Table of the Respondents.

Name (Pseudonym)	Age	Partnership Status
Anna	54	Married
Britta	33	LAT
Clara	44	Single
Doris	41	Single
Eleonore	43	Single
Fanny	50	Single
Greta	35	Single
Hanna	29	Cohabiting
Iris	43	Cohabiting
Julia	39	Cohabiting
Kirsten	36	Single
Lena	33	Cohabiting
Maria	40	Cohabiting
Natalie	43	Single
Paula	43	LAT
Rosemarie	42	Single
Sara	30	Cohabiting
Tina	33	Cohabiting
Ulla	46	LAT
Yvonne	37	LAT
Veronica	37	Single

given in this study, due to research ethical considerations regarding confidentiality.

As in many previous studies on voluntary childlessness, all but one of the informants lived in larger urban areas although many had moved there from the countryside or smaller communities where they grew up (Houseknecht, 1987; Tanturri & Mencarini, 2008; Veevers, 1979). The women constituted a diverse group in terms of education and occupation; physician, actress, author, engineer and project leader are some examples of their occupations. All women interviewed were promised anonymity and that detailed information about them, or their real names, would not be revealed.

The interviews were semi-structured and had a narrative character where the women told their own stories about living a childfree life. The aim of the interviews was to explore the lived experiences of being voluntarily childless and living as a voluntarily childless woman in contemporary Swedish society. The questions asked were based on a thematic interview guide, covering themes such as motives for remaining childfree; attitudes towards them as childfree; how being childfree affected their relationships with partners, friends and family; and their attitudes to contraceptive alternatives, including abortion and sterilisation. Different considerations regarding partner preferences and intimacy goals appeared in the interviews when the women shared their experiences about navigating the dating scene and adopting different relationship initiation strategies. The semi-structured interview style enabled attention to be paid to individual differences in the women's unique experiences. The analysis thus expands on the multifaceted character of childfree women's narratives about partnership formation processes and the themes that emerged.

The empirical data are a small sample and there is no claim that all childfree women share these experiences. The aim is not to generalise these experiences but to provide insights into how a small group of childfree women view partnership formation processes.

Results and Analysis

Partnership Preferences

Despite the fact that 9 of the 21 childfree women were single at the time of the interview, singlehood was not an appealing option for most of them. Instead, the single women looked forward to a status transition into couplehood and described a desire to enter into the partnership formation process. One of the women who most explicitly expressed her desires to transition from her current single status stated clearly: 'I don't enjoy being single. I'd love to meet someone' (*Kirsten*, 36 years, single). The single women all agreed upon the value and the benefits of forming a romantic relationship.

The women who were involved in a relationship with a man at the time of the interview also emphasised the many advantages with forming such a partnership. In the interviews, the women were asked about what was most important in their lives and several of those who enjoyed a romantic relationship typically replied: 'My partner. Definitely. My relationship' (*Ulla*, 46 years, LAT). One of the advantages of being part of an intimate couple relationship was the emotional support it provided. One of the women emphasised the importance of such emotional support that she received from her partner:

> I don't feel different from everybody else or that people question me because I'm childfree or that it's a problem. The reason is that my partner doesn't want kids either, so we have each other and we support each other. When we see screaming kids we exchange looks and we both think: 'Yes! Yes!' [laughter]. (*Iris*, 43 years, cohabiting)

Iris enjoyed the shared, intimate moments with her partner when they confirmed to each other that their choice to forgo parenthood was the right decision, as they did not have to deal with 'screaming kids'. For many of the women interviewed, similarly to Iris, the partner became an important figure in providing the support the women needed due to the stigmatised position that being voluntarily childless still is (Mullins, 2016; Park, 2002; Peterson, 2011).

Ideal Living Arrangements

Although their partnership preferences involved a desire to transition from the single status to couplehood, the women did not pursue marriage. All except one, preferred other partnership forms than marriage, primarily cohabitation. Living as a childfree, cohabiting couple has been described as a living arrangement that allows for almost the same kind of freedom and independence as living alone (Mulder, 2003). Notwithstanding, four of the women had partnership preferences that also excluded cohabitation as an ideal partnership form. Their need for independence and freedom influenced how they practically arranged and organised their intimate and affective relationships. According to these four women, there was an inherent contradiction between keeping their independence while at the same time living together with a man. Fanny, who at the time of the interview was single, explained that her need to be alone was an important motivator for her choice to remain childless, but also for her preference regarding living arrangements with a partner:

> I have this great need to be alone and be on my own. A great, great need. And it just doesn't work with kids. And it's the same with boyfriends. Living apart together is the only option. (*Fanny*, 50 years, single)

Living apart together therefore replaced cohabitation and marriage as a long-term partnership form for these four women. This meant that there were no expectations or desires to transition from living apart together to another type of partnership form. Paula also expressed the advantages of this kind of relationship:

> I'm in 100% control over my own time. I have a real strong need to be alone. That's why we are still living apart together. I need to be in control of my alone time. (*Paula*, 43 years, LAT)

This means that although all women interviewed preferred couplehood, their preferences regarding living arrangements differed slightly. Four of them adjusted their partnership preferences in relation to competing preferences about living an independent life and therefore rejected not only marriage but also cohabitation as an ideal partnership form.

Partner Ideals

Several of the women currently in a relationship described how they considered themselves as fortunate because their partner was also voluntarily childless. It was of utmost importance for these women that their partners shared their intimacy goal; that is had made a choice to remain childfree. These women regarded shared intimacy goals an integral part of what compatibility as a couple meant:

> We've been together for 10 years. I knew long before we met that I didn't want kids. And he doesn't want kids either. That's why we're so compatible. (*Julia*, 39 years, cohabiting)

Yvonne explained that it would be more or less impossible for her to date a man who was already a father because childlessness constituted a fundamental point of attraction for her:

> I've been very careful not to be interested in men with children. It hasn't been that difficult. Somehow, I find men with children so uninteresting. (*Yvonne*, 37 years, LAT)

Most of the seven single women interviewed felt resolute that they would not become involved with a man with intimacy goal that included fatherhood:

> I wouldn't start a relationship with someone who wants children. I'd get out of the relationship immediately if it turned out he wanted children. (*Veronica*, 37 years, single)

Notwithstanding, she continued: 'I would more than welcome children from a previous relationship' (*Veronica*, 37 years, single). The women interviewed, however, voiced different opinions about whether they could become deeply involved with a man who already had children. Some of them experienced it as necessary to expand their partner preferences to encompass also men with already fulfilled intimacy goals concerning parenthood:

> I really want to find true love. If I meet someone it has to be 'the One'. And he has to be 'Mr Right'. He must either have had his kids already or don't want any [laughter]. (*Kirsten*, 36 years, single)

Some of the women had experiences of dating partners who were also fathers and a couple of them were currently, at the time of the interview, involved in such relationships and enjoyed it. Hanna cohabited with a man who had shared custody over children from a previous relationship, and, contrary to the attitude towards children displayed by most of the other women interviewed, she did not see this as problematic. Instead, Hanna described herself as a stepmother to her partner's children and that it was 'marvelous', and that she loved the children (*Hanna*, 29 years, cohabiting).

Timing Partnership Formation

Whether or not their partner preferences excluded or included men with already fulfilled intimacy goals concerning parenthood, the women all emphasised the timing of the partnership formation process. Greta was asked whether or not she would consider dating a man with children and replied:

> I try to avoid that. In theory, it could be an advantage but... no, I don't want that responsibility. I don't want it.

> You could wait to date for 10 to 15 years, when the kids are grown up. They can be nice then. And not too much trouble. They can take care of themselves. That's an option [laughter]. (*Greta*, 35 years, single)

Timing was crucial when initiating a relationship because of how partners' children and childcare responsibilities could affect the relationship and the women's preference for living a childfree life. Young children were considered more problematic than older children: 'I've been lucky and clever and never dated a man with responsibilities for small kids' (*Fanny*, 50 years, single). They thus took into account that childcare responsibilities vary over the life course. For Natalie, it was important to avoid being involved in such care responsibilities and avoid becoming a 'babysitter' for children or grandchildren:

> Well… if he had children when he was young they would be grown up by now. But then there might be grandchildren. I can't risk that [laughter]. I can't risk that. (*Natalie*, 43 years, single)

Eleonore considered it possible to date and live together with a man who had children given that he shared custody of the children with the mother of the children, because that would limit his childcare responsibilities (*Eleonore*, 43 years, single). Some of the women who were cohabitating or dating voluntarily childless men similarly reflected over that they would be prepared to adjust their partner preferences. Paula explained that whether it would work for her to date a man who was a father depended on several different aspects, including the relationship to the mother of the children and how old the children were (*Paula*, 43 years, LAT). Iris shared the view that the age of the child was important and that it would be easier with a teenager than a small child (*Iris*, 43 years, cohabiting).

These women's partner preferences were thus multifaceted and nuanced, taking into account not only their partner ideals but also the social context in which the great majority of men did not share their intimacy goals.

Navigating the Dating Scene

Although the women viewed partnership formation as an essential part of a satisfactory life course, they also associated building and maintaining a significant relationship with a partner with several different challenges and difficulties. The women were aware of that their partner and partnership preferences were strikingly different from the traditional heterosexual relationship that ultimately is expected to lead to marriage and children. That entailed a partner ideal that in many ways defined an exceptional kind of man. Some women therefore felt that their decision to remain childfree jeopardised their chances of dating. Kirsten, for example, described the dating scene as a 'very limited market' (*Kirsten*, 36 years, single). Dating made the women aware of that their intimacy goals diverged from the majority in society. Sara recollected how a date abruptly ended when the subject of children arose:

> Worst was a date where kids were discussed and the guy just said: 'Ok. We can stop right now because I want kids' [laughter]. In hindsight I think that was great. He knew what he wanted and he wasn't afraid of telling me. (*Sara*, 30 years, cohabiting)

To find an exceptional man on a 'limited market' necessitated a special way of navigating the dating scene. Greta explained the dilemma that she faced:

> It's difficult enough to find someone and even more difficult trying to find someone that doesn't want kids when it seems that most people *do* want them. (*Greta*, 35 years, single)

The scarcity of voluntarily childless men meant that the women felt a need to adjust their partner preferences. Notwithstanding preferring a voluntarily childless man, Kirsten realised that she had to be open to compromise about this issue and also consider dating men who already had children:

> Sure, I can become friends with the children but I won't change any diapers [laughter]. I feel that I have to lower my demands. I can't just demand no kids at all because the market is already very limited for me. (*Kirsten*, 36 years, single)

Notwithstanding diverging preferences as regards to the status of their ideal partner, very rarely did the women understand it as possible to live in a relationship where their possibilities to remain childfree were somehow restricted. In order to uphold their own status as childfree women, they adopted specific relationship initiation strategies.

Relationship Initiation Strategies

Replying to the question whether she had any strategies for discussing intimacy goals during a partnership formation process, Clara, who was actively navigating the dating scene, explained that it was not anything that could be negotiated but rather something that a potential future partner had to accept:

> No. No. No. There won't be any kids here. There won't. That's just how it is. Either you want what I want… If you want kids, I'm the wrong person for you. And that scares a lot of men, even if they really don't want kids themselves. (*Clara*, 44 years, single)

Sara, similarly, emphasised how important shared intimacy goals were with reference to the almost existential nature of the issue: 'It's really not something that you can compromise about' (*Sara*, 30 years, cohabiting).

For most of the women interviewed in this study, the childfree decision was already made and no boyfriend, fiancé or husband could affect or change that decision. For these women, it was important to clearly communicate their childfree decision before becoming committed to a relationship. This meant that potential relationships never were pursued if at an early stage of dating it was revealed that intimacy goals diverged. Greta emphasised how fortunate she would consider herself if she could find someone who shared the childfree choice because that meant that the relationship was spared from the strains of difficult discussions and choices. She described her strategy of bringing it up in a previous, now ended relationship:

> We talked about it pretty early on, that none of us wanted kids because it would have been tricky if he had wanted kids. He'd been forced to make a decision. (*Greta*, 35 years, single)

While some women had made sure to discuss their intimacy goals at an initial point in the relationship, others described that luck played a part during the relationship formation process:

> I don't remember how we brought it up for discussion. But I remember that I was very relieved when I realised that he doesn't want kids either. (*Hanna*, 29 years, cohabiting)

For many, an unspoken agreement was considered far too risky and vague. They therefore made a point of talking it over with their partner before agreeing to any more serious commitments:

> It's such a fundamental thing that you have to… otherwise you will regret it bitterly and there is a risk that things will go very wrong in the relationship. You won't be happy and you will blame each other. So there are a lot of costs if you don't. (*Iris*, 43 years, cohabiting)

The women interviewed also shared their experiences concerning such relationship problems. As described below, some relationship problems arose out of lack of communication, misunderstandings or disbelief. Ambivalence concerning intimacy goals also complicated relationship formations. This chapter will therefore end with a discussion of relationship dissolution due to different types of ambivalence.

Ambivalent Intimacy Goals

Some of the women mentioned another, somewhat unexpected, reason for not dating a man who wanted children. Fanny expressed considerable difficulties concerning building and maintaining a relationship with a man. She initially explained her childlessness partly because of her lack of longer and more serious relationships with men: 'I've never really met someone…' (*Fanny*, 50 years, single). In her continuing reflection, however, she reversed the argument, implying she had carefully chosen who she 'had met':

> I've never dated a man who wants kids. I'm sure it's part of it… I think that if I did meet someone that really wanted kids… it would have been problematic. So, it's possible that I subconsciously dated men that don't want… or that I know… it would never happen… I've

> subconsciously dated men I know I'd never want kids with [laughter]. Ever. (*Fanny*, 50 years, single)

Doris, in a similar manner, explained that her reluctance towards dating a man who wanted children was related to a fear that such a relationship could sway her in her decision not to have children. She explained this as a relationship risk:

> When I fall in love... that's one of my weaknesses. I become a damn fool [laughter]. [...] If I meet a man who wants children... I might, even though I don't want, I could let myself be persuaded. And I think that's why I've never lived together with a man because I've somehow known that. I start to realize that now. If I had done that, I might have been a mother today. (*Doris*, 41 years, single)

To remain childfree had thus not been a simple decision for all women. Some expressed their ambivalence about parenthood (see Letherby & Williams, 1999). Paula reflected on whether or not she could date a man who wanted children and implied that dating a partner that did not share her commitment to the childfree lifestyle meant that she could be forced to reconsider her decision:

> You have to think about it because it depends on how much you care for that person. If you are ready to reconsider. If you aren't, then you have to break up and be tough with that decision. My friends have had intense discussions. It's a great strain on the relationship. It's a relief not having to go through that. My current partner doesn't want kids. Otherwise... I don't know. I would have to think about it more. Because then I would have to make a decision. (*Paula*, 43 years, LAT)

Veronica had at one point felt the desire to become a mother and she and her then husband tried to conceive. When the IVF treatments failed to be successful, she started to change her mind about children and reached a decision to remain childfree. She explained how that affected her husband and marriage:

> He wanted to accept my decision but we never really talked about it. Today we are divorced, after one and a half years of marriage. (*Veronica*, 37 years, single)

While Eleonore stated that she would never allow a man to persuade her to have children (*Eleonore*, 43 years, single), not all women had been, or were, as certain about their intimacy goals.

Ambivalent and Undecided Partners

According to the women, men could sometimes also be ambivalent about whether or not they wanted to have children: 'And the guys might not even know what they want either' (*Clara*, 44 years, single). But a man who became involved in a partnership formation process with a voluntarily childless woman sometimes had to figure out his own fertility preferences and make an explicit decision:

> When I met my partner… he hadn't really thought about settling down and said that he didn't mind having children and I confronted him about it and told him that we had to sort that out because I really didn't want kids. And then he said 'no, no, I don't want kids'. 'But you said that you did?' And he explained: 'I just said so because I thought all girls wanted it and I didn't want to scare you away'. (*Maria*, 40 years, cohabiting)

Maria had also considered that her partner might change his mind and that the relationship would have to end because of that:

> You never know. He can change his mind. You never know. It's a chance I have to take. It's up to him if it's important. I totally understand if he wants to be with someone else. That's just how it is. I can't do anything about that. He is not that important that I would consider having children just for him. That would be completely wrong. It would be a violation to the child. (*Maria*, 40 years, cohabiting)

This risk was a particularly relevant concern raised by women in relationships with men who were younger than them. The choice to date a younger man thus came with very real opportunity costs as separation was believed as simply being postponed:

> My boyfriend is six years younger than me and he says he doesn't want kids. But he's really sweet with his friend's

> kid so I think he'll change his mind. (*Yvonne*, 37 years, LAT)

Because women's ability to bear a child is time-limited by their 'biological clocks', whereas men have a less clear biological restriction, the decision to have a child may, for the woman, be decided by the passage of time before the man has resolved his own ambivalence. In relationships where the woman is older than her partner, this is more likely to happen:

> He is two years younger than me and of course it's possible … Men can have children when they're older and he might change his mind. But you never know what will happen. And I've told him if it will be important for him … He knows that I won't change my mind and I will be 40 soon so it's getting too late for me anyway. (*Julia*, 39 years, cohabiting)

Although some of the women interviewed rejected the idea of negotiating their intimacy goals or dating a man who wanted children, the interviews also revealed some rare exceptions. Such negotiations, within the couple, however, in one case resulted in unconventional and painful decisions and realisations:

> We talked about this very early on in our relationship. I felt that he's the only one for me, my last love in life. And he's very honest and told me: 'I can be the only one for you, but you can't be the only one for me'. And we talked and cried a lot and I made it clear: 'Of course, you should have children. But I won't be able to give them to you. It's too late for me. But I won't be standing in your way when you feel that you are ready for your children'. And he felt safe with that. (*Anna*, 54 years, married)

Most women interviewed deemed this type of agreement as impossible or at least highly undesirable. Almost all of the women had past experiences from which they had learnt how difficult it was to become involved with a man who wants children. These experiences had taught them to avoid such involvements in the future. Sara shared her relief of sharing intimacy goals with her current partner: 'Thankfully I've met a man who doesn't want kids' (*Sara*, 30 years, cohabiting). She continued, sharing her experience of having a previous relationship ending due to conflicting intimacy goals: 'It's been a problem in earlier relationships. One boyfriend left me because he wanted kids in the future' (*Sara*, 30 years, cohabiting). Although the dissolution of relationships could be a painful experience, Sara affirmed that the decision was necessary in a situation where partners have conflicting intimacy goals.

Disbelief and Relationship Dissolution

It was of utmost importance for these women that their partner would not try to persuade them to change their decision to remain childfree. What was likewise important for them was that they did not prevent their partner from reaching their intimacy goals. Tina shared her experience from a previous relationship:

> I once dated a man who wanted kids. It was his greatest wish. I felt that as long as we're a couple I prevented him from fulfilling that wish so it didn't work out. (*Tina*, 33 years, cohabiting)

In the end, Tina terminated the relationship with this man, as they were not compatible in this important aspect.

Sometimes, however, the women were mistaken when they thought that they had an understanding with their partner. Even when they had an explicit agreement with their partner not to have children, this was no guarantee that future disagreements would not arise (see Gillespie, 2000). Despite them being explicit about their childfree decision, several of the women had previously been involved with a partner who wanted children and had expected them to change their mind:

> I've dated men who want children. I've told them early on that I don't want any but they think they can make me change my mind. (*Julia*, 39 years, cohabiting)

Two of the women narrated how diverging intimacy goals had destroyed their marriages and ended in divorce. One of the women had married a man thinking they had an agreement about remaining childfree. After the marriage, however, she found out that he disbelieved her commitment to her decision: 'He thought I would change my mind' (*Kirsten*, 36 years, cohabiting). They ended up getting a divorce after being married for seven months because she knew she would never change her mind and she wanted to give him the chance to have children with someone else:

> I insisted on the divorce. Because he loves kids and couldn't imagine a life without them. [...] I didn't see any options. He wanted us to try but I told him: 'But why should we waste each other's time? It's better you find a younger woman that can give you kids' [laughter]. So he didn't have any choice. He had to give in. (*Kirsten*, 36 years, single)

One of the women had an explanation to why some men seemed reluctant to believe the women when they first shared with them that their intimacy goals involved remaining childless:

> Most childless people in their 30s are a bit desperate to find someone to have a kid with. Many of them say they don't want kids and that it's not that much of a deal but people don't believe them – not prospective employers and not prospective boyfriends. You have to be really clear about that this is not on the map. (*Clara*, 44 years, single)

This quote, like many of the earlier ones, illustrates well how deviating from the expected status transitions and having preferences that deviate from the great majority pose challenges for voluntarily childless women and restrict their partnership formation processes.

Concluding Discussion

This chapter has contributed to previous research by investigating voluntarily childless women's preferences regarding partners and partnerships, a topic that has so far been neglected in research on voluntary childlessness and in research on partner preferences. The analysis contributes to the existing body of literature on voluntary childlessness by revealing how remaining single was not, contrary to what has been suggested in previous research (see Dykstra & Hagestad, 2007; Houseknecht, 1987), an appealing option for most of the women interviewed. In sharp contrast to this existing perception, the voluntarily childless women emphasised their desire to form an intimate relationship with a man.

The results, however, also illustrate how those relationship formation processes; that is building and maintaining a romantic relationship with a significant partner, proved to be challenging and problematic for many of these women. Partner formation processes were associated with several different challenges, difficulties and risks (see Lewis, 2006). First of all, being aware of the risks with trying to form and sustain a relationship as a non-mutual couple (see Lee & Zvonkovic, 2014), the women interviewed primarily searched for a partner who also pursued a childfree lifestyle. The problems with finding such a partner were also numerous, most fundamentally the scarcity of childfree men. The women were aware that they were seeking a relationship strikingly different from the expectations on transitioning into a monogamous, heterosexual relationship that ultimately, and ideally, would lead to marriage and children. Becoming part of a relationship where the partners had a mutual agreement to remain childless also involved several different risks. The women described how they had to consider how and when to disclose lack of childbearing intentions. Another risk was not only men's ambivalence regarding childbearing intentions, but also that such intentions can change over time. Risk awareness also existed regarding the possibility that an intimate partner could disbelieve the women's commitment to their childfree decision. Some of the voluntarily childless women had experienced relationships where they had been under the false impression they had a mutual agreement with their partner, while in reality they were a non-mutual couple. In a couple of instances, this false impression led the woman to enter marriage with her partner. The dissonance in these non-mutual couples, however, with only one rare exception, always resulted in the end of the relationship. In that rare exception, however, the dissolution of the relationship was only postponed.

The results highlight how the women's non-conformist fertility behaviour and partnership preferences influenced their partner preferences. Although their ideal 'Mr Right' shared their intimacy goals, the reality of the dating scene made some women adjust their partner preferences to include men who had already fathered children. Some of the women also expressed ambivalence about their commitment to their own intimacy goal and suggested that initiating a relationship with 'Mr Wrong'; that is a man with divergent intimacy goal, could make them sway from their decision. The inconsistency of men's intimacy goals and what the women understood as men's difficulties to articulate and communicate straightforwardly about intimacy goals further complicated relationship initiations and partnership formations.

The analysis in this chapter also contributes to the on-going discussion about gendered preferences concerning work and family. The results suggest that the voluntarily childless women were forced to adjust their partner preferences in relation to their partnership preferences and that their preference to become involved in a partnership formation process was given precedence before the preference for an ideal partner. These results further nuance previous findings about women's preferences and constraints and women's strategies to manage such constraints. Due to these constraints, the women suggested that carefully weighed up, and rational decisions would increase their chances of finding 'Mr Right'.

Acknowledgements

The author wishes to thank the voluntarily childless women and men who made this research possible by their participation. The research was supported by a financial grant from Forte: The Swedish Research Council for Health, Working Life and Welfare. Reviewer comments on an earlier version of the text are gratefully acknowledged.

References

Abma, J. C., & Martinez, G. M. (2006). Childlessness among older women in the United States: Trends and profiles. *Journal of Marriage and Family*, *68*(4), 1045–1056.

Allan, G. (2001). Personal relationships in late modernity. *Personal Relationships*, *8*, 325–339.

Avison, M., & Furnham, A. (2015). Personality and voluntary childlessness. *Journal of Population Research*, *32*, 45–67.

Bartholomaeus, C., & Riggs, D. W. (2017). Daughters and their mothers: The reproduction of pronatalist discourses across generations. *Women's Studies International Forum*, *62*, 1–7.

Bredow, C. A. (2015). Chasing prince charming: Partnering consequences of holding unrealistic standards for a spouse. *Personal Relationships*, *22*, 476–501.

Dykstra, P. A., & Hagestad, G. (2007). Roads less taken: Developing a nuanced view of older adults without children. *Journal of Family Issues*, *28*(10), 1275–1310.

Eurostat. (2015). *People in the EU: Who are we and how do we live?* (Eurostat. Statistical books, 2015 ed.). Luxembourg: Publications Office of the European Union.

Frisén, A., Carlsson, J., & Wängqvist, M. (2014). 'Doesn't everyone want that? It's just a give': Swedish emerging adults' expectations on future parenthood and work/family priorities. *Journal of Adolescent Research*, *29*(1), 67–88.

Gillespie, R. (2000). When no means no: Disbelief, disregard and deviance as discourses of voluntary childlessness. *Women's Studies International Forum*, *23*(2), 223–234.

Hakim, C. (2000). *Work-lifestyle choices in the 21st century: Preference theory*. Oxford: Oxford University Press.

Hakim, C. (2003a). A new approach to explaining fertility patterns: Preference theory. *Population and Development Review*, *29*(3), 349–374.

Hakim, C. (2003b). Public morality versus personal choice: The failure of social attitude surveys. *British Journal of Sociology*, *54*(3), 339–345.

Hakim, C. (2006). Women, careers and work-life preferences. *British Journal of Guidance & Counselling*, *34*(3), 279–294.

Heaton, T. B., Jacobson, C. K., & Holland, K. (1999). Persistence and change in decisions to remain childless. *Journal of Marriage and the Family*, *61*(2), 531–539.

Houseknecht, S. K. (1987). Voluntary childlessness. In M. B. Sussman & S. K. Steinmetz (Eds.), *Handbook of family and marriage* (pp. 369–395). New York and London: Plenum Press.

Kan, M. Y. (2007). Work orientation and wives' employment careers. An evaluation of Hakim's preference theory. *Work and Occupation*, *34*(4), 430–462.

Keizer, R., Dykstra, P. A., & Jansen, M. D. (2007). Pathways into childlessness: Evidence of gendered life course dynamics. *Journal of Biosocial Sciences*, *40*(6), 863–878.

Kemkes-Grottenthaler, A. (2003). Postponing or rejecting parenthood? Results of a survey among female academic professionals. *Journal of Biosocial Science*, *35*(2), 213–226.

Koropeckyj-Cox, T., & Pendell, G. (2007). The gender gap in attitudes about childlessness in the United States. *Journal of Marriage and Family*, *69*(4), 899–915.

Koyama, N. F., McGain, A., & Hill, R. A. (2004). Self-reported mate preferences and 'feminist' attitudes regarding marital relations. *Evolution and Human Behaviour*, *25*, 327–335.

Lee, K.-H., & Zvonkovic, A. M. (2014). Journeys to remain childless: A grounded theory examination of decision-making processes among voluntarily childless couples. *Journal of Social and Personal Relationships*, *31*(4), 535–553.

Letherby, G., & Williams, C. (1999). Non-motherhood: Ambivalent autobiographies. *Feminist Studies*, *25*(3), 719–747.

Lewis, J. (2006). Perceptions of risk in intimate relationships. *Journal of Social Policy*, *35*(1), 39–57.

McRae, S. (2003). Constraints and choices in mothers' employment careers: A consideration of Hakim's preference theory. *British Journal of Sociology*, *54*(3), 317–338.

Mulder, C. H. (2003). The effects of singlehood and cohabitation on the transition to parenthood in the Netherlands. *Journal of Family Issues*, *24*(3), 291–313.

Mullins, A. R. (2016). *'I kid you not, I am asked a question about children at least once a week': Exploring differences in childbearing habitus in pronatalist fields.* Dissertation, University of Central Florida.

Nilsson, K., Hammarström, A., & Strandh, M. (2017). The relationship between work and family preferences and behaviours: A longitudinal study of gender differences in Sweden. *Acta Sociologica*, *60*(2), 120–133.

Park, K. (2002). Stigma management among the voluntarily childless. *Sociological Perspectives*, *45*(1), 21–45.

Park, K. (2005). Choosing childlessness: Weber's typology of action and motives of the voluntarily childless. *Sociological Inquiry*, *75*(3), 372–402.

Persson, L. (2010). Barnlöshet i siffror. In K. Engwall & H. Peterson (Eds.), *Frivillig barnlöshet. Barnfrihet i en nordisk context* (pp. 43–58). Stockholm: Dialogos.

Peterson, H. (2011). Barnfri: En stigmatiserad position. *Sociologisk Forskning*, *48*(3), 5–26.

Peterson, H. (2015). Fifty shades of freedom: Voluntary childlessness as women's ultimate liberation. *Women's Studies International Forum*, *53*, 182–191.

Peterson, H. (2017). 'I will never be a housewife': Refusing to have children in Sweden. *Travail, Genre et Sociétés*, *37*(1), 71–89.

Peterson, H., & Engwall, K. (2013). Silent bodies: Voluntary childless women's gendered and embodied experiences. *European Journal of Women's Studies*, *20*(4), 376–389.

Peterson, H., & Engwall, K. (2015). Missing out on the parenthood bonus? Voluntarily childless in a 'child-friendly' society. *Journal of Family and Economic Issues*, *36*(4), 540–552.

Rijken, A. J., & Merz, E.-M. (2014). Double standards: Differences in norms on voluntary childlessness for men and women. *European Sociological Review*, *30*(4), 470–482.

Sanderson, C. A., Keiter, E. J., Miles, M. G., & Yopuk, D. J. A. (2007). The association between intimacy goals and plans for initiating dating relationship. *Personal Relationships*, *14*, 225–243.

Tanaka, K., & Johnson, N. E. (2016). Childlessness and mental well-being in a global context. *Journal of Family Issues*, *37*(8): 1027–1045.

Tanturri, M. L., & Mencarini, L. (2008). Childless or childfree? Paths to voluntary childlessness in Italy. *Population and Development Review*, *34*(1), 51–77.

Thomas, A. G., & Stewart-Williams, S. (2018). Mating strategy flexibility in the laboratory: Preferences for long- and short-term mating change in response to evolutionary relevant variables. *Evolution and Human Behaviour*, *39*(1), 82–93

Veevers, J. E. (1979). Voluntary childlessness: A review of issues and evidence. *Marriage and Family Review*, *2*(2), 1–26.

Vitali, A., Billari, F. C., Prskawetz, A., & Testa, M. R. (2009). Preference theory and low fertility: A comparative perspective. *European Journal of Population*, *25*(4), 413–438.

Chapter 11

Understanding the Employment Experiences of Women with No Children

Beth Turnbull, Melissa Graham and Ann Taket

Abstract

Whether or not women have children has profound consequences for their employment experiences. Employers may see women with no children as conforming more closely than women with children (and yet not as closely as male employees) to the pervasive 'ideal worker' stereotype of a full-time, committed worker with no external responsibilities. However, managers and co-workers may also perceive women with no children as deviating from prevailing pronatalist norms in Australian and other comparable societies, which construct and value women as mothers and stigmatise and devalue women with no children. Accordingly, women with no children may be rewarded or penalised in different employment contexts at different times according to the degree to which they conform to or deviate from the most salient characteristics associated with the ideal worker and mothering femininity. This chapter explores patriarchal and capitalist configurations of femininities, masculinities and workers as drivers of employment experiences among women with no children. It then discusses empirical research from Australia and comparable countries, in order to elucidate the diversity of employment experiences among women with no children.

Keywords: Employment; women without children; pronatalism; femininities; ideal worker; Australia

Introduction

Whether women have or do not have children has profound consequences for their employment experiences. Much existing research compares the employment outcomes of women with and without children, suggesting women with children are disadvantaged in relation to a range of indicators. While it is important to expose the disadvantage faced by women with children, the foregrounding of their experiences serves to negate the discrimination experienced by all women, as well as silence, invalidate and homogenise the employment experiences of women without children. This chapter applies a feminist lens to the employment experiences of women without children and explores patriarchal and capitalist configurations of femininities, masculinities and workers as key influences. Within this theoretical context, it then positions research from Australia and comparable countries about employment experiences among women without children as agents who perform gendered identities within employment contexts. Given the structures and discourses of patriarchy and capitalism are unique within their political, economic, cultural and social contexts, this chapter focuses on the Australian experience. However, the discussion is likely to be relevant to comparable countries. Illustrative quotations throughout this chapter are from a mixed-methods study conducted in Australia during 2014, in which with 776 women aged 25–44 years without children completed a self-administered questionnaire including closed and open-ended questions (Turnbull, Graham, & Taket, 2016a, 2017).

Theoretical Context: Structures and Discourses of Gender Influencing the Employment Experiences of Women without Children

Patriarchal and capitalist configurations of femininities, masculinities and workers are key drivers of employment experiences (Connell, 1987) among women with no children, although intersections with other power relations, such as class, race, ethnicity, religion, age and ability, produce diverse experiences that cannot be understood by recourse to gender alone (Butler, 2011; Collins, 2000). This chapter conceptualises gender as socially and discursively configured at interacting levels, including how individuals' and groups' performances, identities, opportunities and relationships are shaped by, or resist, the gendered structures and discourses of organisations and societies (Bottero, 2004; Butler, 2011; Connell, 2005c; Skeggs, 1997; Smith, 1987; Wright, 2005).

The power relations of patriarchy and capitalism entail the exercise of power by men over women and capitalists over workers. However, hierarchies also exist within multiplicities of workers, femininities and masculinities (Connell & Messerschmidt, 2005; Gramsci, 1971). Hegemonic configurations of femininities, masculinities and workers contribute to the maintenance of the prevailing patriarchal and capitalist orders (Connell, 2005c; Gramsci, 1971). Such maintenance requires complex relations of hegemony, alliance, compliance, subordination, marginalisation and resistance, between and within hegemonic and alternative femininities and masculinities (Connell, 1987). While Connell (1987) argues for the existence of emphasised rather than hegemonic femininity, Schippers (2007) argues there is a hegemonic configuration of femininity which, 'establish[es] and legitimat[es] a hierarchical and complementary relationship to hegemonic masculinity' (2007, p. 94). Other femininities are constructed against the idealised relationship between dominant masculinity and subordinate femininity (Schippers, 2007). The following sections of this chapter will discuss evidence of configurations of hegemonic and non-hegemonic workers and femininities, and how such configurations influence the employment experiences of women without children.

Societal-level Configurations Influencing the Employment Experiences of Women without Children

In Australian and comparable societies, 'citizen-worker' and pronatalist discourses interact to influence the employment experiences of women without children. From the inception of capitalism, jobs were predicated on the paid productive labour of full-time male workers with no external responsibilities, and the unpaid reproductive labour of full-time wives/mothers caring for husbands/workers and reproducing and nurturing future workers (Acker, 1988; Glenn, 1999). Assumptions that men are breadwinners and women are mothers continue to influence modern femininities and masculinities (Connell, 1987). However, neoliberal restructuring of capitalist economies has resulted in a shift to a 'universal adult worker' model (Lewis & Giullari, 2005; Manne, 2005). Neoliberalism configures hegemonic 'citizen-workers' as full-time paid workers, who achieve citizenship, social worth, self-actualisation and identity through dedication to work (Fryer & Stambe, 2014; Lewis & Giullari, 2005).

Despite being purportedly gender-neutral, feminist scholars argue the citizen-worker is highly gendered. Blair-Loy (2003) has argued the 'work-devotion schema' of the full-time, dedicated employee who derives meaning and identity from paid work, is associated with masculinity; while the 'family-devotion schema', in which fulfilment and meaning are achieved through devotion to and caring for children, husbands and homes, is associated with femininity. These powerful configurations contribute to the constraints within which women 'perform' gender (Blair-Loy, 2003; Butler, 2011; Connell, 1987).

Pronatalist structures, ideologies and discourses, which promote fertility by configuring hegemonic femininity as mothering femininity, are core to the constraints upon women's performances of gender (Gillespie, 2001; Letherby, 1994, 1999). Pronatalism manifests in ideologies, discourses and policies that construct motherhood as a moral, patriotic and economic duty; and cultures perceiving motherhood as natural, innate and inevitable, women's primary identity and role, and essential to women's attainment of maturity, completeness and fulfilment (Gillespie, 2000, 2003; Graham & Rich, 2012a; Letherby, 1994; Park, 2002). Although pronatalism rhetorically values motherhood (Letherby, 1999, 2002), it contributes to hegemonic configurations of submissive, self-sacrificing and caring mothering femininity, in support of the maintenance of hegemonic masculinity and the patriarchal order (Bown, Sumsion, & Press, 2011).

Analyses of government policy, as well as media, professional, scientific, religious and political rhetoric, have found pronatalist discourses are dominant in modern Western societies (Gillespie, 2000, 2001; Letherby, 1999; Peterson, 2014). Studies analysing Australian policies and political and media rhetoric have revealed a strong pronatalist agenda promoting fertility by rewarding, removing obstacles to, or valorising motherhood, and configuring motherhood as feminine, natural and patriotic (Ainsworth & Cutcher, 2008; Baird & Cutcher, 2005; Broomhill & Sharp, 2005; Dever, 2005; Graham, McKenzie, Lamaro, & Klein, 2016; Heard, 2006; Sawer, 2013). On the other side of pronatalism is the policing, silencing and subordination of femininities without children. Pronatalist discourses configure femininities without children as abnormal, unnatural, incomplete and failed femininities who are inferior to hegemonic mothering femininity (Gillespie, 2001, 2003; Letherby, 2002). Analyses of Australian political and media rhetoric have revealed discourses of women without children as selfish, immature, hedonistic, career-focused, blameworthy and failing to contribute to society (Dever, 2005; Graham & Rich, 2012a, 2012b; Heard, 2006;

Sawer, 2013). Stereotypes of women without children as career-oriented, reveal citizen-worker and pronatalist discourses as the two hegemonic discourses influencing configurations of femininities. In the absence of motherhood, neoliberalism configures femininities without children solely as 'career women', who are committed, competitive and ambitious, and have no external responsibilities (Wager, 2000). Such configurations have important implications for the employment experiences of women without children.

Organisational Contexts Influencing Employment Experiences

Societally hegemonic configurations of citizen-workers and mothering femininity interact to influence organisational contexts and individual experiences. This section discusses organisational contexts influencing the employment experiences of women without children.

Although there may be broad similarities between organisations as a result of societal-level configurations, organisations' processes will be unique within their individual contexts. Such contexts include the industries and sectors within which organisations operate, as well as internal processes within organisations (Acker, 1990; Connell, 1987; Gallie, 2007). In relation to internal processes, feminist theorists argue modern organisations are deeply gendered (Acker, 1988; Connell, 1987). Acker (1990) and Connell (2005a) identify processes by which organisations are gendered, including divisions of labour such as physical and occupational segregation; symbolism, culture and discourses; power relations and hierarchies; emotional and human relations; and individual performances of identities. Acker (1990, p. 149) argues these processes construct an 'abstract worker' who exists only for work, and most closely resembles a full-time male worker whose life revolves around his work (Acker, 1990, p. 149). In turn, it is assumed all women are mothers with conflicting external responsibilities (Acker, 1990).

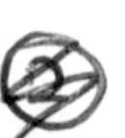

In accordance with Acker's (1990) argument, a wealth of evidence reveals that organisational structures, discourses and cultures configuring the hegemonic 'ideal worker', pervade private and public sector organisations in a wide range of industries (Blair-Loy, 2003; Cahusac & Kanji, 2014; Charlesworth & Baird, 2007; Chesterman & Ross-Smith, 2010; Devine, Grummell, & Lynch, 2011; Lewis & Humbert, 2010; Thornton, 2016). 'Ideal worker' discourses mandate long hours, visibility, availability, devotion and no external commitments (Blair-Loy, 2003; Charlesworth & Baird, 2007; Lewis & Humbert, 2010). The 'ideal

worker' remains a heavily gendered construct. Reflecting Acker's (1990) argument, research suggests assumptions that men are ideal workers devoted to careers, and women are mothers devoted to family, continue to influence women's employment experiences whether or not they have children (Blair-Loy, 2003; Cahusac & Kanji, 2014; Kelan, 2014; Lewis & Humbert, 2010; Pocock, 2003; Wajcman, 1998). Similarly, gender essentialist discourses linked with mothering femininity and breadwinning masculinity, such as submissive, nurturing and empathic femininity and dominant, aggressive, competitive and rational masculinity, influence assumptions about employed women regardless of whether they have children (Broughton & Miller, 2009; Devine et al., 2011). Beyond the ideal worker, there is also evidence in some organisations of 'macho' workplace cultures, which advantage men and disadvantage women, including: 'boys' networks'; the valuing of stereotypically masculine characteristics and devaluing of stereotypically feminine characteristics; and penalising women who fail to conform to gender stereotypes through, for example, being negatively judged as being less likeable and competent than, and not as likely to succeed, as men (Broughton & Miller, 2009; Cahusac & Kanji, 2014; Charlesworth & Baird, 2007; Devine et al., 2011; Genat, Wood, & Sojo, 2012; Kelan, 2014). The organisational structures and discourses of ideal workers, femininities and masculinities outlined in this section facilitate an understanding of the employment experiences among women without children, as discussed in the following section.

Employment Experiences among Women without Children

Societally and organisationally hegemonic configurations of workers and femininities interact to influence the employment experiences of women without children. Femininities without children may in some ways be advantaged within employment due to their perceived capacity to contribute as citizen-workers. Conversely, femininities without children can be stereotyped as career women with no lives outside work, and experience stigmatisation for deviating from hegemonic femininity. This section outlines evidence of positive, mixed and negative consequences influenced by assumptions that women without children are 'ideal workers' and 'deviant' femininities; then explores evidence of diverse performances of employed femininities without children.

'Benefits' of Conforming to the 'Ideal Worker' Stereotype: Employment Participation, Income, Occupational Status and Career Progression

> A work colleague fell ill and someone was needed to fly to Brisbane for three days to cover a conference – not having kids/pets/partner meant I could immediately put up my hand for the opportunity. (ID 224; Undecided about having children; 32 years)

A large body of research provides evidence on the employment participation, income, occupational status and career progression of women without children. Much of this research compares women with and without children, and emphasises the disadvantages faced by women with children. Research about employment participation highlights that women without children are more likely to work in full-time employment than women with children (Gash, 2009). However, broadening the comparison to include men reveals continuing gender differences in employment participation. Australian and international evidence suggests men with children are the most likely to work full-time, followed by men without children, women without children and women with children (Misra, Budig, & Boeckmann, 2011; Travaglione & Chang, 2012).

The majority of evidence from Australia and comparable countries suggests men with and without children are paid more than women, regardless of whether women have children; and that women without children are paid more than women with children (see, for example, Cooke, 2014; Gash, 2009; Parr, 2005; Petersen, Penner, & Hogsnes, 2007; Watson, 2010; Whitehouse, 2002). Such research frequently highlights findings that women without children are paid higher individual incomes than women with children. Such an emphasis disguises the continuing pay gap between men and women. Moreover, comparisons between women with and without children serve to homogenise women without children as high-income earners. In contrast, the authors' research with women without children revealed 16.6% of participants aged 25–44 years, and 17% of participants aged 45–64 years, were paid low or lower-middle incomes, with some women describing low incomes as a barrier to having children (Turnbull et al., 2016a; Turnbull, Graham, & Taket, 2016b).

The pattern of comparing women with and without children continues when shifting the focus to occupational status and career progression, although findings are less consistent. One Australian study found women with no biological children were more likely than women with biological children to work as doctors, lawyers, vets and dentists (Miranti, McNamara, Tanton, & Yap, 2009). Similarly, European research found women without children were more likely than women with children to work in highly skilled professions (Gash, 2009). However, another Australian study found no difference in the likelihood of women without and with children working in professional occupations (Parr, 2005).

Evidence on career progression is similarly inconclusive. Australian research found marital and parental status affected career progression: single employees without children progressed less than married employees with and without children; and single employees with children progressed more than single employees without children (Tharenou, 1999). Overall, marital status affected career advancement more than parental status (Tharenou, 1999). However, this finding may have been influenced by measuring marital status rather than partner status. United States studies have, in contrast, found no differences in the advancement of women with and without children, regardless of marital status (Miree & Frieze, 1999; Schneer & Reitman, 2002). On the other hand, a United Kingdom study found the careers of women without children progressed at similar rates to those of men, and faster than those of full-time and part-time employed women with children (Jacobs, 1999). When shifting the comparison to men and women, a Norwegian study found single women without children were promoted at lower rates than single men without children, while married women with children were promoted at lower rates than married men with children (Petersen et al., 2007).

Beyond measuring employment outcomes, it is essential to explore the perspectives of women without children in order to understand their employment experiences. Research suggests being in a high-status occupation can exclude some women from having children (Baker, 2010; Cannold, 2005; Chesterman & Ross-Smith, 2010; Pocock, 2003; Wood & Newton, 2006). Australian and international studies found that women perceived having children as an impediment to women's (but not men's) career progression in light of the pressure to conform to the 'ideal worker' stereotype, and some women had to sacrifice having children for their careers (Chesterman & Ross-Smith, 2010; Wajcman, 1998; Wood & Newton, 2006).

The body of research on employment participation, income, occupational status and career progression suggests women without children can be advantaged compared to women with children. Such advantages may be influenced by perceptions women without children conform more closely than women with children to ideal worker configurations. However, women without children continue to be disadvantaged compared to men, indicating that having children is not the only factor that disadvantages women in employment. Societally and organisationally hegemonic configurations of mothering femininity influence assumptions that all women are mothers and thus non-ideal workers with external commitments (Wajcman, 1998).

Mixed Consequences of Being 'Ideal Workers' and 'Deviant' Women: Discrimination and Stereotyping

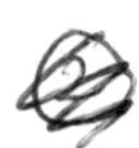

> Because I have a good job and a successful career, people assume I made a choice not to have children because I was too career focused and driven. (ID 416; involuntarily childless; 43 years)

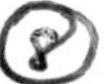

Differences in women and men's recruitment, retention, promotion and remuneration are partially explicable by discrimination against women (Watson, 2010). Evidence suggests women with children face greater discrimination than women without children (Carney, 2009). Studies in Australia and the United States asking undergraduate and postgraduate students to evaluate job applicants, have found participants were more likely to recommend women without children for hiring, promotion and training than women with children (Cuddy, Fiske, & Glick, 2004; Fuegen, Biernat, Haines, & Deaux, 2004; Heilman & Okimoto, 2008). Interestingly, such studies also found participants were more likely to recommend women without children for hiring, promotion and training, than men without and with children (Cuddy et al., 2004; Fuegen et al., 2004; Heilman & Okimoto, 2008). Such recommendations may have been influenced by perceptions that women without children, by sacrificing opportunities to have children, actively demonstrated their commitment to being ideal workers to a degree that exceeded men's default ideal worker status.

In the same series of studies, women without children were rated as more committed (Fuegen et al., 2004; Heilman & Okimoto, 2008), competent (Cuddy et al., 2004; Heilman & Okimoto, 2008), driven (Koropeckyj-Cox, Çopur, Romano, & Cody-Rydzewski, 2015), available (Fuegen et al., 2004) and striving to achieve more (Heilman & Okimoto, 2008) than women with children. In relation to work-related agency, some studies found women without children were rated as more agentic than women with children (Fuegen et al., 2004; Heilman & Okimoto, 2008), while another study found no difference (LaMastro, 2001).

Heilman and Okimoto (2008) conducted two studies comparing women without children to men. The first study found undergraduate students rated women without children as less committed than men without children, but more committed than men with children. The second study found employed postgraduate students rated women without children to be as committed as men without children, but more committed than men with children. Women without children were rated to be equally as competent as men with and without children by undergraduate and postgraduate students. The second study measured additional variables, and found that postgraduate students rated women without children to be equally as agentic as men with and without children, and striving to achieve more than men with children and as much as men without children. While such stereotypes may benefit women without children in terms of career opportunities, stereotypes of being committed and available also feed into assumptions that women without children are solely workers, invalidating their non-work lives. Reflecting this, research from the perspectives of women without children reveals nuanced experiences of discrimination and stereotyping within employment, many of which reflect perceptions of women without children as 'ideal workers' with no external life, interests, commitments or responsibilities. Women without children have described feeling discriminated against in relation to employers': prioritisation of the non-work needs of employees with children; expectations that women without children will cover for people with children by working longer and unsocial hours, inconvenient shifts, weekends and holidays; failure to recognise the non-work responsibilities of women without children; and expectations that women without children will undertake additional work such as supporting colleagues, committee representation and organising meetings, because they are perceived to have more time than women with children (Dixon & Dougherty, 2014; Doyle, Pooley, & Breen, 2013; Peterson & Engwall, 2015; Turnbull et al., 2016a, 2017). Research from Australia, the United Kingdom and the United States further suggests some women felt having no children affected their career opportunities, sometimes due to doubts about their professional credibility and assumptions they could not work with parents or children, sometimes because employers thought employment or promotion was more important for people with children, and sometimes due to assumptions that all women are mothers and women without children would therefore have children in future (see e.g. Dixon & Dougherty, 2014; Kelan, 2014; Rich, Taket, Graham, & Shelley, 2011; Turnbull et al., 2016a).

It is important to acknowledge that, along with stereotypes that can 'benefit' women without children due to their perceived conformance to ideal-worker configurations, employed women without children can also experience negative stereotypes. For example, United States undergraduate students rated professional women without children as less warm than professional women and men with children (Cuddy et al., 2004). Evidence abounds in the broader literature of stereotypes of women without children as less warm, nurturing, fulfilled and feminine than women with children, reflecting stigmatisation of women without children due to their non-conformance to hegemonic configurations of mothering femininity (see e.g. Gillespie, 2000; Letherby, 1999; Rich et al., 2011; Turnbull et al., 2016a, 2016b, 2017).

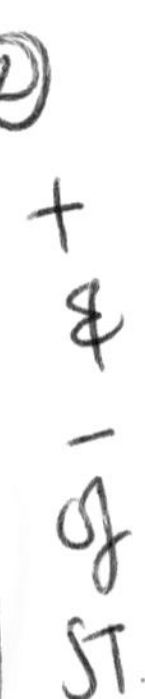

Negative Consequences of Being 'Ideal Workers' and 'Deviant' Women: Work–Life Balance and Access to Employment Benefits

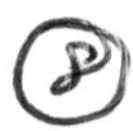

> I've worked full-time hours in condensed days for a number of years … The immediate response from managers, colleagues and clients has always been to think this odd as I don't have children. When I explain to them that there are other dimensions of my life that I pursue during my day off … the response has sometimes been perplexed, sometimes understanding and sometimes quite negatively judgemental. (ID 130; circumstantially childless; 44 years)

Research reveals inequalities in work-life balance and access to employment benefits facilitating work-life balance. Australian studies have found women with children report greater levels of work-life conflict than women without children (see e.g. Chapman, Skinner, & Pocock, 2014; Pocock, Skinner, & Pisaniello, 2010). In contrast, German and New Zealand studies have found no difference in the work-life conflict of women without and with children (Drobnič & Rodríguez, 2011; Haar, 2013), while a United States study found women without children reported less balance between work and home responsibilities than women with children (McNamee & James, 2012).

Comparisons between women without and with children can disguise the reality that women without children can and do experience work-life interference. In the authors' research with Australian women without children aged 25–64 years (Turnbull et al., 2016a, 2016b), participants reported experiencing work-life conflict. In line with this, Australian research suggests women without children work longer hours, and are more likely to prefer working fewer hours, than women with children (Chapman et al., 2014; Pocock et al., 2010). Research in the United States found employees without children were 25% more likely than employees with children to have low control over work hours (Swanberg, Pitt-Catsouphes, & Drescher-Burke, 2005).

The emphasis on promoting work-life balance for people with children can also mean women without children have limited access to flexible working arrangements. An Australian study found, although a quarter of women without children made requests for flexible arrangements, employers refused the requests of people without children at higher rates than people with children, suggesting employers saw the requests of people with children as more legitimate than those of people without children (Skinner & Pocock, 2011). Australian, United States and United Kingdom research similarly found women without children accessed fewer employment benefits than women with children; were more likely than women with children to report difficulties taking time off work for personal matters; and felt work-life policies, such as compassionate leave, carer's leave and flexible working arrangements, were targeted at or only available to employees with children (Bagilhole, 2006; Hamilton, Gordon, & Whelan-Berry, 2006; Swanberg et al., 2005; Turnbull et al., 2016a, 2017).

Positioning such findings within the context of hegemonic configurations of ideal workers and mothering femininity helps to elucidate the work-life experiences of women without children. Work-life balance policies are underpinned by understandings of 'life' as 'family' and 'family' as 'children' (Eikhof et al., 2007). Accordingly, such policies are targeted largely at women with children (Connell, 2005b; Lewis & Giullari, 2005). The prevailing assumption is women without children, who deviate from hegemonic configurations of mothering femininity, contribute solely as citizen-workers (Wager, 2000). While such women may have greater career opportunities, their work-life balance can suffer, as it is assumed they have no external life, responsibilities or interests with which to balance work, and any such responsibilities or interests are challenged or questioned (Smithson & Stokoe, 2005).

Negative Consequences of Being 'Deviant' Women: Workplace Social Interactions

> I cannot say at work that I feel tired if I have not had any sleep – I did this a few times and my colleagues with children made me feel bad – things said were 'at least you weren't up all night with a kid who was vomiting or crying' … [It] is not socially acceptable to say that I was up all night in silence staring at the wall worrying. (ID 089; circumstantially childless; 41 years)

A small but important body of research provides evidence on workplace social interactions experienced by women without children. Studies from Australia, New Zealand, the United Kingdom and Sweden found some women without children described feeling stressed, excluded, invisible, isolated, silenced and unable to contribute in workplaces where conversations about, and images of, families with children were ubiquitous, and conversations about alternative families were not welcome; while others reported experiencing hyper-visibility, such as uninvited and intrusive questioning about having no children, which drove some women to conceal this fact (Baker, 2010; Dixon & Dougherty, 2014). Women without children have also reported experiencing more workplace mistreatment, including exclusion, derogation and coercion, than women with children, men with children and men without children (Berdahl & Moon, 2013). Involuntarily childless women (those who wish to have children, but are unable to do so due to their own infertility (Daniluk, 2001)) have described experiencing workplaces revolving around people with children as exclusive, unsafe and distressing (Malik & Coulson, 2013; Wirtberg, 1999). Some women avoided workplace social interactions and functions as a result of such experiences (Turnbull et al., 2017). Such experiences reveal women without children can have highly negative experiences in workplace social contexts, where women's non-conformance to hegemonic mothering femininity may outweigh their perceived conformance to 'ideal worker' configurations, and result in social isolation and exclusion.

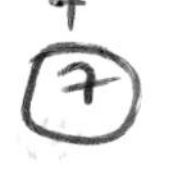

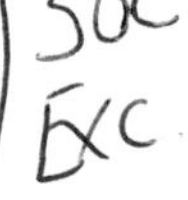

Individual Performances of Femininities without Children

> Career ambition (which I have) as opposed to marriage-and-children ambition (which I happily don't have) is

> viewed poorly. I feel that this really needs to change. (ID 719; voluntarily childless; 32 years)

Women without children are not merely passive receivers of the gendered and classed orders of organisations and societies. Instead, women actively 'perform' gender and class in ways that can be shaped by, or resist, the constraints of organisationally and societally hegemonic configurations of ideal workers and mothering femininity (Butler, 2011). Much of the research revealing how women without children perform gender has been conducted outside the employment context and reveals heterogeneity among women without children. For example, some studies have found involuntarily childless and circumstantially childless women (those who  do not have children due to external circumstances, such as career demands, financial insecurity, having no partner and partner infertility 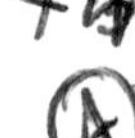 (Cannold, 2005)) can 'internalise' pronatalism and configure themselves as inadequate, incomplete, abnormal, shameful, disempowered, defective, failed and inferior femininities (Culley & Hudson, 2005; Letherby, 1999, 2002; Turnbull et al., 2016a). On the other hand, some involuntarily, circumstantially and voluntarily childless or 'childfree' women (those who freely choose not to have children, and are committed to their choice (Cannold, 2004, 2005; Veevers, 1979)) proactively perform positive femininities challenging hegemonic mothering femininity and emphasising other aspects of their identities (Daniluk, 1991; Doyle et al., 2013; Gillespie, 2003; Letherby, 2002; Maher & Saugeres, 2007; Park, 2002; Peterson & Engwall, 2013; Shaw, 2011; Turnbull et al., 2016a).

Research undertaken in the employment context reflects the diversity among women without children revealed in the broader literature. For example, an Australian study found female senior executives (a minority 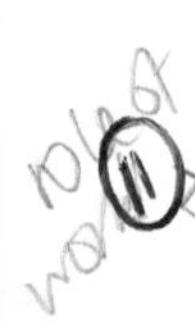 of whom did not have children) felt their work played a central role in their lives and identities (Chesterman & Ross-Smith, 2010). While some women (who might be perceived as circumstantially childless) forewent having children due to career pressures, others (who might be seen as voluntarily childless) had never considered having children in the face of their career devotion (Chesterman & Ross-Smith, 2010). However, in a Swedish study with voluntarily childless women, Peterson (2015) found only one woman identified herself as career-oriented, with the remaining women rejecting career-focused identities and embracing being childfree as providing the freedom to resign from jobs and not pursue a steady career. Thus, it is clear that women perform diverse  femininities without children; while some embrace ideal worker femininities, others perform alternative femininities that conform neither to configurations of the ideal worker nor mothering femininity.

Conclusion

Within the theoretical context of societally and organisationally hegemonic configurations of the ideal worker and mothering femininity, the extant body of research reveals the diverse employment experiences of women without children. Employers may see women without children as conforming more closely than women with children (and yet not as closely as male employees) to the pervasive 'ideal worker' stereotype of a full-time, committed worker with no external responsibilities. However, employers and co-workers may also perceive women without children as deviating from pronatalist configurations of mothering femininity, which construct and value women as mothers and stigmatise and devalue women without children. Accordingly, women without children may be rewarded or penalised in different employment contexts at different times according to the degree to which they conform to or deviate from the most salient characteristics associated with the ideal worker and mothering femininity. Importantly, the imposition of stereotypes of women without children as simultaneously 'ideal workers' and 'deviant women' with high incomes, high-flying careers and no families, interests or lives outside work, homogenises, silences and excludes women without children. It is essential that employers and co-workers challenge hegemonic configurations of ideal workers and mothering femininities within workplaces, which can be damaging to all women, and recognise the legitimacy of and cater to the diverse work and non-work needs of alternative configurations of women without children.

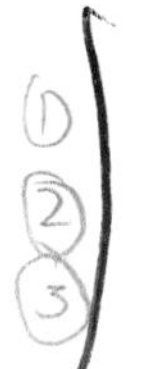

References

Acker, J. (1988). Class, gender, and the relations of distribution. *Signs: Journal of Women in Culture and Society*, *13*(3), 473–497.

Acker, J. (1990). Hierarchies, jobs, bodies: A theory of gendered organizations. *Gender & Society*, *4*(2), 139–158.

Ainsworth, S., & Cutcher, L. (2008). Expectant mothers and absent fathers: Paid maternity leave in Australia. *Gender, Work & Organization*, *15*(4), 375–393.

Bagilhole, B. (2006). Family-friendly policies and equal opportunities: A contradiction in terms? *British Journal of Guidance & Counselling*, *34*(3), 327–343.

Baird, M., & Cutcher, L. (2005). 'One for the father, one for the, other and one for the country': An examination of the construction of motherhood through the prism of paid maternity leave. *Hecate*, *31*(2), 103–113.

Baker, M. (2010). Motherhood, employment and the "child penalty". Paper presented at the Women's Studies International Forum.

Berdahl, J. L., & Moon, S. H. (2013). Workplace mistreatment of middle class workers based on sex, parenthood, and caregiving. *Journal of Social Issues*, *69*(2), 341–366.

Blair-Loy, M. (2003). *Competing devotions: Career and family among women executives*. Cambridge, MA: Harvard University Press.

Bottero, W. (2004). Class identities and the identity of class. *Sociology*, *38*(5), 985–1003.

Bown, K., Sumsion, J., & Press, F. (2011). Dark matter: The 'gravitational pull' of maternalist discourses on politicians' decision making for early childhood policy in Australia. *Gender and Education*, *23*(3), 263–280.

Broomhill, R., & Sharp, R. (2005). The changing male breadwinner model in Australia: A new gender order? *Labour & Industry: A Journal of the Social and Economic Relations of Work*, *16*(1), 103–127.

Broughton, A., & Miller, L. (2009). Women in senior management: Is the glass ceiling still intact. *Industrial Relations & Human Resources Journal*, *11*(4), 7–23.

Butler, J. (2011). *Gender trouble: Feminism and the subversion of identity*. New York, NY: Routledge.

Cahusac, E., & Kanji, S. (2014). Giving up: How gendered organizational cultures push mothers out. *Gender, Work & Organization*, *21*(1), 57–70.

Cannold, L. (2004). Declining marriage rates and gender inequity in social institutions: Towards an adequately complex explanation for childlessness. *People and Place*, *12*(4), 1–11.

Cannold, L. (2005). *What, no baby? Why women are losing the freedom to mother, and how they can get it back*. Fremantle: Curtin University Books.

Carney, T. (2009). The employment disadvantage of mothers: Evidence for systemic discrimination. *Journal of Industrial Relations*, *51*(1), 113–130.

Chapman, J., Skinner, N., & Pocock, B. (2014). Work–life interaction in the twenty-first century Australian workforce: Five years of the Australian Work and Life Index. *Labour & Industry: A Journal of the Social and Economic Relations of Work*, *24*(2), 87–102.

Charlesworth, S., & Baird, M. (2007). Getting gender on the agenda: The tale of two organisations. *Women in Management Review*, *22*(5), 391–404.

Chesterman, C., & Ross-Smith, A. (2010). Good executive, good mother: Contradictory devotions. In S. Goodwin & K. Huppatz (Eds.), *The good mother: Contemporary motherhoods in Australia* (pp. 25–50). Sydney: Sydney University Press.

Collins, P. H. (2000). *Black feminist thought: Knowledge, consciousness, and the politics of empowerment* (2nd ed.). New York, NY: Routledge, 2000.

Connell, R. (2005a). Advancing gender reform in large-scale organisations: A new approach for practitioners and researchers. *Policy and Society*, *24*(4), 5–24.

Connell, R. (2005b). A really good husband: Work/life balance, gender equity and social change. *Australian Journal of Social Issues*, *40*(3), 369.

Connell, R. W. (2005c). *Masculinities* (2nd ed.). Crows Nest: Allen & Unwin.

Connell, R. W. (1987). *Gender & power: Society, the person and sexual politics.* Sydney: Allen & Unwin.

Connell, R. W., & Messerschmidt, J. W. (2005). Hegemonic masculinity: Rethinking the concept. *Gender & Society*, *19*(6), 829–859.

Cooke, L. P. (2014). Gendered parenthood penalties and premiums across the earnings distribution in Australia, the United Kingdom, and the United States. *European Sociological Review*, *30*(3), 360–372.

Cuddy, A. J., Fiske, S. T., & Glick, P. (2004). When professionals become mothers, warmth doesn't cut the ice. *Journal of Social Issues*, *60*(4), 701–718.

Culley, L., & Hudson, N. (2005). Diverse bodies and disrupted reproduction: Infertility and minority ethnic communities in the UK. *International Journal of Diversity in Organisations, Communities and Nations*, *5*(2), 117–125.

Daniluk, J. C. (1991). Strategies for counseling infertile couples. *Journal of Counseling and Development*, *69*(4), 317–320.

Daniluk, J. C. (2001). Reconstructing their lives: A longitudinal, qualitative analysis of the transition to biological childlessness for infertile couples. *Journal of Counseling & Development*, *79*(4), 439–449.

Dever, M. (2005). Baby talk: The Howard government, families, and the politics of difference. *Hecate*, *31*(2), 45–61.

Devine, D., Grummell, B., & Lynch, K. (2011). Crafting the elastic self? Gender and identities in senior appointments in Irish education. *Gender, Work & Organization*, *18*(6), 631–649.

Dixon, J., & Dougherty, D. S. (2014). A language convergence/meaning divergence analysis exploring how LGBTQ and single employees manage traditional family expectations in the workplace. *Journal of Applied Communication Research*, *42*(1), 1–19.

Doyle, J., Pooley, J. A., & Breen, L. (2013). A phenomenological exploration of the childfree choice in a sample of Australian women. *Journal of Health Psychology*, *18*(3), 397–407.

Drobnič, S., & Rodríguez, A. M. G. (2011). Tensions between work and home: Job quality and working conditions in the institutional contexts of Germany and Spain. *Social Politics: International Studies in Gender, State & Society*, *18*(2), 232–268.

Eikhof, D. R., Warhurst, C., Haunschild, A., Ruth Eikhof, D., Warhurst, C., & Haunschild, A. (2007). Introduction: What work? What life? What balance? Critical reflections on the work-life balance debate. *Employee Relations*, *29*(4), 325–333.

Fryer, D., & Stambe, R. (2014). Work and the crafting of individual identities from a critical standpoint. *Australian Community Psychologist*, *26*(1), 8–17.

Fuegen, K., Biernat, M., Haines, E., & Deaux, K. (2004). Mothers and fathers in the workplace: How gender and parental status influence judgments of job-related competence. *Journal of Social Issues*, *60*(4), 737–754.

Gallie, D. (2007). Production regimes, employment regimes, and the quality of work. In D. Gallie (Ed.), *Employment regimes and the quality of work* (pp. 793–795). Oxford: Oxford University Press.

Gash, V. (2009). Sacrificing their careers for their families? An analysis of the penalty to motherhood in Europe. *Social Indicators Research*, *93*(3), 569–586.

Genat, A., Wood, R., & Sojo, V. (2012). *Evaluation bias and backlash: Dimensions, predictors and implications for organisations.* Melbourne: University of Melbourne.

Gillespie, R. (2000). When no means no: Disbelief, disregard and deviance as discourses of voluntary childlessness. *Women's Studies International Forum*, *23*(2), 223–234.

Gillespie, R. (2001). Contextualizing voluntary childlessness within a postmodern model of reproduction: Implications for health and social needs. *Critical Social Policy*, *21*(2), 139–159.

Gillespie, R. (2003). Childfree and feminine understanding the gender identity of voluntarily childless women. *Gender & Society*, *17*(1), 122–136.

Glenn, E. N. (1999). The social construction and institutionalisation of gender and race. In M. M. Ferree, J. Lorber, & B. B. Hess (Eds.), *Revisioning gender* (pp. 3–43). Thousand Oaks, CA: SAGE Publications.

Graham, M., McKenzie, H., Lamaro, G., & Klein, R. (2016). Women's reproductive choices in Australia: Mapping federal and state/territory policy instruments governing choice. *Gender Issues*, *33*(4), 335–349.

Graham, M., & Rich, S. (2012a). Representations of childless women in the Australian print media. *Feminist Media Studies*, *14*(3), 500–518.

Graham, M., & Rich, S. (2012b). *What's 'childless' got to do with it?* Working Paper No. 36. Geelong: Alfred Deakin Researh Institute, Deakin University.

Gramsci, A. (1971). *Selections from the prison notebooks.* London: Lawrence and Wishart.

Haar, J. M. (2013). Testing a new measure of work–life balance: A study of parent and non-parent employees from New Zealand. *The International Journal of Human Resource Management*, *24*(17), 3305–3324.

Hamilton, E. A., Gordon, J. R., & Whelan-Berry, K. S. (2006). Understanding the work-life conflict of never-married women without children. *Women in Management Review*, *21*(5), 393–415.

Heard, G. (2006). Pronatalism under Howard. *People and Place*, *14*(3), 12–25.

Heilman, M. E., & Okimoto, T. G. (2008). Motherhood: A potential source of bias in employment decisions. *Journal of Applied Psychology*, *93*(1), 189–198.

Jacobs, S. (1999). Trends in women's career patterns and in gender occupational mobility in Britain. *Gender, Work & Organization*, *6*(1), 32–46.

Kelan, E. K. (2014). From biological clocks to unspeakable inequalities: The intersectional positioning of young professionals. *British Journal of Management*, *25*(4), 790–804.

Koropeckyj-Cox, T., Çopur, Z., Romano, V., & Cody-Rydzewski, S. (2015). University students' perceptions of parents and childless or childfree couples. *Journal of Family Issues*. doi:0192513X15618993

LaMastro, V. (2001). Childless by choice? Attributions and attitudes concerning family size. *Social Behavior and Personality: An International Journal*, *29*(3), 231–243.

Letherby, G. (1994). Mother or not, mother or what?: Problems of definition and identity. *Women's Studies International Forum*, *17*(5), 525–532.

Letherby, G. (1999). Other than mother and mothers as others: The experience of motherhood and non-motherhood in relation to 'infertility' and 'involuntary childlessness'. *Women's Studies International Forum*, *22*(3), 359–372.

Letherby, G. (2002). Challenging dominant discourses: Identity and change and the experience of'infertility'and'involuntary childlessness'. *Journal of Gender Studies*, *11*(3), 277–288.

Lewis, J., & Giullari, S. (2005). The adult worker model family, gender equality and care: The search for new policy principles and the possibilities and problems of a capabilities approach. *Economy and Society*, *34*(1), 76–104.

Lewis, S., & Humbert, L. (2010). Discourse or reality?: 'Work-life balance', flexible working policies and the gendered organization. *Equality, Diversity and Inclusion: An International Journal*, *29*(3), 239–254.

Maher, J., & Saugeres, L. (2007). To be or not to be a mother? Women negotiating cultural representations of mothering. *Journal of Sociology*, *43*(1), 5–21.

Malik, S. H., & Coulson, N. S. (2013). Coming to terms with permanent involuntary childlessness: A phenomenological analysis of bulletin board postings. *Europe's Journal of Psychology*, *9*(1), 77–92.

Manne, A. (2005). Motherhood and the spirit of the new capitalism. *Arena Journal*, *24*, 37–67.

McNamee, B. G., & James, G. D. (2012). The impact of child-rearing status on perceptual and behavioural predictors of ambulatory blood pressure variation among working women. *Annals of Human Biology*, *39*(6), 490–498.

Miranti, R., McNamara, J., Tanton, R., & Yap, M. (2009). A narrowing gap? Trends in the childlessness of professional women in Australia 1986–2006. *Journal of Population Research*, *26*(4), 359–379.

Miree, C. E., & Frieze, I. H. (1999). Children and careers: A longitudinal study of the impact of young children on critical career outcomes of MBAs. *Sex Roles*, *41*(11–12), 787–808.

Misra, J., Budig, M. J., & Boeckmann, I. (2011). Cross-national patterns in individual and household employment and work hours by gender and parenthood. *Research in the Sociology of Work*, *22*, 169–207.

Park, K. (2002). Stigma management among the voluntarily childless. *Sociological Perspectives*, *45*(1), 21–45.

Parr, N. J. (2005). Family background, schooling and childlessness in Australia. *Journal of Biosocial Science*, *37*(2), 229–243.

Petersen, T., Penner, A., & Hogsnes, G. (2007). *From motherhood penalties to fatherhood premia: The new challenge for family policy*. Berkeley, CA: Institute for Research on Labor and Employment.

Peterson, H. (2014). Absent non-fathers: Gendered representations of voluntary childlessness in Swedish newspapers. *Feminist Media Studies*, *14*(1), 22–37.

Peterson, H. (2015). Fifty shades of freedom. Voluntary childlessness as women's ultimate liberation. *Women's Studies International Forum*, *53*, 182–191.

Peterson, H., & Engwall, K. (2013). Silent bodies: Childfree women's gendered and embodied experiences. *European Journal of Women's Studies*, *20*(4), 376–389.

Peterson, H., & Engwall, K. (2015). Missing out on the parenthood bonus? Voluntarily childless in a "child-friendly" society. *Journal of Family and Economic Issues*, 1–13. doi:10.1007/s10834-015-9474-z

Pocock, B. (2003). *The work/life collision: What work is doing to Australians and what to do about it*. Sydney: Federation Press.

Pocock, B., Skinner, N., & Pisaniello, S. L. (2010). *How much should we work?: Working hours, holidays and working life: The participation challenge*. Adelaide: Centre for Work + Life, University of South Australia.

Rich, S., Taket, A., Graham, M., & Shelley, J. (2011). 'Unnatural', 'unwomanly', 'uncreditable' and 'undervalued': The significance of being a childless woman in Australian society. *Gender Issues*, *28*(4), 226–247.

Sawer, M. (2013). Misogyny and misrepresentation of women in Australian parliaments. *Political Science*, *65*(1), 105–117.

Schippers, M. (2007). Recovering the feminine other: Masculinity, femininity, and gender hegemony. *Theory and Society*, *36*(1), 85–102.

Schneer, J. A., & Reitman, F. (2002). Managerial life without a wife: Family structure and managerial career success. *Journal of Business Ethics*, *37*(1), 25–38.

Shaw, R. L. (2011). Women's experiential journey toward voluntary childlessness: An interpretative phenomenological analysis. *Journal of Community & Applied Social Psychology*, *21*(2), 151–163.

Skeggs, B. (1997). *Formations of class & gender: Becoming respectable*. London: Thousand Oaks.

Skinner, N., & Pocock, B. (2011). Flexibility and work-life interference in Australia. *Journal of Industrial Relations*, *53*(1), 65–82.

Smith, D. E. (1987). *The everyday world as problematic: A feminist sociology*. Toronto: University of Toronto Press.

Smithson, J., & Stokoe, E. H. (2005). Discourses of work–life balance: Negotiating 'genderblind' terms in organizations. *Gender, Work & Organization*, *12*(2), 147–168.

Swanberg, J. E., Pitt-Catsouphes, M., & Drescher-Burke, K. (2005). A question of justice: Disparities in employees'access to flexible schedule arrangements. *Journal of Family Issues*, *26*(6), 866–895.

Tharenou, P. (1999). Is there a link between family structures and women's and men's managerial career advancement? *Journal of Organizational Behavior*, *20*(6), 837–863.

Thornton, M. (2016). Work/life or work/work? Corporate legal practice in the twenty-first century. *International Journal of the Legal Profession*, *23*(1), 13–39.

Travaglione, A., & Chang, J. (2012). A demographic analysis of breadwinner and domestic childcare roles in Australia's employment structure. *Labour & Industry: A Journal of the Social and Economic Relations of Work*, *22*(4), 361–378.

Turnbull, B., Graham, M. L., & Taket, A. R. (2016a). Social exclusion of Australian childless women in their reproductive years. *Social Inclusion*, *4*(1), 102–115.

Turnbull, B., Graham, M. L., & Taket, A. R. (2016b). Social connection and exclusion of Australian women with no children during midlife. *Journal of Social Inclusion*, *7*(2), 65–85.

Turnbull, B., Graham, M. L., & Taket, A. R. (2017). Pronatalism and social exclusion in Australian society: Experiences of women in their reproductive years with no children. *Gender Issues*, *34*, 333–354.

Veevers, J. E. (1979). Voluntary childlessness. *Marriage & Family Review*, *2*(2), 1–26.

Wager, M. (2000). Childless by choice? Ambivalence and the female identity. *Feminism & Psychology*, *10*(3), 389–395.

Wajcman, J. (1998). *Managing like a man: Women and men in corporate management*. University Park, PA: Pennsylvania State University Press.

Watson, I. (2010). Decomposing the gender pay gap in the Australian managerial labour market. *Australian Journal of Labour Economics*, *13*(1), 49–79.

Whitehouse, G. (2002). Parenthood and pay in Australia and the UK: Evidence from workplace surveys. *Journal of Sociology*, *38*(4), 381–397.

Wirtberg, I. (1999). Trying to become a family; or, parents without children. *Marriage & Family Review*, *28*(3–4), 121–133.

Wood, G. J., & Newton, J. (2006). 'Facing the wall' – 'Equal' opportunity for women in management? *Equal Opportunities International*, *25*(1), 8–24.

Wright, E. O. (2005). Foundations of a neo-Marxist class analysis. In E. O. Wright (Ed.), *Approaches to class analysis* (pp. 4–30). Cambridge: Cambridge University Press.

Chapter 12

Gender Congruity, Childlessness and Success in Entrepreneurship: An Intersectional Bourdieusian Analysis

Natalie Sappleton

Abstract

The growth in women's entrepreneurship that has been witnessed recently in regions such as the USA has been lauded by scholars and policymakers alike. However, women continue to start businesses in sectors that reflect the kind of work that women do in the home, such as cooking, cleaning and catering. Research shows that women's 'choices' for female-typed businesses are driven by their need to accommodate domestic responsibilities – that is, caring for children. This raises questions about whether women without such responsibilities are freer to start businesses in the types of industries (e.g. high technology) that have long been dominated by men. Furthermore, given pronatalist assumptions, there are questions about the extent to which childfree women operating businesses in male-dominated sectors are perceived as legitimate by their business relations. Taking these questions as a starting point, this chapter examines the way in which the intersections of *parental status* (mother/other) and *gender role (in)congruence* (congruent/incongruent) make the entrepreneurial experiences of women working in male-dominated/masculinised industries and sectors qualitatively different from the experiences of women working in female-dominated/feminised industries. Focus is upon the resources (i.e. social capital) that women entrepreneurs are able to secure from their social network, for the ability to secure such resources is a prerequisite to business success.

Keywords: Entrepreneurship; business ownership; entrepreneurial segregation; social capital; social networks; gender role congruity

Introduction

This chapter offers a critical interrogation of the way in which individuals' – and especially women's – socially constructed and structural intersectional identities shape their experiences of self-employment and entrepreneurship.[1] More specifically, the chapter is concerned with the way in which the intersections of *parental status* (mother/other) and *gender role (in)congruence* (congruent/incongruent) make the entrepreneurial experiences of women working in male-dominated/masculinised industries and sectors qualitatively different from the experiences of women working in female-dominated/feminised industries in terms of the resources that they are able to secure from their social networks.

Three empirical observations suggest that an attempt to address this topic is worthwhile. First, there has been a substantial increase in childlessness worldwide since the 1970s. In the US, for instance, childlessness among women aged between 40 and 44 reached 15.1% in 2012 (up from 10.2% in 1976) (Monte & Mykyta, 2016), while in India, the proportion of women between the ages of 35 and 39 that are not mothers doubled from 3.86% in 1981 to 7.28% in 2011 (Sarkar, 2016).

Second, at the same time, the labour force participation of women has increased and there has been an upsurge in the proportion of entrepreneurial roles occupied by women, albeit in feminised industries (Jyrkinen, 2014). However, the extent to which these developments are interconnected with one another has not fully been explored in the extant literature. Given the broader observation that motherhood acts as a structural impediment to occupational advancement for women generally (Cahusac & Kanji, 2014), it is likely that growing childlessness is somehow linked to the growth of women in entrepreneurship.

Third, occupational segregation by gender – the concentration of men and women into occupations and occupational hierarchies dominated by members of one gender – has invidious and insidious consequences for gender inequalities (Acker, 2012). For instance, it is one of the primary causes of the gender pay gap, and since it helps to reinforce

---

[1]Debate continues on the semantic reconcilability of the terms 'self-employment' and 'entrepreneurship' (see Iversen, Jørgensen, & Malchow-Møller, 2007; Jonsson, 2014 for good overviews of the debate). By using these terms interchangeably in this chapter, I do not suggest that they are in fact synonymous, but rather that the key arguments presented herein have implications for both entrepreneurs and self-employed persons.

societal stereotypes about the 'proper' roles for men and women it has self-reproducing effects (Acker, 2012). The evidence that entrepreneurial segregation contributes to inequality in similar ways to sex segregation in employment is plentiful. Women earn less than men in self-employment and business ownership, with segregation making a significant contribution to earnings disparities (Hundley, 2001; Lowrey, 2005). Revenues and profitability are higher in masculine industries, female-typed industries have higher rates of firm turnover and firms in sectors such as manufacturing, construction and computer services have better chances of survival than those in the competitive retail and services industries (Bird & Sapp, 2004; Dahlqvist, Davidsson, & Wiklund, 2000; Brüderl & Preisendorfer, 1998; Brüderl & Rolf, 1992; Robb & Watson, 2012; Schmidt & Parker, 2003).

Breaking down gender segregation in entrepreneurship could therefore help boost efforts to achieve societal equality. However, there is some evidence elsewhere in the occupational literature that women who do undertake work in demanding masculinised industries often sacrifice childbearing and childrearing, for work in those sectors is incommensurate with parenthood for women (Wood & Newton, 2006). Furthermore, in remaining childfree, these women are often perceived negatively by those with whom they interact because of pronatalist beliefs (see Chapter 11 of this volume). Little is known about whether women entrepreneurs have similar experiences. This provides impetus for an exploration into the impact of the intersections of parental status and role congruity in the context of entrepreneurship.

Drawing on an intersectionalist feminist epistemology, and using a Bourdieusian understanding of the concept of social capital, this chapter describes the results of a study that examines if, and how, parental status and gender role congruity interact to impact ability of women and men entrepreneurs to raise the resources from their social networks that they need to support their business enterprises. The next section justifies this focus on social networks and resource acquisition.

Social Networks, Social Capital and Resource Acquisition

The formation of a new business entity has been likened to piecing together a jigsaw puzzle. Prospective entrepreneurs are tasked with identifying, accessing, mobilising and assembling resources in order to successfully create a viable venture. Budding entrepreneurs are advised that the foremost important task facing them is the 'identification and engagement of resources that will make it possible for you to turn your dream into a reality' (Brush, Carter, Gatewood, Greene, & Hart, 2004, p. 1). The people that a business owner knows, or their *social network*, may be able to directly or indirectly provide the assistance, support, information and other necessary resources that they need. Other people are said to be so crucial to the entrepreneurial project that entrepreneurship should be treated as inherently social activity, 'embedded in a social context, channeled and facilitated or constrained and inhibited by people's positions in social networks' (Aldrich & Zimmer, 1986, p. 4).

Social networks, then, are not important in and of themselves, but because they allow business owners to locate and access what Bourdieu (1986, p. 86) termed *social capital*:

> ...the sum of the resources, actual or virtual, that accrue to an individual or a group by virtue of possessing a durable network of more or less institutionalized relationships of mutual acquaintance and recognition.

However, it is crucial to distinguish resource *accessibility* (i.e. the ability to reach those parties that hold the resources necessary for the business enterprise) from resource *appropriability* (i.e. the ability to capture the resources held by those parties for use in the business enterprise) (Tata & Prasad, 2008). In other words, merely having a well-endowed social network is not enough; entrepreneurs must *convince* members of their social networks to supply them with social capital. Business owners draw on their *role performance* as a means of establishing their legitimacy as entrepreneurs, and it is this performance that is used to convince network members to supply resources. It is contended here that parental status and role congruity both constitute key aspects of that role performance. Next, the concept of performance is clarified and role congruity theory is justified as a theoretical framework.

Role Performance, Role Congruity, Parental Status and Workplace Outcomes

Sociologists view gender as a performative act, as exemplified in de Beauvoir's axiom that 'one is not born but becomes a woman' (de Beauvoir, 1949, p. 267). Individuals 'do' gender by performing certain clusters of gender-appropriate and socially sanctioned behaviours – described by Linton (1936) as *roles*. Importantly, while these roles are not innate, but artificially created by society, 'once the differences have been constructed, they are used to reinforce the "essentialness" of gender' (West & Zimmerman, 1991, p. 24). Gender role congruity theory, proposed by Nieva and Gutek (1980), argues that women are idealised to fulfil *communal* roles, while *agentic* roles are assigned to men. Communality refers to the extent to which an individual is sensitive, empathetic, cares for others, helpful, nurturing and kind (Rosener, 1990). Agentic traits relate to self-sufficiency, self-confidence, aggression and control. Women and men that conform to such roles are rewarded, while those that deviate from them are punished, penalised and pressured to conform (Nieva & Gutek, 1980). Both motherhood and occupations are societally driven roles that are used to produce, maintain and uphold the gender order.

Motherhood is both socially constructed and interwoven into the dominant institutional, sociopolitical and cultural frameworks of societies, giving rise to *pronatalism* – a gendered system that encourages and normalises childbearing among women (Phoenix & Woollett, 1991). For women, motherhood is seen as an innate and natural activity that reinforces womanhood so that 'woman = mother = woman' (Ramsay & Letherby, 2006, p. 40). The normativity of pronatalism is a reflection of the prevailing essentialist gender order which serves to render women that (voluntarily or involuntarily) pursue alternative paths as deviant, or what Gotlib (2016, p. 327) refers to as '*unwomen*'.

Similarly, occupational roles play an important part in reinforcing gendered societal beliefs because organisations are effectively gendered substructures 'in which gendered assumptions about women and men, femininity and masculinity, are embedded and reproduced and gender inequalities perpetuated' (Acker, 2012, p. 215). According to gender role congruity theory, by undertaking gender-congruent occupational roles, women and men reproduce and reinforce societal expectations (Nieva & Gutek, 1980). Women undertake occupational roles that are extensions of the home-making role and which facilitate conformity to the feminine ideal of the nurturing, caring woman. For instance, the vast majority of Western working women are employed in just five broad occupational categories known as the five Cs: cleaning, catering, caring, cashiering and clerical work (Ruth Eikhof, 2012). Men dominate managerial positions – roles which uphold their traditional status as breadwinners and which are commensurate with the ideology of hegemonic masculinity that emphasises power, ambition and stewardship.

The empirical literature confirms that individuals that violate these gender norms, such as women who rise to senior management positions, and 'stay-at-home dads' can expect to be vilified socially (Jyrkinen, 2014; Sappleton & Takruri-Rizk, 2008).

Acker (2012) argues that organisations are imbued with norms and values that produce expectations about worker behaviours, such as the time of arrival, the way in which they should dress and how work should be undertaken. This *organisational logic*, however, is not gender neutral. Rather, it is 'implicitly built on the image of a gender neutral, abstract worker who has no body and no obligations outside the work place: this worker is unencumbered' (Acker, 2012, p. 218). Men are better able to conform to this ideal because the gendered society does not expect men to assume primary responsibility for childrearing. Furthermore, this logic is intensified in male-dominated organisations. Women who violate gender prescriptive stereotypes by taking up careers in male-dominated fields are further pressurised to 'manage like a man' (Acker, 2012, p. 216) and adopt male career patterns because those occupations have been designed to accommodate heteronormative masculine norms (Wajcman, 1999). Childlessness may be one way in which this performance is enacted. For instance, one survey of 1,000 North American managers found that 62% of male managers had children at home, compared to just 20% of their women counterparts (Brett & Stroh, 1999), while Wajcman (1999, p. 143), observes that for women, 'childlessness is a precondition of a successful management career' for 'the job consumes most waking hours and dominates life in every respect' (p. 156).

Some studies have adopted what McCall (2005) describes as an *intra-categorical* approach, comparing the workplace experiences of mothers and women who are childless (Kahn et al., 2014; Kmec, 2011; Jyrkinen, 2014; Ramsay & Letherby, 2006). This strand of research reveals that non-mothers have qualitatively different workplace experiences compared to mothers (and indeed, fathers). Both Ramsay and Letherby (2006) and Jyrkinen (2014), for instance, observe that non-mothers in gendered organisations are expected to increase their workplace commitment in order to counterbalance the perceived lower commitment of mothers, causing conflict between these groups of women. However, as pointed out by Monte and Mykyta (2016), while mothers experience a workplace penalty in terms in pay and promotion prospects, non-mothers may experience a 'bonus'. Childfree women have better economic outcomes compared to mothers in terms of their pay levels and their wealth in later life (Plotnick, 2009). Moreover, childfree women are more likely than women with children to be in managerial positions

(Monte & Mykyta, 2016), so that when compared to the wider category of women, childfree women could be described as what Crenshaw (1989) called 'otherwise privileged'.

In sum, this literature demonstrates the paradox that 'dominant societal discourses favour having children, while not having children is privileged in the workplace' (Rick & Meisenbech, 2016; p. 217). In broader society, childlessness is cast as a deviant act and women who voluntarily choose to remain childfree are vilified as 'unnatural, unwomanly, uncreditable and undervalued' (Rich, Taket, Graham, & Shelley, 2011, p. 226). However, in the workplace, these women are 'otherwise privileged' because they are better able to conform to what Acker (2012) described as the notion of the 'ideal worker' who is committed to the employer, can extend their working hours, and does not take time off to accommodate family matters. The 'unwomaning' of childless managerial women strips them of their performed gender and casts them as 'man-like', as exemplified by the disdain felt towards these women by some working mothers in the Ramsay and Letherby (2006) and Jyrkinen (2014) studies, and their ability to accomplish positions that women with children are unable to achieve. The observation that childless women may be both privileged and marginalised contingent upon the context 'reminds us that individuals within an intersectional space (i.e. of two overlapping categories) may be experiencing something significantly different to those occupying one of the categories' (McBride, Hebson, & Holgate, 2015, p. 336).

Parental Status, Role Congruity and Entrepreneurship

Although Acker (2012) theorises an interconnection between management, gender segregation and childlessness, far less attention has been paid in the empirical literature to the intersections of parental status and role congruity in the entrepreneurial arena. However, drawing on insights from the managerial literature, there is reason to suspect that women who undertake entrepreneurship in male-dominated business sectors have different experiences of parenthood and social networking compared to women who start firms in sectors such as childcare and cleaning. Monte and Mykyta's (2016) analysis of US Census data shows that childless women are significantly more likely to be found in STEM (Science, Technology, Engineering and Mathematics) occupations than women with children, and that childlessness is an effective predictor of managerial attainment. Research conducted in a host of male-dominated occupations has demonstrated that women who are either in, or aspire to senior positions are less likely to be married than their male colleagues, and that they tend to have levels of childlessness that are higher than average (Wood & Newton, 2006; Brett & Stroh, 1999; Wajcman, 1999; Hoobler, Wayne, & Lemmon, 2009; Wright, 2016). Wood and Newton (2006) carried out interviews with 10 women and 10 men middle managers on their negotiation of the work and family nexus, their attitudes towards childrearing and childrearing choices. Although the authors did not report information on the types of sectors, occupations and organisations in which the interviewees worked, they did conclude that the choice to be a mother or remain childless is 'generated contextually in a social field in which discourses and symbolic meanings are refracted through material dimensions' (Wood & Newton, 2006, p. 355).

Wajcman (1999) reported on the results of qualitative interviews with 20 women and men managers, including those working in male-dominated/masculinised industries such as computing, chemicals and oil and gas extraction. The men managers tended to have female partners who took responsibility for looking after the home, while the women tended to have partners that worked full-time. Consequently, many of the women undertook a 'second shift' of housework after completing paid work. The interviews led Wajcman (1999, p. 156) to conclude that the women managers 'have mostly given up the opportunity to have children in order to pursue their careers'. Interestingly, this sacrifice is often in vain as many women in these industries do not advance to the senior positions to which they aspire, suggesting that the gendered organisational logic (Acker, 2012) continues to act as an impediment to the progression of women. Acker (2012, p. 218) explains this by pointing out that

> [E]mployers may be reluctant to hire women for jobs, usually male-dominated and defined, in which the worker is expected to be unencumbered. *This reluctance may be important in the continuing sex segregation of jobs* (emphasis mine).

Conceptual Framework

Women who go into entrepreneurship often do so as a means of balancing their work and domestic responsibilities (McGowan, Redeker, Cooper, & Greenan, 2012). However, only certain types of entrepreneurship – businesses which start small, stay small and serve local markets (e.g. hairdressing, beauty and cleaning enterprises), are reconcilable with motherhood. Yet even the demands of these businesses can lead women entrepreneurs in gender role-congruous industries to be perceived by society as 'bad mothers' (Duberley & Carrigan, 2013). Women that remain childfree in these sectors may realise success as an entrepreneur, but are otherwise viewed by pronatalist society as 'bad women'.

Because of gendered notions about the 'proper' role of women in business,

> a woman entrepreneur within a male-dominated industry or culture may carry the invisible-yet-cumbersome baggage of sex-based stereotypes when she attempts to secure resources, develop business networks, and gain legitimacy for her business venture. (Godwin, Stevens, & Brenner, 2005, p. 624).

Drawing on the work of Acker (2012), it can be surmised that those that are also mothers are perceived by their networks as lacking the ability to invest the time and energy that a business in masculinised industries demands, so that these women are construed as 'bad entrepreneurs'. Remaining childfree may be a way for women business owners in gender-incongruent forms of entrepreneurship to overcome gendered expectations of their occupational/societal role. Yet, acceptance of such gender non-conforming acts bring about a 'double bind' for these women. On the one hand, these women are in a better position to be able to invest energy and effort in their businesses, and their networking/resource-seeking activities. However, as violators of conventional stereotypes of both the occupational and societal role, these women may also be vilified by their networks when it comes to their attempts to appropriate resources, so that role-incongruent non-mothers are simultaneously privileged (in the workplace) and marginalised (in society) as a consequence of their childfree state. This conceptual framework is depicted in Table 1.

Table 1. The Implications of the Intersections of Role (In)Congruity and Parental Status for Women Entrepreneurs' Experiences.

	Parental Status	
Role Congruity	**Mother**	**Childless**
Incongruous	Bad entrepreneur	Privileged and marginalised
Congruous	Bad mother	Bad woman

Methods

Data Collection

Data for this chapter are taken from a wider study of women and men business owners of firms in gender-typical and atypical business sectors (Sappleton, 2013). Invitations to participate in an online questionnaire were distributed to 700 randomly selected women and men business owners of firms in the construction (male-dominated), sound recording (male-dominated), childcare (female-dominated) and publishing (integrated) sectors in New York City. The entrepreneurs were identified through the *Dun & Bradstreet's Selectory* and *ReferenceUSA* databases and email addresses were purchased from *ReferenceUSA* or located through an online search. Two hundred and fifty-five completed and useable questionnaires were submitted, equivalent to a response rate of 38.1%, discounting bouncebacks and refusals. Data from 90 male business owners and 78 female business owners in the sound recording, construction and child day-care sectors is drawn upon for the purposes of this chapter.

Data and Variables

Dependent Variable

Like entrepreneurship itself, 'success' is a heavily contested term in the empirical literature on entrepreneurship and gender. Ever since women first began to take up self-employment in significant numbers in the 1980s, researchers have attempted to compare the relative performance of women- and men-owned firms, generally concluding that the latter outperform the former in terms of variables such as longevity, profitability and growth (Robb & Watson, 2012; Rosa, Carter, & Hamilton, 1996; Srinvasan, Woo, & Cooper, 1994; Zolin, Stuetzer, & Watson, 2013). However, some critics of the so-called 'underperformance hypothesis' have argued that the definition of the key construct 'success' is, in itself, gendered (Headd, 2003; Justo, DeTienne, & Sieger, 2015; Reavley & Lituchy, 2008). Many women are 'pushed' into self-employment out of necessity, for instance, while others deliberately begin lifestyle-oriented businesses, which they do not wish to grow beyond a personally manageable size so that they may balance domesticity with career (Fleck, Hegarty, & Neergaard, 2011; Morris, Miyasaki, Watters, &

Coombes, 2006; Reichborn-Kjennerud & Svare, 2014). Thus, measuring success in terms of financial and economic outcomes renders invisible those (mainly, but not only) women, who enter entrepreneurship for alternative reasons.

Embracing an inclusive and feminist understanding of the notion of success, then, the dependent variable is defined as success in acquiring resources. This gauges the extent to which owners were successful in their attempts to secure resources from network members. Respondents were asked whether they had attempted to secure, and had managed to secure 21 different financial, informational, emotional and tangible resources. Examples of such resources were loans or business investment advice, legal assistance, help securing new contracts, physical resources and emotional support. Resources successfully obtained from networks were coded 1; unattained resources were coded 0. Resources that were not obtained because respondents did not require them (e.g. where respondents had no employees and therefore did not require assistance in finding staff, or where childless owners did not require help with childcare) are treated as not sought, coded −1 and specified as missing data. The measure of total resources acquired is expressed as a percentage and was calculated in the following way: *Total resources obtained/ Total resources sought*100.*

Independent Variables

Gender congruity of business sector is a dichotomous variable so that an individual owning a gender-congruent business is coded as 0, while a business owner of a gender-incongruent firm is coded as 1. *Parental status* is a dichotomous variable, whereby an individual that is the parent of at least one child is coded 1, and childfree individuals are coded as 0.

Control Variables

Following the recommendations of Rouhani (2014), efforts are made to integrate an intersectional approach into the analysis. Specifically, data was gathered on the *age* of the business owner, their *sexual orientation* (0 = non-heterosexual, 1 = heterosexual) and their *ethnicity* (0 = non-White, 1 = White/Caucasian). In addition, data were gathered on the age of the firm (in months) and *marital status* from a set of pre-given categories.

Method of Analysis

In order to explore the propositions suggested in the conceptual framework, an exploratory approach to data analysis is employed. In the first instance, descriptive statistics are yielded in order to describe the sample as a whole, as well as disaggregated by gender and role congruity of business sector. Next, bivariate analyses are used to compare resource acquisition according to the independent variables. Finally, linear regression analysis on the female sample is performed to order to explore the interplay between gender role congruity and parental status, taking into consideration multiple dimensions of intersectionality.

Analysis

The Sample

Demographic and firm characteristics are supplied in Table 2. There are some interesting patterns worth highlighting. New York City is famously described as a 'melting pot' so it is perhaps unsurprising that the sample is diverse in terms of ethnicity. However, patterns of ethnicity differ according to gender congruity of sector. In general, it seems that a greater proportion of incongruent than congruent owners in this sample are from ethnic minorities. For example, just 4.3% of owners of gender-congruent businesses describe themselves as Black/African-American compared to 12.9% of owners of gender-incongruent firms. And, 71% of congruent owners are White/Caucasian compared to 55.3% of incongruent owners. Overall, 44.7% of incongruent owners are non-White compared to 28.7% of congruent owners.

Although patterns of reported sexual orientation are comparable among the male and female sample, these patterns differ when the gender role congruity of the firm is considered. A greater proportion (93.7%) of men entrepreneurs in the gender-role-congruent sectors than men in the incongruent sector (48.3%) describe themselves as heterosexual. Over one-quarter of male owners in the incongruent (i.e. childcare) industry describe their sexual orientation as gay; in comparison, 84.3% of owners in the gender-role-congruent describe themselves as heterosexual.

Table 2. Demographic and Firm Characteristics.

	All	Women-owned	Men-owned	Congruent	Female-owned	Male-owned	Incongruent	Female-owned	Male-owned
Mean age (years)	44.8	43.5	46.2	45.8	43.0	47.1	42.9	42.8	43.2
Ethnicity (%):									
Asian/Asian-American	10.3	13.2	7.4	5.3	6.5	4.8	17.6	21.4	10.3
Middle Eastern	6.2	5.8	6.6	8.5	12.9	6.3	2.4	0	6.9
Black/African-American	10.3	11.6	9.1	4.3	6.5	3.2	12.9	10.7	17.2
White/Caucasian	61.6	59.5	63.6	71.3	71.0	71.4	55.3	53.6	58.6
Hispanic/Latino	5	5	5	3.2	3.2	3.2	4.7	3.6	6.9
Other ethnicities***	6.6	9.9	8.3	7.4	0	11.1	7.1	10.7	0
% Run a firm before	58.4	50.4	68.6	62.8	54.8	66.7	67.1	64.3	72.4
% with degree or above	62.9	73.5	52.5	53.8	83.3	39.7	65.9	64.3	69.2
Sexual Orientation (%)									
Heterosexual	75.3	76.9	77.7	88.3	77.4	93.7	64.2	73.1	48.3

Table 2. (*Continued*)

	All	Women-owned	Men-owned	Congruent	Female-owned	Male-owned	Incongruent	Female-owned	Male-owned
Gay/Lesbian	14.9	16.2	13.2	7.4	16.1	3.2	25.9	19.2	37.9
Others**	9.8	6.9	9.1	4.3	6.5	0	9.9	3.8	6.9
Mean hours of work	49.6	47.0	52.2	52.8	45.1	56.4	47.7	47.7	47.6
% Married or cohabiting	68.8	63.5	74.1	73.0	78.6	70.5	61.0	57.1	69.2
% with children	40.1	40.9	39.3	41.4	60.7	32.2	39	28.6	61.5
Has employees (%)	81.3	73.6	89.1	89.1	83.9	91.8	72.9	64.3	89.7
Mean no. of employees	21.99	12.86	30.49	30.82	7.10	40.85	19.35	17.891	17.30
Mean firm age (months)	161.21	140.46	181.61	184.24	134.81	205.43	130.21	128.54	133.45

Notes: **Includes bisexual and 'other' categories but excludes refusals and missing; *** includes Indian, Native American, 'Other' category.

Gender, Role Congruity and Parental Status

For the full sample, there are few gender differences in terms of parental status, but large gaps when gender role congruity is considered. Twice as many role congruent women (60.7%) as men are parents (32.2%) $\chi^2(1) = 6.36$, $p < 0.05$, but twice as many incongruent men (61.5%) as women (28.6%) have children, $\chi^2(1) = 8.11$, $p < 0.01$. The differences are starker when the data is disaggregated by gender and role congruity (Table 3). In the first evidence of support for the propositions stated in the conceptual framework, childfree women entrepreneurs are overrepresented in the gender-role-incongruent sectors, compared to the role congruent sectors, $\chi^2(1) = 8.21$, $p < 0.05$. There are also differences in parental status for men entrepreneurs according to role congruity of sector, $\chi^2(1) = 6.78$, $p < 0.05$.

Table 4 compares the sample in terms of gender, gender role congruity, parental status and success in acquiring resources. First, it is noteworthy that on the whole, men entrepreneurs seem to be more

Table 3. Gender, Role Congruity and Parental Status.

	Women Entrepreneurs		**Men Entrepreneurs**	
	Incongruent	**Congruent**	**Incongruent**	**Congruent**
Parent	16 (29)	14 (64)	14 (64)	22 (32)
Non-parent	40 (71)	8 (36)	8 (36)	46 (68)
Total	56	22	22	68

Note: Percentages (rounded) shown in parentheses.

Table 4. Gender, Role Congruity, Parental Status and Success in Acquiring Resources.

	Women Entrepreneurs		**Men Entrepreneurs**	
	Congruent	**Incongruent**	**Congruent**	**Incongruent**
Parent	98.27	66.58	98.76	90.04
Non-parent	91.13	62.99	96.49	96.54
Total	95.46	74.22	97.22	94.04

Note: Mean success rates shown. Rounded figures.

successful at leveraging resources from their networks compared to their female counterparts, regardless of whether or not they are in congruent or incongruent business sectors. This suggests that parenthood is not as salient a characteristic for men as for women when it comes to resource acquisition. For women entrepreneurs, there were stark differences in success in resource acquisition, when parental status and role congruity were considered. Considering the gender-role-congruent sectors, women who do not have children are less likely to be able to leverage resources from their networks than women who have children, with their success rate just over 91%, compared to a success rate for parents of 98.27%. However, in *t*-tests, the difference does not reach statistical significance, $t(27.38) = -1.434$, $p = 0.163$. Women in the incongruent sectors, both parents and non-parents, are the least successful of any group when it comes to their ability to acquire resources. These women were successful in leveraging resources from their networks just 74.22% of the time, compared to a success rate of 95.46% for gender-role-congruent women, 94.04% for role-incongruent men and 97.22% for role-congruent male entrepreneurs.

Taking parental status into consideration, the differences are even more stark. Women entrepreneurs in the incongruent business sectors who are parents recorded a resource acquisition success rate of 66.58%. Those that were not parents recorded a success rate of just 62.99%, and the differences between the groups were statistically significant, $t(26) = -3.23$, $p < 0.05$. This would suggest that women entrepreneurs who enter male-dominated/masculinised business sectors and remain child-free incur a double penalty imposed by their social networks.

Regression Analysis

Finally, linear regression analysis is performed in order to test the resilience of the finding for women entrepreneurs, controlling for demographic characteristics and one measure of human capital. The enter method is used, with the variables forced into the model in two blocks. The first block contains the control variables. Dummy variables are created for sexual orientation (0 = not heterosexual, 1 = heterosexual) and ethnicity (0 = white, 1 = non-white). Two other control variables are included – age of entrepreneur squared, in order to account for the diminishing impact of entrepreneur age on perceived levels of experience and maturity, and a binary variable measuring whether the entrepreneur had any previous experience running a firm (0 = yes, 1 = no), since this is likely to exert an impact on their ability to successfully network. The second block contains the independent variables measuring role congruity and parental status, as well as an interaction term in order to explore combined, as well as independent effects.

The significant *F*-test suggests that model one is a good fit. Just one of the control variables – age squared – is found to exert a significant impact on the ability of women entrepreneurs to leverage resources from their networks, but the effect size appears to be small. None of the other variables have any influence on success rates. When the independent variables are added to the analysis in model two, also a good model, age squared remains significant. Both parental status and role congruity are statistically significant, confirming the earlier findings. However, the interaction term, parental status* role congruity is not statistically significant in this model (Table 5).

Discussion and Conclusions

There is something of a celebratory tone in the recent literature on female self-employment and entrepreneurship, especially that which has been published in the North American context and pertaining to North American women. These women, it is argued, are taking up entrepreneurship at such a quickening pace that it has even been suggested that gender disparities in entrepreneurial rates are soon to be a thing of the past. Furthermore, it has been lauded that self-employed women are more ethnically and racially diverse than ever before, and suggestions are that these women have the potential to correct the pay gap that plagues their employed sisters.

However, the majority of women continue to take up self-employment and entrepreneurship in sectors and industries that are both dominated by women, and which reflect the types of work that women do, both paid and unpaid. One reason for this is that the industries in which men entrepreneurs dominate tend to be less accommodating to domestic responsibilities. This would suggest that women who do take up entrepreneurship in role-incongruous sectors are more likely to remain child-free than their counterparts who are operating businesses which are traditional for their gender. Furthermore, it is not known whether parental status has an impact on the 'success' and performance of businesses for either role-congruent or incongruent women. Resource acquisition is an important measure of success, because without the appropriate resources, businesses will rarely survive. Furthermore,

Table 5. Summary of Linear Regression Analysis.

Variables	**Model 1**			**Model 2**		
	B	**SEB**	***β***	***B***	**SEB**	***β***
(Constant)	60.777***	14.544		68.392***	13.263	
Sexual orientation	1.776	6.322	0.031	1.877	5.059	0.033
Ethnicity	−8.902	5.568	−0.173	−6.801	4.435	−0.133
Age^2	0.014***	0.004	0.406	0.014***	0.003	0.409
Experience	0.950	5.784	0.018	−1.402	4.609	−0.026
Parental status				16.407*	7.453	0.323
Role congruity				−19.369**	6.700	−0.375
Parental status* role congruity				−11.347	10.062	−0.176
F of the model	4.146**			11.974***		
R^2	0.189			0.510		
Adjusted R^2	0.144			0.467		

Note: Because of missing data, $n = 78$. $^{*}p < 0.05$, $^{**}p < 0.01$, $^{***}p < 0.001$.

resource appropriability is determined by the perceived legitimacy of entrepreneurs, suggesting that it is important to consider characteristics that impact perceptions of legitimacy among network members. Therefore, in this chapter, I have explored the parental status of women (and men, for comparison), in role-congruent and incongruent entrepreneurial sectors, and the impact that this has upon their ability to acquire social capital from their social networks.

The analysis finds some support for the proposed conceptual framework (Table 6). Mothers in role-incongruent sectors have relatively low rates of success in resource acquisition, suggesting that network members see them as 'bad entrepreneurs'. Success rates are considerably stronger (and equivalent to male rates) for mothers operating firms in the childcare (i.e. role-congruent) sector, so these women are able to use their role as entrepreneurs, undertaking the kind of work that women do to acquire legitimacy in the eyes of their network members. In spite of pronatalist norms, there is no evidence from this sample that business network members see these women as bad mothers. However, alternative results might be yielded from a study of friends and other social contacts. Childless women in the role-congruous sector are also relatively successful in extracting resources from their networks. Again, there is insufficient data in this study to explore whether these women are perceived to be 'bad women'. It is noteworthy, however, that childless women in the role-incongruous sector have the lowest success rates of all four samples. It was suggested that these women might be simultaneously privileged and marginalised because of their childfree status in sectors traditionally viewed as masculine. In fact, when it comes to the acquisition of resources, these women are even less successful than their counterparts who are mothers. Thus, this chapter finds heightened

Table 6. Summary of the Intersections of Role (In)Congruity and Parental Status for Women Entrepreneurs' Success Rates.

	Parental Status	
Role Congruity	**Mother**	**Childless**
Incongruous	Bad entrepreneur (66.58)	~~Privileged and~~ Marginalised (62.99)
Congruous	~~Bad mother~~(98.27)	~~Bad woman~~(91.13)

levels of marginalisation and exclusion from social networks for role-incongruous mothers.

Undoubtedly, workplace gender inequality is a challenging and multifarious problematic that necessitates multilayered and complex ontologies. However, as pointed out by Knapp (2005, pp. 258–259), 'the questions concerning inequalities among women cannot be answered by looking at *women*' (emphasis in original). Rather, what is required is intra-categorical as well as inter-categorical analysis that takes into account the diversity of women's experiences, the relationality of different groups and the way in which the conditions of women's experiences are constituted in specific cultural, economic, symbolic and socio-historical conditions contexts (McBride et al., 2015). The literature on childlessness emphasises the negative impact that childlessness can have upon women in pronatalist societies. Focusing on entrepreneurs, this chapter has shown that it is important to consider cultural contexts when discussing questions pertaining to social outcomes. In this study, both mothers and non-mothers seemed to be penalised by their social networks for their social choices. Mothers were penalised if they started businesses in sectors that are not deemed to be socially appropriate for women (and indeed, mothers). Non-mothers were similarly less able to leverage social capital from their networks. In contrast, men did not seem to experience these penalties, regardless of business location or parental status.

Although there are limitations to this study in terms of the type of data collected and the level of analysis, in general, this study provides a springboard for further analysis of the roles played by gendered workplaces and social networks in determining outcomes for childless women and mothers alike.

References

Acker, J. (2012). Gendered organizations and intersectionality: Problems and possibilities. *Equality, Diversity and Inclusion: An International Journal, 31*(3), 214–224.

Aldrich, H., & Zimmer, C. (1986). Entrepreneurship through social networks. In D. L. Sexton & R. W. Smilor (Eds.), *The art and science of entrepreneurship* (pp. 3–23). Cambridge, MA: Ballinger.

Bird, S. R., & Sapp, S. G. (2004). Understanding the gender gap in small business success. *Gender & Society, 18*(1), 5–28.

Bourdieu, P. (1986). The forms of capital. In J. G. Richardson (Ed.), *Handbook of theory and research for the sociology of education* (pp. 241–258). New York, NY: Greenwood Press.

Brett, J. M., & Stroh, L. K. (1999). Women in management: how far have we come and what needs to be done as we approach 2000? *Journal of Management Inquiry*, *8*(4), 392–398.

Brüderl, J., & Preisendorfer, P. (1998). Network support and success of newly founded businesses. *Small Business Economics*, *10*(2), 213–225.

Brüderl, J., & Rolf, P. Z. (1992). Survival chances of newly founded business organizations. *American Journal of Small Business*, *57*(2), 227–242.

Brush, C., Carter, N. M., Gatewood, E., Greene, P. G., & Hart, M. M. (2004). *Clearing the hurdles: Women building high-growth businesses*. Upper Saddle River, NJ: Financial Times Prentice Hall.

Cahusac, E., & Kanji, S. (2014). Giving up: How gendered organizational cultures push mothers out. Gender. *Work & Organization*, *21*(1), 57–70.

Crenshaw, K. (1989). Demarginalising the intersection of race and sex: A black feminist critique of antidiscrimination doctrine, feminist theory and antiracist politics. *The University of Chicago Legal Forum*, *1*, 139–167.

Dahlqvist, J., Davidsson, P., & Wiklund, J. (2000). Initial conditions as predictors of new venture performance: A replication and extension of the Cooper et al. study. *Enterprise and Innovation Management Studies*, *1*(1), 1–17.

de Beauvoir, S. (1949). *The second sex*. New York, NY: Bantam Books and Alfred A. Knopf.

Duberley, J., & Carrigan, M. (2013). The career identities of 'mumpreneurs': Women's experiences of combining enterprise and motherhood. *International Small Business Journal*, *31*(6), 629–651.

Fleck, E., Hegarty, C., & Neergaard, H. (2011). The politics of gendered growth. *International Journal of Gender and Entrepreneurship*, *3*(2), 164–173.

Godwin, L. N., Stevens, C. E., & Brenner, N. L. (2005). Forced to play by the rules? Theorizing how mixed-sex founding teams benefit women entrepreneurs in male-dominated contexts. *Entrepreneurship: Theory & Practice*, *30*(5), 623–642.

Gotlib, A. (2016). 'But you would be the best mother': Unwomen, counterstories, and the motherhood mandate. *Journal of Bioethical Inquiry*, *13*(2), 327–247.

Headd, B. (2003). Redefining business success: Distinguishing between closure and failure. *Small Business Economics*, *21*(1), 51–61.

Hoobler, J. M., Wayne, S. J., & Lemmon, G. (2009). Bosses' perceptions of family-work conflict and women's promotability: Glass ceiling effects. *Academy of Management Journal*, *52*(5), 939–957.

Hundley, G. (2001). Why women earn less than men in self-employment. *Journal of Labor Research*, *22*(4), 818–828.

Iversen, J., Jørgensen, R., & Malchow-Møller, N. (2007). Defining and measuring entrepreneurship. *Foundations and Trends® in Entrepreneurship*, *4*(1), 1–63.

Jonsson, P. O. (2014). What's in a name? On language, concept formation, and the definition disputes in the entrepreneurship literature. *Cultural Science Journal*, *7*(1), 1–22.

Justo, R., DeTienne, D. R., & Sieger, P. (2015). Failure or voluntary exit? Reassessing the female underperformance hypothesis. *Journal of Business Venturing*, *30*(6), 775–792.

Jyrkinen, M. (2014). Women managers, careers and gendered ageism. *Scandinavian Journal of Management*, *30*, 175–185.

Kahn, J. R., García-Manglano, J., & Bianchi, S. M. (2014). The motherhood penalty at midlife: Long-term effects of children on women's careers. *Journal of Marriage and Family*, *76*(1), 56–72.

Kmec, J. A. (2011). Are motherhood penalties and fatherhood bonuses warranted? Comparing pro-work behaviors and conditions of mothers, fathers, and non-parents. *Social Science Research*, *40*(2), 444–459.

Knapp, G. A. (2005). Race, class, gender: Reclaiming baggage in fast travelling theories. *European Journal of Women's Studies*, *12*(3), 249–265.

Linton, R. (1936). *The study of man*. New York, NY: Appleton-Century.

Lowrey, Y. (2005). *US sole propriertorships: A gender comparison 1985–2000*. Washington, DC: US Small Business Administration, Office of Advocacy.

McBride, A., Hebson, G., & Holgate, J. (2015). Intersectionality: are we taking enough notice in the field of work and employment relations? *Work, Employment and Society*, *29*(2), 331–341.

McCall, L. (2005). The complexity of intersectionality. *Signs: Journal of Women in Culture and Society*, *30*(3), 1771–1800.

McGowan, P., Redeker, C. L., Cooper, S. Y., & Greenan, K. (2012). Female entrepreneurship and the management of business and domestic roles: Motivations, expectations and realities. *Entrepreneurship & Regional Development*, *24*(1/2), 53–72.

Monte, L. M., & Mykyta, L. (2016). *The occupational attainment of mid-career childless women, 1980–2012*. Paper presented at the Work and Family Researchers Network (WFRN) Conference, Washington, DC.

Morris, M. H., Miyasaki, N. N., Watters, C. E., & Coombes, S. M. (2006). The dilemma of growth: Understanding venture size choices of women entrepreneurs. *Journal of Small Business Management*, *44*(2), 221–244.

Nieva, V. F., & Gutek, B. A. (1980). Sex effects on evaluation. *The Academy of Management Review*, *5*(2), 267–276.

Phoenix, A., & Woollett, A. (1991). *Motherhood: Social construction, politics and psychology*. Thousand Oaks, CA: Sage.

Plotnick, R. D. (2009). Childlessness and the economic well-being of older Americans. *Journals of Gerontology Series B: Psychological Sciences and Social Sciences*, *64*(6), 767–776.

Ramsay, K., & Letherby, G. (2006). The experience of academic non-mothers in the gendered university. *Gender, Work & Organization*, *13*(1), 25–44.

Reavley, M. A., & Lituchy, T. R. (2008). Successful women entrepreneurs: A six-country analysis of self-reported determinants of success? More than just dollars and cents. *International Journal of Entrepreneurship and Small Business*, *5*(3–4), 272–296.

Reichborn-Kjennerud, K., & Svare, H. (2014). Entrepreneurial growth strategies: The female touch. *International Journal of Gender and Entrepreneurship*, *6*(2), 181–199.

Rich, S., Taket, A., Graham, M., & Shelley, J. (2011). 'Unnatural', 'unwomanly', 'uncreditable'and 'undervalued': The significance of being a childless woman in Australian society. *Gender Issues*, *28*(4), 226–247.

Rick, J. M., & Meisenbach, R. J. (2016). Social stigma, childfree identities, and work-life balance. In E. F. Hatfield (Ed.), *Communication and the work-life balancing act: Intersections across identities, genders, and cultures*. New York: Lexington Books.

Robb, A. M., & Watson, J. (2012). Gender differences in firm performance: Evidence from new ventures in the United States. *Journal of Business Venturing, 27*(5), 544–558.

Rosa, P., Carter, S., & Hamilton, D. (1996). Gender as a determinant of small business performance: Insights from a British study. *Small Business Economics, 8*(6), 463–478.

Rosener, J. B. (1990). Ways women lead. *Harvard Business Review, 68*(6), 119–125.

Rouhani, S. (2014). Intersectionality-informed quantitative research: A primer. *American Journal of Public Health, 103*(6), 1082–1089.

Ruth Eikhof, D. (2012). A double-edged sword: Twenty-first century workplace trends and gender equality. *Gender in Management: An International Journal, 27*(1), 7–22.

Sappleton, N. (2013). *The segregation stereotyping bind: Social networks and resource acquisition among men and women business owners in gender typical and atypical sectors*. PhD thesis, Manchester Metropolitan University.

Sappleton, N., & Takruri-Rizk, H. (2008). The gender subtext of science, engineering, and eechnology (SET) organizations: A review and critique. *Women's Studies, 37*(3), 284–316.

Sarkar, K. (2016). Fertility transition in India. Emerging significance of infertility and childlessness. In A. R. B. K. Singh (Ed.), *India 2016: Population transition* (pp. 87–102). Bhopal: MLC Foundation.

Schmidt, R. A., & Parker, C. (2003). Diversity in independent retailing: Barriers and benefits – The impact of gender. *International Journal of Retail & Distribution Management, 31*(8), 428–439.

Srinvasan, R., Woo, C. Y., & Cooper, A. C. (1994). Performance determinants for male and female entrepreneurs. Paper presented at the Proceedings of the 14th Annual Entrepreneurship Research Conference, Babson College, MA.

Tata, J., & Prasad, S. (2008). Social capital, collaborative exchange and microenterprise performance: The role of gender. *International Journal of Entrepreneurship and Small Business, 5*(3–4), 373–388.

Wajcman, J. (1999). *Managing like a man: Women and men in corporate management*. Cambridge: Polity.

West, C., & Zimmerman, D. H. (1991). Doing gender. In S. Farrell (Ed.), *The social construction of gender*. Newbury Park, CA: Sage.

Wood, G. J., & Newton, J. (2006). Childlessness and women managers: 'Choice', context and discourses. *Gender, Work & Organization, 13*(4), 338–358.

Wright, T. (2016). *Gender and sexuality in male-dominated occupations*. London: Palgrave Macmillan.

Zolin, R., Stuetzer, M., & Watson, J. (2013). Challenging the female underperformance hypothesis. *International Journal of Gender and Entrepreneurship, 5*(2), 116–129.

SECTION V
NATIONAL PERSPECTIVES ON CHILDLESSNESS

Chapter 13

Is There Voluntary Childlessness At All in Hungary?

Ivett Szalma and Judit Takács

Abstract

We chose to analyse Hungarian childlessness in order to map whether there is any voluntary childlessness at all in a society which is characterised by strong traditional family values and the widely accepted social norm that everyone should become a parent.

To answer to this question, we applied both quantitative and qualitative methods. First, we analysed the first three waves of the Hungarian panel survey 'Turning Points of the Life Course' conducted in 2001, 2004 and 2008. The focus is on men and women who were childless in 2001 and were still childless in 2008. To have a better understanding of the background of the quantitative results, we have also analysed 55 life-history interviews conducted with heterosexual men and women, who were recruited by using chain-referral sampling.

According to the qualitative findings the categorisation of childless people is quite fluid. For example, *postponers* became definitely childless while some originally voluntarily childless respondents became parents. However, the qualitative analysis allowed us to understand the mechanism behind this. In addition, using mixed methods also highlighted some inconsistencies between the qualitative and quantitative results.

Keywords: Voluntary childlessness; mixed methods; post-socialist country; traditional family attitudes; postponers; Gender differences

Introduction

Historically, childlessness has been associated with two main determinants: sterility and celibacy, but these traditional causes cannot explain the increasing proportion of childlessness among the younger generations of Europeans. Moreover, the developments in biotechnology and medical procedures have made it possible to an unprecedented extent for individuals who would previously have remained childless, such as individuals with medical problems, single women or same-sex couples, to experience parenthood with the help of artificial insemination, *in vitro* fertilisation and surrogate motherhood (see, e.g. Bartels, 2004; Hudson, Culley, Rapport, Johonson, & Baharadwaj, 2009). Thus, besides the traditional causes of infertility and childlessness, we have to consider previously unknown or unthinkable (post)modern features such as the transformation(s) of intimacy towards plastic sexuality and the pure relationship (Giddens, 1992), or increasing demand for private and public gender equality (Wood & Newton, 2006). In this context, parenthood, and especially motherhood, can be seen as an overly demanding commitment, which does not necessarily seem to be a very attractive lifestyle option for young Europeans.

Social scientists have started to devote increasing attention to this issue from the late twentieth century, especially in the English-speaking world since the 1970s (Bloom & Pebley, 1982; Bloom & Trussell, 1984; De Jong & Sell, 1977; Houseknecht, 1979; Veevers, 1973), when the proportion of voluntarily childless people started to increase in Western societies and being 'childfree' (Gillespie, 2003) became a non-stigmatised lifestyle option. However, in central Eastern Europe there have been only a limited number of empirical studies focusing specifically on childlessness; see, for example, Hašková (2010, 2011) and Mynarska, Matysiak, Rybińska, Vignoli, and Tocchioni (2013) for Czech and Polish findings – while it can be expected that – at least partly – different reasons contribute to the development and increase of childlessness in Central Eastern Europe than in the West.

This assumption can be supported by the different popularity levels of childless life; that is, childfree by choice, in different countries of Europe. By analysing Eurobarometer data Miettinen and Szalma (2014) found that the average rate of people aged 18–40 who are childfree by choice in Europe is about 1–6%. However, major differences can be observed among the countries. While the rate of those opting for living childfree is constantly around 8–10%, for example, in Austria, Luxembourg, Germany and Switzerland, it is below 2% in Central and

Eastern Europe.[1] In addition, Spéder and Kapitány (2014) point out another significant difference regarding fertility: according to their results a higher rate of planned children are born in Western European countries than in the Central and Eastern European countries of their study (Hungary, Bulgaria and Georgia). We believe the reasons are the major structural and cultural changes that affected the post-socialist societies in the past 20–30 years; due to the high speed of changes, postponing childbearing seemed a rational decision.

Mynarska et al. used sequence analysis on Polish panel data and examined how various life events such as graduation, joining the labour market and forming a relationship affect women's choice of a childfree life. By comparing Poland and Italy they found that similar life paths lead to childlessness in both countries, however, an insecure labour market position was a typical life path element only in Poland (Mynarska et al., 2013). Hašková (2011) used both qualitative and quantitative data to map what factors might have led to the increase of childlessness in the Czech Republic. She found that value changes (greater individualisation and personal fulfilment) as well as the increase of uncertainties, among others in connection with decreased social security and higher labour market uncertainty, made their contributions.

Male childlessness has received less attention than female childlessness within the literature related to fertility patterns. Most research studies of childlessness tend to focus on women (see, e.g. Graham, Hill, Shelly, & Taket; Mynarska et al., 2013; Szalma & Takács, 2012), while it has been shown that childlessness rates – both total and voluntary childlessness – are higher among men than among women in almost all European countries (Miettinen & Szalma, 2014).

---

[1]In Hungary, little attention has been devoted to the empirical study of childlessness, although the quantitative study Population Policy Acceptance Study (PPAS) conducted in 14 European countries between 2002 and 2005, involving more than 34,000 participants, did examine the issue of childfree life by choice as well. Research results show that the rate of people childfree by choice is on average less than 10% in the countries examined. However, while this rate remained below 5% in Cyprus, Slovenia and Lithuania both among men and women and only among women in Poland, Hungary and Estonia, Western European respondents had much higher rates. In Germany, 15.4% of women and 22.5% of men, in the Netherlands 12.5% of women and 17.5% of men, while in (the Flemish part of) Belgium 10.4% of women and 15.3% of men wanted no children. In addition, it was also revealed that choices to refuse childbearing were largely influenced by doubts about the future in Estonia, Germany, Hungary, Rumania and Cyprus (European Commission, 2007, pp. 47–48).

The focus of our chapter is Hungary where the very low fertility rate – that is, below 1.5 births per woman from the mid-1990s onwards – projects a demographically unsustainable population. Such a low level of fertility seems to be a reflection of constrained individual agency and weak capabilities for having and caring for children, linked to economic uncertainties and incoherence of public versus private sphere gender equity (Hobson, Fahlén, & Takács, 2014; Takács, 2013). Additionally, survey data show that the proportion of childless people is increasing within the Hungarian population: the most recent Hungarian census data indicated an increase in the childlessness rate of women over 41 from 7.8% to 11.2% between 2001 and 2011 (Kapitány, 2015), although there is no evidence of any short-term increase in biological or disease-related infertility (Simó, 2006). In this chapter, we focus on both men and women. To gain a rich, detailed picture of the reasons for voluntary childlessness we use both qualitative and quantitative analyses.

Quantitative Analysis

There are three main aims of our quantitative analysis. First, we explore the incidence of voluntary childlessness among Hungarian men and women. Second, we analyse the rate of postponing and voluntarily childlessness men and women who became parents within the examined time period of seven years. Finally, we investigate what kinds of factors can lead to childlessness (or more precisely: the prolongation of a childless life period) among those men and women who – according to their self-assessment – were not prevented from having children by their own or their partner's health constraints.

Methods

In the course of our empirical analysis, we used the first and third waves of the panel study Turning Points of the Life Course ('*Életünk fordulópontjai*') conducted by the Demographics Research Institute of the Central Statistical Office of Hungary within the Generations and Gender Survey (GGS) in 2001, 2004 and 2008; and we applied descriptive statistics, multinomial logistic regression models as methodological tools. The first GGS data collection wave of 2001 reached 16,364 persons, representative of the Hungarian population aged between 18 and 75 years. The sample of the third wave comprised a total of 10,641 people, with the reduction due to respondents dying, refusing answers and other causes of attrition.[2]

We used the panel survey questions directed at the number of own children, highest level of education (primary school, vocational school, secondary school or university), employment status, relationship status (being single, married or cohabiting), demographic background variables (gender, age and settlement type),[3] religiosity and attitudes in connection with family life. Taking into account that the income level of respondents is difficult to measure, we opted for examining whether respondents (or their partners) own an apartment.[4]

We have also created and applied a Traditional Family Attitudes (TFA) index by using principal component analysis with the following variables: (1) 'It is right and proper if, for the husband, work is the more important, while, for the wife, the home and the children, even when both are working?'; (2) 'A child should submit in everything to their parents and respect them, even if they do not deserve that'; (3) 'With a good profession and a good workplace, women are right if work is more important to them than having more children'; (4) 'There are, of course, parental responsibilities, but one should not give up life goals because of children'. Replies to all four statements were measured on a three-point scale (agree, disagree and unsure). In the case of the first two statements, agreement expresses the acceptance of traditional family-related attitudes, while for the other two statements, disagreement signals the same. We coded the responses to the statements accordingly. High values of the TFA index indicate an acceptance of traditional forms of family life and low values their rejection.

---

[2]In the third wave, attrition due to ageing was corrected with a sub-sample consisting of young(er) people. Since the present research only examined those who were older than 30 in 2001 and took part in all three waves, we did not use this sub-sample in our study.

[3]Age was measured as a categorical variable with the following categories (in 2001): aged 30–34, 35–40 and 41–45 for women, and aged 33–39, 40–44 and 45–50 for men.

[4]This was necessary not only because many respondents would not state their real income (the proportion of those refusing to answer usually being very high), but also because in those cases where respondents live in one household with their parents or other relatives, it is difficult to separate them, or the actual personal income is less relevant. Including the question whether respondents own an apartment was also supported by the fact that almost 90% of all apartments in Hungary are privately owned, and for most young Hungarians, getting their own apartment is a precondition for having children (Szalma, 2010).

Regarding our analytical strategy, as a start we wanted to find out more about those who were childless postponers or voluntarily childless compared with parents in 2001. We applied slightly different age categories for women and men partly because of the gendered differences regarding the mean ages at first childbearing (KSH, 2014), and partly because the question about future childbearing intentions ('Do you intend to have a/another child?') was put only to female respondents aged 45 or younger, and to male respondents aged 50 or younger. Thus we focused only on women aged 30–45 and men aged 33–50 who did not have children. Then we divided the childless respondents into three groups: the postponers, the voluntarily childless and the childless due to reproductive health problems.[5] We considered those respondents 'postponers' who had no children of their own in 2001 and answered 'yes' to the question 'Do you intend to have a /another child?', and at the same time had indicated that there were no health problems standing in the way of having children. We placed those childless respondents into the 'voluntarily childless' category who had answered 'no' to the question 'Do you intend to have a child?', and indicating no health problems at the same time. The 'childless due to reproductive health problems' group included those childless respondents who indicated that their decision regarding not having children depended on their own or their partner's health.

As a first step of analysis, we examined descriptive statistics. Then we examined those people who belonged to different childless categories in 2001 to assess how many of them had become parents by 2008. We created a dichotomous dependent variable by assigning the value of 0 to those who remained childless between 2001 and 2008, and assigning 1 to those who entered parenthood in the examined time period. Finally, we applied multinomial logistic regression on the Hungarian GGS data of 2001 to determine whether respondents belonging to the postponers or the voluntarily childless categories have any particular characteristics when compared with parents of similar ages. We chose this method because it allows us to predict the probabilities of the different possible outcomes of a categorically distributed dependent variable (types of childlessness) given a set of independent variables (such as age, religiosity, educational level, having paid work, family status, settlement type, having own apartment, traditional family-related attitudes and the view

[5]We could not include '(hetero)normatively prescribed childlessness' (of same-sex partners) as an additional category because of the lack of empirical data.

on the importance of having a child together for a happy marriage). Since we used only the first wave of the panel data in this phase, for internal consistency we applied the cross-sectional weight of the Hungarian survey rounds.

Results

First, we examined the number of respondents who belonged to a different childless category in 2001. Table 1 provides an overview of the number of respondents according to these three different childlessness categories while Table 2 shows the proportion of parenthood and childlessness by categories.

We can see (in Tables 1 and 2) that postponers form the largest group among childless men as well as women. In the 2001 sample, 87.8% of women aged 30–45, and 84.5% of men aged 35–50 had already entered parenthood. The proportion of voluntarily childless men (5%) was about twice as high as the proportion of voluntarily childless women (2.7%), while 8.7% of women and 9.3% of men could be categorised as postponers and 1% of respondents reported that they cannot have children because of their own or their partner's health-related problems.[6]

Since the last decades of the twentieth century, most Hungarians tended to postpone their childbearing to later ages; for example, women became mothers in their early 20s in 1970, but the age of first motherhood had shifted to their mid-20s by 1995, while in 2009 most women experienced first motherhood only in their early 30s (OECD, 2014). Timing of childbearing at a later age can lead to an increase in the childlessness rate because those who plan to have a child at later ages might have given up these plans or run out of time (i.e. that time period when childbearing might still be possible biologically) (Szalma & Takács, 2014). The biological timespan for having children and the social norms for childbearing intervals do not always fully coincide with each other. According to 2006 European Social Survey findings the latest acceptable age for becoming a mother is 39 in Hungary, while men should not have children after the age of 45.7 (Paksi & Szalma, 2009).

[6]The 1% seems to be an underestimation of infertility. The underestimation can derive from the reluctance of respondents to report this type of intimate information. It can also derive from the lack of awareness of their own fertility problems: for instance, some postponers might not be aware of their reproductive health problems before they actually try to have a child.

Table 1. Categories of Childlessness Among Women Aged 30–45 and Men Aged 33–50 in 2001.

	Childless Male Respondents Aged 33–50 (*n* = 521)			**Childless Female Respondents Aged 30–45 (*n* = 280)**		
	Postponers	**Childless due to reproductive health problems**	**Voluntarily childless**	**Postponers**	**Childless due to reproductive health problems**	**Voluntarily childless**
Health problem	No	Yes	No	No	Yes	No
Intention to have a child	Yes	NA	No	Yes	NA	No
Number of cases	381	28	112	198	20	62

Source: Generations and Gender Survey for Hungary, first wave (2001), authors' calculation.

Table 2. Proportion of Parenthood and Childlessness by Categories, Among Men Aged 35–50 and Women Aged 30–45 in 2001.

	Women		**Men**		**Total**	
	%	*N*	%	*N*	%	*N*
Has children	88	2,674	76	2,004	83	4,712
Postponers	7	214	16	422	11	624
Childless due to reproductive health problems	3	91	3	79	3	170
Voluntarily childless	2	60	5	132	3	170
Total	100	3,039	100	2,637	100	5,676

Source: Generations and Gender Survey for Hungary, first wave (2001), authors' calculation.

At the same time, younger people tend to be somewhat more permissive regarding their norms for the latest acceptable age to have a child than older people: Hungarian Eurobarometer data indicated 41 years as the latest socially acceptable age for entering motherhood by the younger cohort (aged 25–39) and 40.3 years by the older cohort (aged 40–65), while it was 46.9 for fatherhood according to the younger cohort, and 45.9 years according to the older cohort (Testa, 2006). The changing perception of childbearing age norms does not only reflect greater tolerance towards various individual life strategies, but as previous Hungarian studies indicate, it can also affect the actual childbearing age (Spéder & Kapitány, 2007).

Due to the nature of our quantitative survey data, it is impossible to determine whether the respondents were voluntarily childless from the beginning of their fertility career or if they stated that they did not want any children because they had given up on becoming parents at a certain point in their life. In the latter case, the re-interpretation of unfulfilled plans as a conscious choice might help to decrease cognitive dissonance. However, this can work the other way around as well: some of those respondents who were categorised as postponers perhaps did not want to become parents at all, but due to the internalised pressure about the 'parenting directive'; that is, the widely accepted social norm in Hungary that everyone should become a parent, they did not want, or dare to admit their intention to remain childless. Table 3 provides an overview of the rates of becoming a (non-)parent by 2008 according to the different childlessness categories of 2001.

By examining our 2008 sample, we can see that only 22% of the female respondents, defined as postponers in 2001, were able to realise their childbearing intentions in the examined time period. Since even the youngest women from this group became 37 by 2008, it can be assumed that the rate of entering parenthood would not improve considerably in the future as the probability of becoming a first-time mother after the age of 37 is quite low. Among postponer men, only 14% became fathers by 2008. However, men's average age at the birth of their first child tends to be higher than women's, and men do not have to face such a constraining 'biological deadline' (neither social, nor institutionalised) regarding their fertility, so in theory they can have a greater chance of entering parenthood later in their life course than women. The fact that seven women and two men who previously (in 2001) belonged to the voluntarily childless category became parents by 2008 can well illustrate the fluid nature of childlessness categories: in these cases (because of the quantitative nature of our data), we can only assume that changing

Table 3. Becoming a (Non-)Parent by 2008 According to the Different Childlessness Categories of 2001.

	Becoming a (Non-) parent by 2008	**Childless Respondents in 2001**		
		Postponers	**Childless Due to Reproductive Health Problems**	**Voluntarily Childless**
Women (childless and aged 30–45 in 2001)	Still childless in 2008	$N = 155$ (78%)	$N = 17$ (85%)	$N = 55$ (89%)
	Became a mother by 2008	$N = 43$ (22%)	$N = 3$ (15%)	$N = 7$ (11%)
$N = 280$		198	20	62
Men (childless and aged 33–50 in 2001)	Still childless in 2008	$N = 342$ (90%)	$N = 27$ (96%)	$N = 110$ (98%)
	Became a father by 2008	$N = 39$ (10%)	$N = 1$ (4%)	$N = 2$ (2%)
$N = 521$		381	28	112

Source: Generations and Gender Survey for Hungary, first and third waves (2001 and 2008), authors' calculation.

preferences and circumstances or contraceptive failure[7] led to their parenthood.[8]

In order to explore the specific features when comparing postponers with those having children in the same cohorts we have applied multinomial logistic regression analysis, using respondents who were parents in the first GGS round as a reference group. In Table 4, we have summarised the impacts of the basic socio-demographic variables, such as belonging to a certain age group, highest level of education, settlement type, partnership status, religiosity, as well as having one's own apartment, the view about the importance of having a child together for achieving a happy marriage and traditional family-related attitudes on the female and male postponers and voluntarily childless categories.

Outcomes of our analysis show that women belonging to the older age groups were significantly less likely to belong to the postponer category than younger women. This result is consistent with previous research findings (Berrington, 2004; Heaton, Jacobson, & Holland, 1999; Schoen, Astone, Kim, Nathanson, & Fields, 1999), which were conducted in Western European contexts. The similarity between the Western European and the Hungarian trends indicates that the mean age of women at first birth has increased in both types of society in the past decades.[9] Regarding men, with the progress of age the chance of postponement – similarly to the case of women – decreases; older age groups of men were significantly less likely to be postponers (and more likely to be childfree articulators) than younger men in 2001.

Women with higher levels (of secondary and especially tertiary level) of education were a lot more likely to be postponers than their lower-educated counterparts. A somewhat similar but much less pronounced tendency could be detected among men, while men with

[7]Including the case when socio-economically disadvantaged families cannot afford reliable contraceptive methods such as contraceptive pills or condoms.

[8]There were three women and one man who became parents in 2008 even though they were categorised in 2001 as belonging to the childless due to reproductive health problem group. This might be explained for instance by medical interventions or re-partnering (between 2001 and 2008): if the choice of not having children (in 2001) was made because of the previous partner's health problem. However, due to the limited explanatory potential of our survey data, we cannot be sure about the exact reasons.

[9]According to the OECD Family Database, the mean age of women at childbirth started to increase in the mid-1990s in Hungary, and we can find a similar trend in many Western European countries, including the United Kingdom, Germany, Spain and Finland.

Table 4. Impacts of Different Variables on the Types of Childlessness in 2001.

	Female Respondents (30–45)		**Male Respondents (33–50)**	
Variables	**Postponers**	**Voluntarily childless**	**Postponers**	**Voluntarily childless**
Age group: 30–34/33–39	Ref.	Ref.	Ref.	Ref.
Age group: 35–39/40–44	–1.76***	0.01	–0.89***	–0.16
Age group: 40–45/45–50	–3.83***	0.53	–1.32***	0.59*
Religiosity: 'not believing in God'	Ref.	Ref.	Ref.	Ref.
Religiosity: 'believe in God'	0.12	0.07	0.01	–0.16
Highest level of education: primary school	Ref.	Ref.	Ref.	Ref.
Highest level of education: vocational school	–0.01	–0.22	–0.44*	–0.38
Highest level of education: secondary education	0.54*	–0.16	0.49^	–0.21
Highest level of education: university	1.24***	0.25	0.59^	–0.63
Not having paid work	Ref.	Ref.	Ref.	Ref.
Having paid work	1.05***	–0.07	0.1	–0.25
Family status: single	Ref.	Ref.	Ref.	Ref.
Family status: living in cohabitation	–0.47*	–0.92*	–1.7***	–1.64***
Family status: living in marriage	–2.36***	–2.41***	–3.3***	–2.82***
Settlement type: village	Ref.	Ref.	Ref.	Ref.

Settlement type: town	−0.32	−0.22	0.04	−0.09
Settlement type: capital	0.01	0.02	0.36	−0.01
Not having own apartment	Ref.	Ref.	Ref.	Ref.
Having own apartment	0.06	−0.51^	−0.2	−0.41^
Traditional family attitudes	−0.08	0.05	0.09	−0.12
For a happy marriage, it is not important to have a child together (Values: 1–2)	−0.79*	1.38**	−0.49	−0.25***
For a happy marriage, it is not SO important to have a child together (Value: 3)	Ref.	Ref.	Ref.	Ref.
For a happy marriage, it is important to have a child together. (Values: 4–5)	−0.68	−0.2	−0.7	−1.77*
Number of observations	*2,285*		*2,139*	
LR chi^2 *(57)*	*541.45*		*724.84*	
Pseudo R^2	*0.24*		*0.28*	
Log likelihood	*−843.43*		*−948.47*	

Source: Generations and Gender Survey for Hungary, first wave (2001), authors' calculation.
Note: B coefficients in Multinomial Regression Analysis; Reference Group: Parents. Ref., Reference Group.
^$p<0.1$; *$p<0.05$; **$p<0.01$; ***$p<0.001$.

vocational school background were the least likely to be postponers. Regarding the voluntarily childless, educational level has not shown any significant effect, which was a slightly unexpected result as voluntary childlessness is often associated with higher levels of education, leading to increased opportunities of self-realisation, for instance, in the context of employment. Having paid work indeed significantly increased the chance of postponement for women whose employability in the Hungarian labour market – characterised by very limited parent-friendly flexibility – can be seriously constrained by having children. At the same time (because of the highly gendered nature of family practices that can largely 'free' men from adjusting their work-life balance after having children) employment did not have the same effect on men in the context of having children.

Living in a partnership significantly decreased the chances of being a postponer as well as that of voluntary childlessness for both genders especially in the case of marriage (but also in the case of cohabitation). Being partnered as a very strong predictor of entering parenthood is a result that reaffirms the findings of several previous studies (Berrington, 2004; Heaton et al., 1999; Schoen et al., 1999; Szalma & Takács, 2012, 2014).

Having their own apartment was shown to somewhat decrease the chance of belonging to the voluntarily childless categories for both men and women, a result that coincides with previous Hungarian research findings that having one's own apartment is regarded as a necessary precondition of having children (Szalma, 2010). Since the quantitative survey data of the Hungarian GGS rounds do not allow us to find out exactly what might be in the background of negative childbearing intentions, we cannot exclude the possibility that our voluntarily childless category, at least to a certain extent, overlaps with involuntary non-parenthood, associated with a historically well-known inequality pattern, consisting of people who cannot afford to have children or even establish a stable relationship because of financial reasons. An alternative hypothesis might be that people without an apartment have a more flexible mobile lifestyle, and are less willing to have children.

Regarding settlement type, religiosity and traditional family-related attitudes we have not found any significant effect, which might be due to the low number of cases. However, regarding the importance of having a child within marriage was shown to have a significant effect; when compared with parents, voluntarily childless women agreed more, while female postponers – in a somewhat self-justifying manner – tended to agree less with the importance of having children for a happy marriage. At the same time, voluntarily childless men tended to disagree with this view much more than those male respondents who had already become fathers by 2001.

The above analysis showed that there is a very low rate of voluntary childlessness in Hungary. Furthermore, the different childlessness categories have a fluid nature: some of the voluntarily childless men and women became parents while many of the postponers will probably remain childless forever. With the quantitative analysis we could not detect the decision-making mechanisms behind these transitions (and non-transitions) and we were not able to underpin the expected positive association between high education and voluntary childlessness. In order to understand voluntary childlessness better in the Hungarian context we also apply qualitative analysis in the next part of our chapter.

Qualitative Analysis

The main aim of our qualitative analysis is to examine childlessness patterns in Hungary on the basis of recently collected qualitative data more closely. The Hungarian qualitative data analysis is based on in-depth life-history interviews conducted with 30 heterosexual men aged and 25 heterosexual women within the *FamiliesAndSocieties* FP7 project between 2015 and 2016. The interviewees were recruited by advertising in print and social media as well as applying the snowball method, when that was possible. We chose only such individuals who did not have any biological children and were not living together with children in their household at the time of the interview. However, we did not exclude those individuals who used to have experience of living together with children (having lived together with their partner's children in a certain period) before the interview. As for partnership status, we did not apply any restrictions. Our selection criteria included lower (but not upper) age limits, which were 50 in the case of men and 40 in the case of women.[10] We considered only people with heterosexual orientation as we believe that childlessness of people

[10]Our aim was to focus on those childless men and women who will probably remain childless. Since having children is very rare among men above 50 and among women above 40 according to statistical data (KSH, 2014) we chose these age limits.

with same-sex orientation is a specific theme that should be examined by taking into consideration those discriminative policies that push them or most of them into a state of 'socially prescribed childlessness' in many countries, including Hungary.

Finally, our sample included interviewees from different geographical areas within Hungary: 17 men and 10 women were from Budapest, the capital, four men and five women from smaller towns and nine men and 10 women from small villages of about 3,000 residents (see Table 5 and Table 6). There were three educational subgroups among them: 10 men and seven women with low level of education (i.e. lower than completed secondary school), eight men and seven women with medium-level education (i.e. having a secondary school leaving exam) and 12 men and 11 women who were highly educated (i.e. having a university degree, including two men and four women with a doctoral degree). Regarding marital status, most men (23) and seven women were single, one man and three women were married, three men and two women were divorced, one man and 11 women had a cohabiting partner and two men and two women had a LAT (living together apart) relationship.

Our interview guideline covered five main topical areas: childhood, opinion about modern family changes (having children alone, raising children by same-sex couples), employment history, partnership history and future plans. Furthermore, we also asked some intimate questions about sexual life in the form of a self-administered questionnaire. Thus, we gained rich retrospective biographical narratives of the respondents, especially focusing on their private and family life. During the interviews, respondents talked about their experiences, desires and intentions regarding childbearing. Using these narratives, we identified all passages related to age, employment status, financial situation, partnership, physical well-being and childbearing desires or intentions. The richness of the textual data allowed us to study the relationship between people with different backgrounds and their fertility choices in detail, and enabled us to reconstruct the various mechanisms which could lead to their childless lifestyles. Focusing on both men and women allowed us to understand the gender differences in childlessness trajectories better.

Voluntary Childlessness among Women

The media and public opinion often magnify the phenomenon of voluntary childlessness. Our sample included three women who were voluntarily

Table 5. Sample Composition of Male Interviewees.

Educational Level		**Marital Status**		**Geographical Areas**		**Age Groups**	
Low	10	Single	23	Capital	17	50–55	10
Medium	8	Married	1	Town	4	55–60	12
High	12	Divorced	3	Villages	9	Over 60	8
Total	30	Cohabiting partner	1	Total	30	Total	30
		Living in LAT	2				
		Total	30				

Table 6. Sample Composition of Female Interviewees.

Educational Level		**Marital Status**		**Geographical Areas**		**Age Groups**	
Low	7	Single	7	Capital	10	40–45	10
Medium	7	Married	3	Town	5	45–60	10
High	11	Divorced	2	Villages	10	Over 60	5
Total	25	Cohabiting partner	11	Total	25	Total	25
		Living in LAT	2				
		Total	25				

childless. The underlying reason was not their choice of career over motherhood in spite of the fact that all of them were highly educated. Elisabeth[11] explained her choice of living without children in the following way: 'Actually I've never been thrilled by the idea of pampering a small child … It's alien to me' (Elisabeth, 47, college education, from the countryside).

Meanwhile Emma – who has a PhD and works at a university as a lecturer – was also sure that: 'I don't want any children and I have never had these kinds of feelings'; she never analysed the reasons. She mentioned different types of arguments against having children such as:

> It is terribly hard to raise a child – your life will be totally messed up … and … I have financial concerns about bringing up a child – it is hard to make ends meet even for myself.

In addition, she expressed her worries about finding a good school for the child in present-day Hungary. As for her partnerships, she said that she doesn't trust men. It is partly due to her father finding another woman immediately after her mother's death. Additionally, she always feels that 'men try to grab me, capture me or keep me by having children'. However, she added that she is aware of that this kind of stereotype works the other way around as well, usually men are afraid of being captured by a woman because of a child.

Our third interviewee, Annie, who works as a human rights lawyer, would fit the stereotype of career woman because she works very hard and travels a lot because of her job. However, she emphasised that the reason for not having children is not her career. She works a lot because she enjoys it very much. She thinks that the reason for not having children is related to the fact that she had an awful relationship with her mother. Additionally, her mother kept telling her that she would be a terrible mother.

Previous research has emphasised the importance of a partner's support when choosing to be childfree (Gillespie, 2003). Annie was divorced but her decision not to have children played a role in her divorce. She was not satisfied with her relationship, while her husband

[11]Interviewees are referred to with the use of pseudonyms (in order to protect their anonymity), followed by their age at the time of conducting the interview.

didn't want a divorce. 'Finally my husband agreed to a divorce because he wanted to have a child, although I wanted to divorce because of other things'. Now she lives in a LAT relationship and her partner is aware of that she doesn't want any children. However, if she did become pregnant despite using contraceptives, she would keep the child, not because of him, but because of moral issues, but she emphasised: 'I do not want that to happen'.

Emma is single but she desires to have a proper partner. She highlighted that while her counterparts (single women in their 40s) desire to have a child so they try to find a man for this project, her aim is slightly different: 'For me to have a partner would be bloody important'. Although she does not have a desire to have children she also mentioned that if she became pregnant, she would keep the child.

Elisabeth lives in cohabitation. She had a serious relationship previously that ended because her partner wanted children, Elisabeth later intentionally chose a partner who did not have such wishes. Her present partner does not want to have children because he already has one child from a previous relationship.

Most of the interviewees did not report any prejudice or discrimination in their workplace or private lives because of being childless (voluntarily or involuntarily). Only some higher-educated women had experience of being discriminated because of not having any children. For example, Emma said the following:

> Don't you have any children? Oh dear! Sometimes these kinds of utterances slip out of people's mouth. It is not painful for me, but when they ask me whether I have a husband that is painful for me. I feel that even those who don't have any children but have husbands have higher social prestige than those who have neither husbands nor children. Thus we are the lowest caste in this society.

In spite of the fact that Emma stated that the social expectation to have children does not hurt her, she admitted having two protecting mechanisms against these prejudices. On the one hand, she has the feeling that she has fulfilled life without children because of her interesting jobs and having many friends. On the other hand, her sister has done an above-average reproductive job: 'My sister has four children and we share almost the same genome so it is just like if I had reproduced myself as well'.

Another higher-educated but not voluntarily childless woman described a less direct prejudice affecting her as a childless single woman. She found it difficult to book a hotel or go out in a restaurant by herself in Hungary because people would look at her as a weird person. She does not have the same experience in Western European countries:

> 'Abroad you do not feel that you are despised because you are alone in a restaurant or in a hotel, childless and single women are more equal there than in Hungary. I believe that having children is not a moral category' – as it is considered in Hungary. Thus her defensive tactic is to go abroad for recreation instead of staying in Hungary.

Lower-educated and older interviewees did not report any prejudice. They found it reasonable and acceptable to work on bank holidays and do the overtime instead of their colleagues who do have children: 'Those who have children never work in the Christmas holidays but we (those who have not children) find it absolutely acceptable' (Nora, 45 years old lower-educated, blue-collar worker living in the countryside).

We did not find any women who can be defined as voluntarily childless among lower-educated women. Many women, especially among the oldest ones, who originally wanted to have children, reported feelings of strong regret and pain due to their lack of children:

> If I could restart my life I would do a lot of things differently. And I would insist on having children because to lead a fulfilled life, a woman needs a child. It was a big mistake that I didn't become a mother. Unfortunately, I am not able to correct it now. (Jelena, 70 years old, lower-educated retired)

It is partly because in their old age they can experience loneliness practically to its full extent, and because their youth was characterised by even more familistic norms than today (so they could see themselves as more deviant than their younger childless peers).

In our study on female childlessness in Hungary, we rarely found references to intentional childlessness or a preference for leading a child-free lifestyle (Szalma & Takács, 2014). These few voluntarily childless women were all highly educated and their intentional childlessness could be interpreted in the context of being occupied with life goals other than having children.

Voluntary Childlessness among Men

Our sample included altogether 30 men, and 12 of them were voluntarily childless. When interviewing childless men, we had the impression that they were more comfortable with discussing their intentional childlessness than the female interviewees. Some of the interviewed men, especially the highly educated ones talked about their childfree lifestyle almost as an achievement. One of them, a 50-year-old single man living in the countryside said that he enjoys himself in children's company but this good relationship with children never led him to aspire to have his own child: 'My life project is not about having children'. Another well-educated man pointed out that not everybody was born to have children: 'I don't feel that I miss out on anything because of not having children' (53, divorced single, Budapest).

We also found an interviewee, Jonas, who expressed his explicit aversion to having children:

> None of my girlfriends ever tried to persuade me to have children as it was so obvious that I abhor children ... it would have been like trying to force meat eating on a determined vegetarian. (52, highly educated, Budapest divorced)

When he was 40 and still living in a marriage Jonas decided to have a vasectomy to avoid having children. His aim was not having children, but he also considered gender equality:

> I know it might sound a bit ironic. However, I find it incredibly outrageous that 95% of the Hungarian middle class want to limit the number of their children, but 90% think that it is the women's responsibility even if that is to the detriment of their health.

We found various other reasons behind the examined men's decisions not to have children. One of them, Lucas, a 50-year-old, highly educated artist pointed out that he is simply not a suitable person to have children:

> I cannot take responsibility at all. However, I can entertain children and I can tell them stories and they would probably learn lots of important things from me. But I am

> not able to take them anywhere on time. I am even not able to manage my life. I have had problems with everyday time management ever since my childhood. I could never have been a soldier or a doctor.

A man with a medium-level education, living alone in Budapest, stated that his care activities scared him away from having children:

> The reason [for not wanting to have children] is partly connected to my grandma's story … because I have seen her suffering a lot and I am terribly scared of seeing someone suffering … so I knew that having children would cause me non-stop anxiety on a daily basis … so if the child is not around, I would be nervous or if they are around I would worry whether they will be sick or what would happen to them.

We have also encountered a case where a 50-year-old man with medium education admitted that he has been having drug problems for many years. He reported that taking drugs has changed his way of thinking about life, and even in the period when he stopped taking drugs for a few years, he was not content with what many people would consider a decent life: 'I believed that happiness can be achieved by working hard, having a house and children. I have worked hard, and I had a house but I felt like a droid'. Finally, he realised that he did not want any children because he would not be happy while having a child.

References to voluntary childlessness also came up in the narratives of men with lower education, although they did not articulate their views as clearly as their higher-educated counterparts did. For example, one of them just simply stated that 'I did not have any particular intention to have children' (55, lower-educated, village, living in LAT), while another expressed his view that it is not motherhood that makes a woman a woman, and added that 'even if I could start my life all over again I wouldn't decide otherwise … regarding not having children' (60, single, village, primary school).

As for partnerships, we can see voluntarily childless men living in different forms of partnerships: three live or used to live in marriage at the time when they decided not to have any children, three live in cohabitation, one in a LAT relationship and five of them are single. For example, Jonas lived in a marriage when he decided to have a vasectomy. His wife desired to have a child so she had to choose between staying with him and not have any children, or leaving him. Finally, she decided to stay with him, although they split up later. According to Jonas, there was a connection between her abandoned desire to have a child and their spoilt relationship: 'If my wife had satisfied her child-rearing ambition our other types of problems wouldn't have worsened and we wouldn't have divorced'.

Andrew, a 58-year-old, highly educated man works as an engineer. He is not against having children, he just never felt that he was ready to have one. When his wife wanted to have children unexpectedly, he decided to divorce. Shortly after his divorce, he moved in with his new partner who had three children already. For his new partner, it was not important to have a common child because she already had her own. Meanwhile he enjoyed living together with children. He described that

> (Children) communicate with me in a different way than with their parents. I would say that they are more honest with me because they are sure that I will not tell their secrets to anybody.

Hugo, a 55-year-old, taxi driver with a medium level of education had never lived together with a woman, however, he has a long-term LAT relationship. He said that his personality foreshadowed that he would have neither children nor a wife: 'I haven't liked being together with somebody continually since my childhood … I meet my girlfriend twice or three times a week and that is enough for me'. Hugo assumed that his girlfriend did not want any children, but she has some excuses: 'It was not up to her that she doesn't have any children. She had to nurse her grandma for more than 20 years … while I do not have any such loophole'.

As two voluntarily childless women emphasised there is a situation where they would not refuse to have a child: they would not choose to abort their embryo if they became pregnant by accident. We found similar cases among men, too. For example, Jonas mentioned that life could bring a situation when one must live together with a child: when his mother-in-law died, her sister-in-law with a mental disorder was left alone. He then agreed that the girl should live with them until they could find a proper care-home for her. The other case is that of Martin, a well-educated white-collar worker who has lived together with his partner for more than 20 years. His partner definitely wanted to have children, but he never desired to have one. However, after living together for some years he gave in. He described his feeling in the following way:

> I took some years from her life so it was only fair that I accepted her will and helped her to achieve her aim. It is another story that in the end she didn't have any children.

As among women, where we found some highly educated women who reported prejudice because they did not have any children, we detected similar patterns among men. There were only two men who mentioned prejudice because they did not have any children. One is Lucas who said:

> I am asked whether I have children or not as if it would be a defect that I don't have any. Unknown people ask me and assume that I am gay, sterile, impotent or drug addicted because I don't have any children. I find this a complete nonsense.

The other one is Romeo who is a single, highly educated man living in the countryside. According to him, 'In the countryside people look at you strangely because you do not have a wife and children at a certain age so there is some gossip about me as well'.

Men also have some tactics to defend themselves against prejudice. Romeo, for example, tries to keep a distance from the local people in the village where he lives: he does not make any friends there. While Martin said that when people ask about his family situation he always adds that 'unfortunately' he does not have children; when he uses this emotional expression, people stop asking him about this topic because they feel that it must be a sad topic for him.

Conclusion

In the present study, we have tried to answer our main question – *Is there voluntary childlessness at all in Hungary?* – by applying quantitative and qualitative methods. This question is important because Hungary belongs to the countries with strong traditional family values and the widely accepted social norm that everyone should become a parent. However, Hungarian survey data show that the proportion of childless people is increasing. Our quantitative analysis highlighted that the group of persons childless due to reproductive health problems is the smallest one. The largest group consisted of postponers, followed by a smaller group of voluntarily childless respondents. Meanwhile, we were unable to examine the social phenomenon of heteronormatively prescribed childlessness empirically – a relevant feature for instance for Hungarian same-sex couples with child-rearing intentions – because of the lack of data to be analysed.

Based on our GGS data sets, we cannot tell the full story of Hungarian childlessness. However, we can see that the definition of different types of childlessness can become fluid: many postponers failed to realise their fertility intentions while some of the voluntarily childless men and women became parents within the examined time period of seven years. Our qualitative analysis allows us to understand the mechanism behinds these transitions. Voluntarily childless men and women are able to adjust their intentions to their possibilities by agreeing to live together with children if life brings some inevitable situation such as a non-intended pregnancy or the necessity to care for the partner's children.

We perceived some inconsistency between the findings of the quantitative and qualitative analyses. While we did not find any positive association between educational level and voluntary childlessness using GGS data, we did find this association on the basis of our qualitative data among women. However, it should be noted that preference for a childfree lifestyle was expressed not only by highly educated men, as was the case for women, but also by men with lower levels of education. As for preference of a childfree lifestyle we cannot be sure whether these issues are more relevant in the case of lower-educated men than in that of lower-educated women or perhaps lower-educated men felt socially less restricted and were only more ready to 'admit' that these issues might play a part in their childlessness than lower-educated women.

However, when we asked whether they experienced any prejudice related to their childlessness we can see similar patterns in the responses of the two genders: only higher-educated women and men reported prejudice based on their not having any children. Meanwhile, men constructed tactics that can defend them by controlling the outside world (keeping their distance or pretending not to have any children because of some health-related issues). Tactics developed by women were slightly different: they tried to defend themselves without controlling the outside world (reassuring themselves that their life is fulfilled without children and, for instance, concentrating on the fact that their genome is reproduced through their siblings' children).

Another inconsistency between the qualitative and quantitative results is related to the importance of partnership status. Based on the survey analysis, we found that voluntarily childless people are under-represented among those who live in a cohabiting relationship (cohabitation or marriage). Our interview analysis showed that voluntarily childless men and women can live in different types of partnerships and only some of them are single. However, partnered voluntarily childless women found it more important to have their partners' support for their decisions than voluntarily childless men did.

Our study has some limitations such as the low number of cases. However, we believe that this chapter contributes to a better understanding of an under-researched field of enquiry, especially in the post-socialist countries. In Hungarian society, family practices such as postponing the birth of a first child and the increase in childless people have changed more rapidly (starting from the 1990s) than in Western societies where the changes started from the 1970s with the emergence of the Second Demographic Transition. However, it seems that ideas change slowly; most Hungarians would like to have children, especially women – at least so they say. The results of the quantitative analysis showed that many postponers are not able to realise their plans. These unsuccessful scenarios are mainly related to the lack of a partner – which is a common reason in many societies. However, in Hungary – and probably in many other post-socialist countries – the financial difficulties and uncertainties on the labour market can play an important role as well.

This study also highlights the importance of using mixed methods in analysing childlessness related issues. We consider our present work a starting point for further investigations, which should proceed with comparative analysis to delve deeper into patterns of (voluntary) childlessness in Central and Eastern Europe.

Acknowledgment

The research leading to these results has received funding from the NKFIH Research Project No. 123789.

References

Bartels, D. M. (2004). Brave new families: Modern health technologies and family creation. In *Handbook of contemporary families*. Sage Publications.

Retrieved from http://sage-ereference.com/hdbk_contempfamilies/Article_n28.html. Accessed on October 15, 2009.

Berrington, A. (2004). Perpetual postponers? Women's, men's and couple's fertility intentions and subsequent fertility behaviour. *Population Trends*, *117*, 9–19.

Bloom, D. E., & Pebley, A. R. (1982). Voluntary childlessness: A review of evidence and implications. *Population Research and Policy Review*, *1*, 203–224.

Bloom, D. E., & Trussell, J. (1984). What are the determinants of delayed childbearing and permanent childlessness in the United States? *Demography*, *21*(4), 591–611.

De Jong, G. F., & Sell, R. R. (1977). Changes in childlessness in the United States: A demographic path analysis. *Population Studies*, *31*(1), 129–141.

European Commission. (2007). *Population policy acceptance study – The viewpoint of citizens and policy actors regarding the management of population related change*. Luxembourg: Office for Official Publications of the European Communities. Retrieved from http://cordis.europa.eu/documents/documentlibrary/100124311EN6.pdf. Accessed on March 10, 2015.

Giddens, A. (1992). *The transformation of intimacy. Sexuality, love and eroticism in modern societies*. Stanford: Stanford University Press.

Gillespie, R. (2003). Childfree and feminine: Understanding the gender identity of voluntarily childless women. *Gender and Society*, *17*(1), 122–136.

Graham, M., Hill, E., Shelly, J., & Taket, A. (2013). Why are childless women childless? Findings from an exploratory study in Victoria, Australia. *Journal of Social Inclusion*, *4*(1), 70–89.

Hašková, H. (2010). Fertility decline, the postponement of childbearing and the increase in childlessness in central and Eastern Europe: A gender equality approach. In R. Crompton, S. Lewsi, & C. Lyonette (Eds.), *Women, men, work and family in Europe* (pp. 76–85). London: Palgrave Macmillan.

Hašková, H. (2011). The role of work in fertility plans of childless men and women in their thirties. In V. Cuzzocrea & J. Laws (Eds.), *Value of work: Updates on old issues* (pp. 149–158). Oxford: Inter-Disciplinary Press.

Heaton, T. B., Jacobson, C. K., & Holland, K. (1999). Persistence and change in decisions to remain childless. *Journal of Marriage and Family*, *61*(2), 531–539.

Hobson, B., Fahlén, S., & Takács, J. (2014). A sense of entitlement? Agency and capabilities in Sweden and Hungary. In B. Hobson (Ed.), *Worklife balance. The agency & capabilities gap* (pp. 57–91). Oxford: Oxford University Press.

Houseknecht, S. K. (1979). Timing of the decision to remain voluntarily childless: Evidence for continuous socialization. *Psychology of Women Quarterly*, (1), 81–96.

Hudson, N., Culley, L., Rapport, F., Johonson, M., & Baharadwaj, A. (2009). Public perceptions of gamete donation. *Public Understanding of Science*, *18*(1), 61–77.

Kapitány, B. (Ed.). (2015). Terjed a gyermektelenség Magyarországon [Increasing childlessness in Hungary]. *Korfa Népesedési hírlevél*, *XV*(1), 1–4.

KSH [Central Office of Statistics]. (2014). *Demográfiai Évkönyv, 2013* [Demographic yearbook, 2013]. Budapest: KSH.

Miettinen, A., & Szalma, I. (2014). Childlessness intentions and ideals in Europe. *Finnish Yearbook of Population Research*, *49*, 31–55. http://ojs.tsv.fi/index.php/fyp/article/view/48419. Accessed on March 10, 2015.

Mynarska, M., Matysiak, A., Rybińska, A., Vignoli, D., & Tocchioni, V. (2013). *Diverse paths into childlessness over the life course*. Zeszyty Naukowe, Instytutu Statystyki i Demografii, Szkoła Główna Handlowa, ISID Working Papers 34. http://kolegia.sgh.waw.pl/pl/KAE/struktura/ISiD/publikacje/Documents/Working_Paper/ISID_WP_34_2013.pdf. Accessed on March 10, 2015.

OECD. (2014). *OECD family database*. Paris: OECD. Retrieved from www.oecd.org/social/family/database. Accessed on August 2, 2014.

Paksi, V., & Szalma, I. (2009). Mikor vállaljunk gyereket? [When should we have children?]. *Szociológiai Szemle*, *3*, 92–116.

Schoen, R., Astone, N. M., Kim, Y. J., Nathanson, C. A., & Fields, J. M. (1999). Do fertility intentions affect fertility behavior? *Journal of Marriage and the Family*, *61*(3), 790–799.

Simó, T. (2006). *Ha nem jön a baba: a meddőség okai és kezelése* [*If there is no baby coming: The causes and treatment of infertility*]. Budapest: New Age Média Kft.

Spéder, Z., & Kapitány, B. (2007). *Gyermekek: Vágyak és tények. Dinamikus termékenységi elemzések* [*Children: Desires and facts. Dynamic fertility analyses*]. Budapest: KSH Népességtudományi Kutatóintézet.

Spéder, Z., & Kapitány, B. (2014). Failure to realize fertility intentions: A key aspect of the post-communist fertility transition. *Population Research and Policy Review*, *33*(3), 393–418.

Szalma, I. (2010). Attitűdök a házasságról és a gyermekvállalásról. [Attitudes towards marriage and childbearing]. *Demográfia*, *53*(1), 38–67. Retrieved from http://www.demografia.hu/letoltes/kiadvanyok/Demografia/2010_1/Demografia_2010_1_Szalma.pdf

Szalma, I., & Takács, J. (2012). A gyermektelenséget meghatározó tényezők Magyarországon. [Factors influencing childlessness in Hungary]. *Demográfia*, *55*(1), 44–68. Retrieved from http://www.policy.hu/takacs/pdf-lib/2012_Szalma_Takacs_Gyermektelen_Demografia_F.pdf

Szalma, I., & Takács, J. (2014). Gyermektelenség – és ami mögötte van. Egy interjús vizsgálat eredményei. [Qualitative study of childlessness from Hungary]. *Demográfia*, *57*(2–3), 109–137. Retrieved from http://demografia.hu/kiadvanyokonline/index.php/demografia/article/view/2477/2334

Takács, J. (2013). Unattainable desires? Childbearing capabilities in early 21st century Hungary. In L. S. Oláh & E. Fratczak (Eds.), *Childbearing, women's employment and work-life balance policies in contemporary Europe* (pp. 179–206). New York, NY: Palgrave Macmillan.

Testa, M. R. (2006). *Childbearing preferences and family issues in Europe*. Brussels: European Commission.

Veevers, J. E. (1973). Voluntary childlessness: A neglected area of family study. *The Family Coordinator*, *22*(2), 199–205.

Wood, G. J., & Newton, J. (2006). Childlessness and women managers: 'Choice', context and discourses. *Gender, Work and Organization*, *13*(4), 338–358.

Chapter 14

Stigma and Childlessness in Historical and Contemporary Japan

Kimiko Tanaka and Deborah Lowry

Abstract

Japanese women's life courses have changed dramatically in recent history. Yet, transformation of the meanings and experiences of childlessness did not follow a linear, one-dimensional path. Childlessness in Japan today – strongly influenced by Western, modern education after the World War II – can indeed be interpreted as a form of liberation from a restrictively gendered life-course. However, in Japan's pre-modern period, there were in fact alternative paths available for women to remain childless. As Japan became nationalised and the meanings of Japanese womanhood shifted, childlessness became increasingly stigmatised and notably, stigmatised across social classes.

This chapter provides concise accounts of the social meanings of marriage and fertility from the Tokugawa period through the Meiji period and continues with analysis of pressures faced by contemporary Japanese women who are childless. Also highlighted are the particular socio-demographic contexts which have brought involuntary childlessness, too, into the realms of public discussion and expected action on the part of the government. Through its account of the Japanese context, this chapter emphasises the larger theoretical, sociological argument that the historically placed social construction of childlessness – and thus, of the experiences and identities of childless women – always occurs through particular intersections of cultural, political-economic and demographic conditions.

Keywords: Social stigma; childlessness; Japanese family; intersectionality; social construction of family; motherhood imperative

Introduction

Feminist literature has long highlighted the stigma associated with a woman's choice to remain childfree (Hird, 2003; Letherby, 2002; Lisle, 1999; Morell, 1994; Park, 2002; Reti, 1992; Whiteford & Gonzalez, 1995). Much of this work focuses on Western societal definitions of womanhood, macro-level trends, women's rationale for various reproductive choices and individual experiences of stigma (Blackstone & Stewart, 2012). Less emphasised are the particular socio-historical factors shaping childfree stigma; how individual experiences are structured by class, age and national identity, and how reproductive privilege and oppression may coexist (Collins, 2000). In this chapter, we examine social meanings and contexts of women's childlessness in Japan from the pre-modern Tokugawa period (1600–1868) to the present day.

This historical overview of Japan's shifting motherhood norms illustrates how childfree stigma is a characteristic of the social structures; in this case, a product of intersecting processes of Confucian patriarchal culture, industrial capitalism, international politics and Western influence. This broader geographical and sociological perspective lends insight into the conditions under which childfree stigma flourishes or languishes. Also suggested is the role that an individual woman's class, family roles and place of origin played in influencing her reproductive obligations (and opportunities). This chapter begins with a description of family arrangements and attitudes during Japan's Tokugawa period (1603–1868), the Meiji period (1868–1912) characterised by the rapid modernisation, the Taisho period (1912–1926) marked by further modernisation with continuation of influence, the Showa period (1926–1989) of great post-war socio-economic change and the Heisei period (1989–present). A discussion of the role of contemporary reproductive technologies in formulating modern-day childfree stigma precedes a summary of the cultural and political forces structuring motherhood imperatives in Japan's recent history.

Family and Motherhood in Japan's Tokugawa Period (1603–1868)

Japanese sense of self was inextricably tied to hierarchical social relations, and particularly to the stem family or *ie* (Inoue, 1991). The practice and concept of *ie* emerged from the aristocracy in the Heian period (794–1185) and became a unit of social organisation for the elite class that led to 'strengthening primogeniture and weakening women power' (Fauve-Chamoux & Ochiai 2009, p. 19). The *ie* depended on the continuation of the family line through the male offspring of the family (Inoue, 1991; Keyser & Kumagai, 1996). Such morality defined the role of women as a tool for producing a male child to support the *ie* economy and undoubtedly intensified social stigma for women who failed to do so. It is important to note that the *ie* during the Tokugawa period was a functional unit based on economic activities intended to sustain the *ie* over generations (Keyser & Kumagai, 1996). The *ie* included not only family members, but also employees who contributed to the *ie* economy but whom were not related to the family by blood or marriage (Inoue, 1991). The succeeding head of the *ie* was necessary to the support of all members.

Initially, the *ie* was practised only among the privileged, such as aristocrats of the and samurai warriors (Takeya, 2008), and some historians argue that the *ie* only became a fully established unit for ordinary people during the course of the Tokugawa period as it moved towards the Meiji period (Fauve-Chamoux & Ochiai, 2009). Prior to this time, the *ie* was not the major unit of social and family life among peasants and merchants (Fauve-Chamoux & Ochiai, 2009).

It was during the Tokugawa period that the *Onna Daigaku (The Great Learning for Women)* was authored by the seventeenth century moralist Ekken Kaibara. Kaibara applied Confucian ethics to argue that women were obligated by filial piety to honour in-laws and obey their husbands (Kaibara & Takaishi, 1908). One of his well-known statements is '*yomeshite sannen ko nakiwa saru*', meaning that a childless woman should leave her husband's *ie* after three years of marriage. (Kaibara & Takaishi, 1908). Infertility meant absence of descendants to perform ritual services for the deceased family members, which resulted in violating the norm of filial piety (Muraoka, 2004).

Confucian values were certainly not new to Japanese society, but *Onna Daigaku* re-invoked and highlighted these ideas specifically to emphasise women's moral duty to reproduce. This development occurred in concert with the increasingly widespread *ie* system. During this era, women were often blamed for infertility of the couple, and men were publicly allowed to have mistresses to gain a male successor (Takeya, 2008). Among the justifications for divorce stated in the book was infertility – unless the woman consented to adopting a child. Notably, adoption was a widely accepted method for infertile couples to forward the *ie*. Childless women of the privileged obeyed the head of household (her father-in-law or her husband) in deciding who to adopt as a successor of the *ie*. The adoptee was not necessarily the male child of relatives; rather, he might be a trusted young employee (Hayes & Habu, 2011). Of course, adoption for the sake of perpetuating the *ie* differs from contemporary Western adoption in which an emphasis is placed on forming emotional attachments in the way done with a biological child (Hayes & Habu, 2011).

Women's reproductive obligation to the extended family in a Confucian culture is likely familiar to many readers. However, of significance is the fact that these strong reproductive imperatives had applied mainly to women of the privileged classes (Imai, 2002). Among the remaining 90% of the population, there was great variety in family structures and dynamics. Subservience to the husband was not necessarily demanded of women in lower classes (Imai, 2002). Women in peasant households worked in the fields along with men, and people tended to prioritise work before marriage (Imai, 2002). There was greater flexibility in gender roles, artisan and merchant households shared productive and reproductive work, and women even participated in social protests (Imai, 2002). Rural towns and villages also had some power in limiting childbearing, as people in towns and villages shared responsibility for annual taxes that dominated rice payments. In order to limit population growth, local officials might restrict marriage for the second and third sons, or order couples to adopt a child (Ishizaki, 2015). Although women still did not exercise autonomy in determining whether to become mothers, any of these policies might have mitigated social stigma surrounding childlessness within these social strata.

After centuries of warring states ruled by competing feudal lords, the Tokugawa (Edo) period had brought 250 years of stability to Japan. The era and its developments were crucial to establishing a foundation for Japan's later rapid modernisation. In efforts to exterminate Christianity – seen by leaders as a foreign threat to their power – samurai warriors carried out village investigations and rural populations were ordered to complete *shūmon aratame cho* or religious investigation registers (Cornell & Hayami, 1986). These registers became important demographic resources through which to understand families during this period.

Records show that during this era, age norms for people to marry and have a child was far from universal, and childlessness was not uncommon among people who were not entitled to perpetuate an *ie*. Based on records from the Higo clan, chances of marriage for an eldest son with enough wealth were great (89%) (Kito, 2007). However, proportions of unmarried men were high for men who were not eldest sons (81.1%) and for those who were in subordinate positions serving the privileged (89.5% for men and 70.6% for women) (Kito, 2007). Many rural men and women who were not entitled to succession worked in the city and lived in a merchants' house. Due in particular to migration of young men to cities, Edo (today's Tokyo) was full of single and temporal workers, and the city had markedly unbalanced sex ratios (Nawata, 2006). The Edo culture also accelerated the commodification of young single women through public and private prostitution (Imai, 2002). These women were portrayed in *ukiyoe* art and literature that emphasised the female body as an object of sexual desire. Women who made their living by selling flowers, books and teas on the streets, as well as maids and wet nurses of merchant households were often depicted sensually (Imai, 2002).

In short, there was marked diversity in the life courses of Japanese women – and thus reproductive expectations – before and during the Tokugawa period (Shirai, 2004). Certainly, producing a successor was important in a Confucian context, but in earlier years, this was the case most particularly among the elite classes. Wives of the privileged lived and worked within the *ie*, where childlessness was not tolerated. Although women from all social strata were severely restricted and objectified, the particular stigma of childlessness was not simply gendered, but also a classed phenomenon further influenced by the social location and birth order of a woman's husband.

The Motherhood Imperative and the Political Economy of the Meiji Period (1868–1912)

To protect Japan from foreign influence, the Tokugawa leaders had barred trade with Western nations. But the growth in Western powers towards the end of the Tokugama period pushed Japan to open its doors. Thus, the ensuing Meiji Period witnessed increasing levels of both modernisation and nationalism. A drive to expand the Japanese population engendered the view of motherhood as a way for women to serve the nation (Nemoto, 2008).

Industrial capitalism continued to develop throughout the Meiji period. These political-economic shifts influenced fertility values and behaviours in both urban and rural settings. In the cities, a new urban middle class emerged as more men could attain stable employment to support independent families. The wives of these 'salarymen' followed the duties of diligent housewives and managers of the home; good wives and wise mothers (*ryosai kenbo*). The *ryosai kenbo* (good wife, wise mother) ideology had become the major focus of higher education for women as reflected in slogans such as 'the woman is the key of the home' (Cwiertka, 1998; Takeya, 2008). Marriage and motherhood became important life events for urban, educated women (Shirai, 2004) as the ideal described in *Onna Daigaku* became a major influence on female students (Koyama, 2012). At the same time, ideas about domesticity and a woman's duty to create a happy home were introduced to Japan through Protestant mission schools. The *ie* was legally recognised in the Meiji Civil Code (Fauve-Chamoux & Ochiai, 2009); however, influenced by Western concepts of modern family, the code officially defined the *ie* as a unit based only on blood and marriage (Matsuki, 2016). During this era, the magazine *Seito*, published by educated women interested in planned births, attempted to initiate discussion about contraceptives. But the Japanese government, declaring the topic lewd, banned reference to contraceptives in books and magazines (Ishizaki, 2015) and women who questioned the *ryosai kenbo* ideology, including the view of children as divine gifts, became increasingly marginalised (Ishizaki, 2015).

In villages, ownership of farms was transferred to individuals, and this decentralisation of property resulted in less emphasis on fertility control at the town and village levels. With fewer formal restrictions, numbers of impoverished farmers with large families increased. Based on historical records, Ishizaki (2015) claims that many rural women were interested in contraceptive methods, but their voices were ignored by strong social norms of regarding children as destined from the gods. Still, during the Meiji period, in the event that a couple failed to produce biological children, it was still common to adopt and raise a child from relatives. Examining the 1870 Tama household register of 33 villages in the South-Tama region (west of Tokyo today), Kurosu and Ochiai (1995) found that 11% of the male population was adopted. Notably, the majority of adoptions in South-Tama were *adult* adoptions made to ensure the succession of the family line, by either adopting sons of a reproductive age, or through recruiting 'adopted' sons-in-law in the case of having only daughters. The progeny of the 'adopted' son-in-laws would follow the lineage of the adopting family rather than the natal family of the sons-in-law. Thus, motherhood imperatives in both rural and urban areas remained strong, but alternatives to carrying on the family line (beyond biological reproduction) existed particularly in more traditional rural settings that were insulated from Western influence.

Finally, during the Meiji era, a drive to expand the Japanese population engendered the view of motherhood as a way for women to serve the nation (Nemoto, 2008). As Japan industrialised and nationalised further, and with government attempts to unify the nation, the legalisation of the *ie* system was the '*invention* of the Meiji government and was the Japanese counterpart of the modern family' (Ueno, 2009, p. 109) characterised by 'the worship of domesticity; the exclusion of women from productive labour; the birth of childhood, and the formation of the concept of "motherhood"'(Ueno, 2009, p. 109). Reproduction could be a way for all Japanese women to contribute to society. Still, alternatives to parenthood existed. Many members of the 'excess' rural population moved to urban areas, leaving home without a strong responsibility to have children. Despite high mortality in cities due to disease and infection, the Meiji urban population did not decrease owing to migration of these single men and women (Ishizaki, 2015; Kito, 2007). According to the 1888 historical record of the city of Tokyo, the percentage of married persons was only 35.2% among men aged 15–59 years old, and 48% among women between 20 and 39 years old (Kito, 2007). Cities were full of poor rural migrants (Kagaya, 2014) and many people remained single and childless. This childless population diminished as the Japanese economy expanded in ensuing years. Although inaccessibility to marriage and parenthood reflected strong economic disadvantage, there is no evidence of childlessness itself being stigmatised among lower classes who had little resources by which to support progeny. Childlessness and childfree stigma can still thus be seen as classed phenomena in the Meiji period, as urban educated women felt particular pressure to demonstrate their value and patriotism through becoming mothers.

Taisho and Showa Eras: Economic Development, Childfree Stigma and Resistance

The World War I further stimulated industrial capitalism as Japan moved into the Taisho era (1912–1926). Industrialisation had increased employment opportunities for both men and women and the proportion of the married population grew (Ishizaki, 2015). By 1920 in Tokyo, for example, 45.5% of men between 15 and 59 years old and 72.2% of women between 20 and 39 years old were married (Kito, 2007). (Men were more likely to be single due to their relatively higher migration rate to the city.) Increasingly, working-class households engaged in division of labour in which the husband worked outside and wives tended to children and perhaps low-wage, non-technical work at home (Ishizaki, 2015). Such gendered division of labour became standardised during the Taisho era, and increased salaries allowed these families to send male children to high schools to acquire skills. Many of these working-class daughters were now educated for marriage, and the majority of their marriages were arranged between *ie*. Increasingly, women from a variety of walks of life followed the edicts of the *Onna Daigaku* to be submissive to their *ie* (Shimada, 2002). In 1920, only 2.2% of men and 1.8% of women remained never married by age 50, and economic stability allowed early marriage as well (27.4 years for men and 23.2 years for women for the first marriage) (National Institute of Population and Social Security Research, 2012b). In short, the effects of industrial capitalism included greater standardisation of life courses. These emerging life-course norms promoted more general stigmatisation of women who refused marriage and motherhood. There were movements to free women from the structural constraint of the *ie* and Confucianism, but they were eventually 'swallowed by the aggressive nationalism of Showa centred around the emperor' (Sugiyama-Lebra, 1998, p. 212).

As Japan moved towards the Showa era (1926–1989) and approached the World War II, the Ministry of Health and Welfare created the slogan 'give birth and multiply for the nation' (Nemoto, 2008). By 1940, a system was in place to reward families with many children (Kano, 2004). Women were encouraged to produce a son for the family and for the emperor (Kano, 2004; Nemoto, 2008; Takeya, 2008). A woman's worth was measured by her ability to produce a son and to raise children who would obey their father and the emperor (or 'the father of the nation'). Women were educated to be good wives and mothers for the country as well as the family and ideal woman embodied 'a patriotic version of Confucian womanhood' (Sugiyama-Lebra, 1998, p. 212). With reproduction a patriotic duty, unmarried women were assumed to be infertile, harmful for the household and less than ideal community citizens (Takeya, 2008). In some religion circles, 'unlucky' unmarried women were not invited to weddings, and infertile women were asked to leave the community for fear that local land would become barren. Although age at marriage increased, even less than 2% of population remained unmarried at age 50 during this period (National Institute of Population and Social Security Research, 2012b). As in the past, it was still custom for infertile couples to adopt a child from relatives since the male succession of the family line is at the heart of the *ie* system.

After the World War II, Japanese society went through dynamic transformations influenced by the West. Although the *ie* was no longer enforced by the government, post-war economic expansion reinforced a norm for people to marry and have at least two children. It became standard for women to retire from any waged employment upon marriage and to devote all energies to support of their households and children. Once children entered schools, women might engage in part-time waged work. Such life-cycle of women's employment is called the M-shaped curve of women's employment (Sugimoto, 2010). At the same time, women increasingly received Western liberal education no longer based on *ryosai kenbo* (good wife, wise mother). By the 1970s, a women's liberation movement had formed in Japan and some women found the opportunity to break from isolation and openly expressed their anger at an oppressive society that obligated women to duties of home and motherhood (Ogino, 2014). While the *ie* system continued to influence Japanese families – for example, by giving the eldest sons greater power and responsibility in taking care of parents and the house – Japanese lifestyles became diversified and younger generations rejected the view that parenthood was a prerequisite to full adulthood (Oishi, 2007). Reflecting such trends, the proportion of women who had never married by age 50 began to rise steeply after 1975, increasing from 3% to 19% between 1970 and 2000 (Retherford, Ogawa, & Matsukura, 2001).

As a larger portion of women acquired higher levels of Western liberal education, a 'good marriage' no longer required a wife to be full-time caretaker of family members and producer of offspring. Moreover, women who acquired stable employment could find an alternative to the standard life-course of marriage and then motherhood (Shimada, 2002). People became more likely to seek relationships for self-fulfilment and they postponed marriage if they did not find a suitable mate. Values related to premarital sex, cohabitation and divorce also played a role in reducing the attractiveness of marriage (Matsuo, 2003). These viewpoints very much reflect the influence of contemporary Western social norms and contrast sharply with the values of earlier periods when marriage and reproduction represented obligations defined by collective interests.

Childfree Stigma and the Technological Imperative in Heisei Era Japan

Because an overwhelming majority of childbirth continues to occur within marriage in contemporary Japan, an understanding of the conditions affecting today's childfree social stigma is incomplete without attention to marriage trends. Between 1970 and 2000, age at first marriage in Japan rose from 24.2 to 27 years for women and 26.9 to 28.8 years for men (Raymo, 2003). Between 1995 and 2014, the average age of first childbirth increased from 27.5 years to 30.6 years (Ito, 2015). By 1999, fertility rates had declined to 1.34 and they remain around this figure (Atoh, Kandiah, & Ivanov, 2004). Today, Japan is well known for its demographic characteristics of late marriage, less marriage and low fertility (Retherford et al., 2001; Tanaka & Iwasawa, 2010).

Despite increasing portions of childfree women, childlessness remains stigmatised. Questions such as 'Are you married?' and 'Do you have a child?' are traditional forms of greetings still used by older generations. Of course, the pressures of the motherhood imperative are not consistent throughout the biography (Kayama, 2016). Relatively young women are encouraged to participate in the labour force, but after a certain age they will face questions such as, 'Are you really okay with not having kids?' 'Who will support you after you retire?' or 'You were born a woman, why remain childless?' Childfree women may experience more criticism than their male counterparts due to enduring cultural norms holding women primarily responsible for producing heirs (Matsubayashi, Hosaka, Izumi, Suzuki, & Makino, 2001). Kayama (2016) refers to such questions and ensuing advice as 'non-mama' harassment (p. 76); a type of harassment that receives far less attention than other forms of gender harassment faced by women. But there is no formal recognition of 'non-mama' harassment, and it is possible that the general public receives such commentary positively, as reflective of the persistent belief that raising a child is always a precious, destined experience for all women (Kayama, 2016). To be childfree, then, continues to suggest failure to fulfil the responsibilities of womanhood.

The tenacious social primacy of motherhood over other pursuits is reflected in workforce dynamics. Approximately 80% of Japanese women with regular full-time employment continue to resign from waged work when they marry (Nemoto, 2008). Women with full-time jobs continue to face discrimination by being demoted or transferred to a 'less stressful' division that would ostensibly facilitate work-family life balance (Kobayashi, 2013). Those holding part-time or temporary work may find their employer unwilling to renew their contract (Kobayashi, 2013). Since the early 1990s, the Japanese government has implemented parental leave policies and childcare services to enable women to more easily combine labour force participation with motherhood. However, these policies do not target women in all occupations and have been labelled failures (Goldstein, Sabotka, & Jasilioniene, 2009). The government has responded to maternity harassment through posters and brochures emphasising the illegality of demoting or firing women on the basis of pregnancy or motherhood. However, many women continue to face significant challenges in balancing work and family without adequate resources and support from families, communities and their employers (Kobayashi, 2013). These conditions of gender inequality in opportunities and wages perpetuate a cycle in which many women rely on marriage (and by strong association, motherhood) (Nemoto, 2008). Choosing to avoid marriage in hopes of remaining childfree may thus threaten a woman's material security.

In Japan's twenty-first century, more than political economy and continuity of traditional gender inequalities may be at work in support of childfree stigma, however. Japan is distinct in the extent and speed of its population aging and population decline, and demographic reports consistently warn of the rising old-dependency ratio (calculated by dividing the aged population by the population of the working-age group) from 36.1% in 2010 to 50.2% by 2022, estimated to reach 78.4 by 2060 (National Institute of Population and Social Security Research, 2012a). The demographic crises would be mitigated by increases in the national total fertility rate. The influences of this demographic context and the widespread public concern about Japan's low birth rates cannot be overlooked in efforts to understand the newest iterations of social pressure surrounding a woman's choice to remain childfree.

Reproductive Technologies Replace Adoption Alternatives

Developments in reproductive technologies represent an additional social context shaping childfree experiences and stigma in contemporary Japan. As in the case of many social phenomenon, infertility has come to be understood as a medical condition to be treated by medical personnel. In Japan, *in vitro* fertilisation (IVF) and other procedures have become a popular approach to solving the 'problem' of infertility, replacing to a large extent the tradition of adopting a child from relatives. (Declining fertility rates make it unusual to find relatives with many children due.) By the year 2003, 466,900 people were annually visiting fertility clinics to receive treatment (Ito, 2015). Regardless of which partner is infertile, responsibilities associated with receiving infertility treatments often fall disproportionately upon women. The characteristics of these modern treatments in fact reflect and support traditional expectations of the woman as the primarily responsible party in reproductive efforts. In addition to enduring the invasive nature of some procedures, women must make arrangements that do not unduly interrupt their work schedules, their spouse's work schedules and the governmental regulations for subsidised infertility treatment. The Japanese government offers subsidies for couples whose wives are younger than 43 years old, and up to 15,000 *yen* (approximately 1,450 USD) may be provided per IVF procedure up to 10 times over 5 years (Ito, 2015). Although the initial procedures such as ovulation induction are covered by national health insurance, artificial insemination and IVF are not covered. This subsidy thus helps to make the option more attractive but, at costs of 300,000–500,000 *yen* (Ito, 2015), the patient's financial burden remains heavy. Moreover, the result and the length of treatment cannot easily be predicted.

Governmental encouragement for reproduction in contemporary times continue to support pronatalism that 'saturates women's consciousness and chokes off the options that are subjectively available to them' (Meyers, 2001, p.764). Childfree women continue to be labelled deviant, and they feel marginalised in the pronatalist culture. Recently, *Weekly Toyo Keizai* magazine published a feature titled, 'The truth of childlessness – Is it a sin to live without a child?' to claim that pronatalist programs are making childless people uncomfortable and some people experience '*konashi*-harassment' (harassment towards childless people) at work (Saito, 2016). Although the *ie* system was abolished, its custom continues to influence Japanese family including Japanese family graves; many of them are requiring succession of the family line requiring the descendants to take care of the ancestral spirit. As younger Japanese are more likely to become the only child in the household, pressures to become parents due to support from the medical industry and government may become even stronger, leaving less room to be childfree as a choice that is not accompanied by heavy social stigma.

Discussion and Conclusion

Confucian culture has been offered as a primary explanatory factor behind women's historical subordination in East Asian societies (Li, 2000), thus, it may be tempting to assume that it underlies past and contemporary childfree stigma in Japanese society. However, historical variances in social pressures for women to become mothers suggest that attributing motherhood pressures to traditional culture – a constant through much of Japan's history – is overly simplistic. Industrial capitalism in the Meiji period promoted the isolation of women in domestic private spheres, and the influence of the West likewise helped to shift familial structures away from communal and extended networks that allowed for variation in the reproductive lives of women to nuclear family structures that put pressure on all women to be mothers. Even within an increasingly industrial society, economic inequalities and migration had allowed for childlessness among working-class women when nationalism and strong demographic pressures were absent. Of course, none of these scenarios provided reproductive autonomy for individual women, but they did foster a degree of diversity in social expectations and the life courses of Japanese women. The historical, cross-cultural case of Japan also lends support to observations that motherhood imperatives are experienced differently across social strata (Riegle, 2015).

We suggest that childfree stigma associated with societal attitudes linking womanhood with motherhood (Hird & Abshoff, 2000; Ireland, 1993), should neither be assumed to be constant across time nor a phenomenon destined to decline with economic development, Westernisation or 'modern values'. On the contrary, it was primarily in Japan's Showa era – amid the intersection of industrial capitalism, missionary influence regarding family norms and Japanese nationalism – that a particularly strong motherhood imperative and ensuing general stigma emerged. Even then, the 'problem' of childlessness could be solved by adopting a child from relatives or by accepting that childlessness as the destiny of those who could not afford to establish households. In today's Japan, with medical improvements, views of infertility as a disease that can be treated, and declined fertility rates that reduce the options of adopting a child from relatives, pressure on women to be mothers remains strong. As in Western nations, Japanese women may associate being childfree with the freedom to pursue powerful social roles and a wider range of lifestyles, but it comes with high social costs. While the government claims to be fostering an environment that will allow couples to have an ideal number of children, motherhood continues to be a chief virtue, reflected in the remarks of former prime minister Yoshiro Mori that childless women are unworthy and should be denied public pensions (Morioka, 2011).

Social stigma is not inherent in individuals but resides in social structures and relations of power (Goffman, 1963; Link & Phelan 2001; Scambler 2006). As such, a full understanding of the factors affecting the strength and contours of childfree stigma requires examination of multiple sociological factors. In illustrating some of the social contexts that have historically shaped childfree stigma in Japan, this chapter aims to encourage similar attention in other settings to intersections of cultures, global politics, economies, demographic conditions and individual social location in formulating childfree experiences and stigma.

References

Atoh, M., Kandiah, V., & Ivanov, S. (2004). The second demographic transition in Asia? Comparative analysis of the low fertility situation in East and South-East Asian countries. *The Japanese Journal of Population*, *2*(1), 42–75.

Blackstone, A., & Stewart, M. D. (2012). Choosing to be childfree: Research on the decision not to parent. *Sociology Compass*. doi:10.1111/j.1751-9020.2012.00496.x

Collins, P. H. (2000). *Black feminist thought: Knowledge, consciousness, and the politics of empowerment*. New York, NY: Routledge.

Cornell, L., & Hayami, A. (1986). The Shumon aratame cho: Japan's population registers. *Journal of Family History*, *11*(4), 311–328.

Cwiertka, K. (1998). How cooking became a hobby: Changes in attitude toward cooking in early twentieth-century Japan. In S. Linhart & S. Frühstück (Eds.), *The culture of Japan as seen through its leisure* (pp. 41–58). New York, NY: State University of New York.

Fauve-Chamoux, A., & Ochiai, E. (2009). Introduction. In A. Fauve-Chamoux & E. Ochiai (Eds.), *The stem family in Eurasian perspective: Revisiting house societies, 17th–20th centuries* (pp. 1–50). Bern: Peter Lang.

Goffman, E. (1963). *Stigma: Notes on the management of spoiled identitiy*. Englewood Cliffs, NJ: Prentice-Hall.

Goldstein, J., Sabotka, T., & Jasilioniene, A. (2009). *The end of the 'lowest-low' fertility?* Working Paper of the Max Planck Institute for Demographic Research. Retrieved from www.demogr.mpg.de/papers/working/wp-2009-029.pdf

Hayes, P., & Habu, T. (2011). *Nihon no yoshiengumi*. Tokyo: Akashi Shoten.

Hird, M. J. (2003). Vacant wombs: Feminist challenges to psychoanalytic theories of childless women. *Feminist Review*, *75*(1), 5–19. doi:10.1057/palgrave.fr.9400115

Hird, M. J., & Abshoff, K. (2000). Women without children: A contradiction in terms? *Journal of Comparative Family Studies*, *31*(3), 347–366. Retrieved from http://search.ebscohost.com/login.aspx?direct=true&db=a9h&AN=3999529&lang=es&site=ehost-live

Imai, S. (2002). The independent working woman as deviant in Tokugawa Japan, 1600-1867. *Michigan Feminist Studies*, *16*. Retrieved from http://quod.lib.umich.edu/cgi/t/text/text-idx?cc=mfsfront;c=mfs;c=mfsfront;idno=ark5583.0016.005;rgn=main;view=text;xc=1;g=mfsg

Inoue, K. (1991). *Macrthur's Japanese constitution: A linguistic and cultural study of its making*. Chicago, IL: University of Chicago Press.
Ireland, M. S. (1993). *Reconceivnig women: Separating motherhood from female identity*. New York, NY: Guilford.
Ishizaki, S. (2015). *Kingendai Nihon no Kazokukeisei to Shusseijisuu*. Tokyo: Akashi Shoten.
Ito, M. (2015). The true cost of fertility treatment in Japan. *Japan Times*, June 20. Retrieved from https://www.japantimes.co.jp/life/2015/06/20/lifestyle/true-cost-fertility-treatment-japan/#.Wow4YKinHIU
Kagaya, M. (2014). Meijino hinkon wo meguru jojyutsu: Rekishi teki bunmyaku kara yomitoku. *Bungaku Kenkyuronshu*, *32*, 19–32.
Kaibara, E., & Takaishi, S. (1908). *Women and the wisdom of Japan*. New York, NY: Dutton.
Kano, M. (2004). *Feminism and society in contemporary Japan*. Tokyo: Yuhikaku.
Kayama, R. (2016). *Non mama toiu ikikata*. Tokyo: Gentosha.
Keyser, D., & Kumagai, F. (1996). *Unmasking Japan today*. London: Praeger Press.
Kito, H. (2007). *Jinko de miru Nihonshi*. Tokyo: PHp editors group.
Kobayashi, M. (2013). *Umasenai Shakai*. Tokyo: Kawade Shobo Shinsha.
Koyama, S. (2012). *Ryosai kenbo: The edcuational ideal of 'good wife, wise mother' in modern Japan*. Boston: BRILL.
Kurosu, S., & Ochiai, E. (1995). Adoption as an heirship strategy under demographic constraints: A case from nineteenth-century Japan. *Journal of Family History*, *20*(3), 261–288. doi:10.1177/036319909502000303
Letherby, G. (2002). Childless and bereft?: Stereotypes and realities in relation to 'voluntary' and 'involuntary' childlessness and womanhood. *Sociological Inquiry*, *72*(1), 7–20. doi:10.1111/1475-682X.00003
Li, C. (2000). Can confucianism come to terms with feminism? In C. Li (Ed.), *The sage and the second sex: Confucianism, ethics, and gender* (pp. 2–12). Peru, IL: Carus Publishing Company.
Link, B. G., & Phelan, J. C. (2001). Conceptualizing stigma. *Annual Review of Sociology. Sociol*, *27*, 363–385. doi:10.1146/annurev.soc.27.1.363
Lisle, L. (1999). *Without child: Challenging the stigma of childlessness*. New York, NY: Routledge.
Matsubayashi, H., Hosaka, T., Izumi, S., Suzuki, T., & Makino, T. (2001). Emotional distress of infertile women in Japan. *Human Reproduction (Oxford, England)*, *16*(5), 966–969. doi:10.1093/humrep/16.5.966
Matsuki, H. (2016). Ikuji no shakaika wo saikochiku suru. In *Hybrid na oyako no shakaigaku* (pp. 15–41). Tokyo: Seikyusha.
Matsuo, H. (2003). *The transition to motherhood in Japan: A comparison with the Netherlands*. West Lafayette, IN: Purdue University Press.
Meyers, D. T. (2001). The rush to motherhood: Pronatalist discourse and women's autonomy. *Signs*, *26*(3), 735–773.
Morell, C. M. (1994). *Unwomanly conduct: The challenges of intentional childlessness*. New York, NY: Routledge.
Morioka, M. (2011). Umanai sentaku to shakaiteki jyuyou. *Bulletin of Studies on Education and Gender*, 21–36.

Muraoka, K. (2004). Funin to Dansei wo meguru Mondai-kei. In *Funin to Dansei* (pp. 101–150). Tokyo: Seikyūsha Library.
National Institute of Population and Social Security Research. (2012a). *Population projections for Japan*. Retrieved from http://www.ipss.go.jp/site-ad/index_english/esuikei/econ2.html
National Institute of Population and Social Security Research. (2012b). *Population statistics 2012*. Tokyo. Retrieved from http://www.ipss.go.jp/syoushika/tohkei/Popular/P_Detail2012.asp?fname=T06-23.htm&title2=%95%5C%82U%81%7C23+%90%AB%95ʐ%B6%8AU%96%A2%8D%A5%97%A6%82%A8%82%E6%82я%89%8D%A5%94N%97%EE%81i%82r%82l%82%60%82l%81j%81F1920%81%602010%94N
Nawata, Y. (2006). Rekishiteki ni mita Nihon no jinkou to kazoku. *Rippou to Chosa*, *10*(260), 90–106.
Nemoto, K. (2008). Postponed marriage: Exploring women's views of matrimony and work in Japan. *Gender & Society*, *22*(2), 219–237. doi:10.1177/0891243208315868
Ogino, M. (2014). *Onna no karada: feminizumuigo*. Tokyo: Iwanami shinsho.
Oishi, T. (2007). Josei ga ikikata wo erabu toiukoto. In E. Matsuoka (Ed.), *Umu, Umanai, Umenai* (pp. 11–32). Tokyo: Koudansha Gendai Shinsho.
Park, K. (2002). Stigma management among the voluntarily childless. *Sociological Perspectives*, *45*(1), 21–45. doi:10.1525/sop.2002.45.1.21
Raymo, J. M. (2003). Premarital living arrangements and the transition to first marriage in Japan. *Journal of Marriage and Family*, *65*(2), 302–315.
Retherford, R. D., Ogawa, N., & Matsukura, R. (2001). Late marriage and less marriage in Japan. *Population and Development Review*, *27*(1), 65–102. doi:10.2307/2695155
Reti, I. (1992). *Childelss by choice: A feminist anthology*. Santa Cruz, CA: Herbooks.
Riegle, A. L. (2015). *Economic and racial differences in women's infertility experiences*. Doctoral dissertation, Iowa State University.
Saito, M. (2016). Konashi fu-fu no nakanaka rikai sarenai jittai (Reality of childless couples). *Toyo Keizai Online*, July. Retrieved from http://toyokeizai.net/articles/-/125569?page=2
Scambler, G. (2006). Sociology, social structure and health-related stigma. *Psychology, Health & Medicine*, *11*(3), 288–295. doi:10.1080/13548500600595103
Shimada, A. (2002). *Nihon no feminism*. Tokyo: Hokujyu Shuppan.
Shirai, C. (2004). Dansei Funin no Rekishi to Bunka. In *Funin to Dansei* (pp. 151–192). Tokyo: Seikyusha.
Sugimoto, Y. (2010). *An introduction to Japanese society*. Cambridge: Cambridge University Press.
Sugiyama-Lebra, T. (1998). Confucian gender role and personal fulfillment for Japanese women. In W. H. Slote & G. A. De Vos (Eds.), *Confucianism and the family* (pp. 209–227). Albany, NY: SUNY Press.
Takeya, K. (2008). Funin wo meguru shakaiteki haikei to sono gensetsu. *Kyoiku-Houhou No Tankyu*, *11*, 25–32.

Tanaka, K., & Iwasawa, M. (2010). Aging in rural Japan – Limitations in the current social care policy. *Journal of Aging & Social Policy*, *22*(4), 394–406.

Ueno, C. (2009). *The modern family in Japan: Its rise and fall.* Melbourne, Australia: Trans Pacific Press.

Whiteford, L. M., & Gonzalez, L. (1995). Stigma: The hidden burden of infertility. *Social Science and Medicine*, *40*(1), 27–36. doi:10.1016/0277-9536(94)00124-C

Chapter 15

The Effects of Childcare Arrangements on Childlessness in Germany

Nazli Kazanoglu

Abstract

Over the last two to three decades, European welfare states have witnessed fundamental changes in both family and labour market structures with many more women being in the paid labour market. While this was seen to address previous problems linked to women's disadvantage, it has also been argued to give rise to new risk and social inequalities, including falling fertility rates and increasing childlessness. Research has identified the lack of affordable childcare as a key factor in childlessness leading to a strong EU focus on early childhood education and care. Since 2000, the EU has played a more proactive role in policies and initiatives aimed to address decreasing fertility rates with greater pressure for convergence among member states. However, there has continued to be a large degree of variation between countries. This chapter thus examines the case of Germany which has one of the highest levels of childlessness in Europe. It focuses on the intersection between childlessness and childcare provision in Germany and analyses the existing childcare arrangements with a view to understand how they influence childlessness. Particular attention is given to the role of the German government as the main actor in the process to explore ideology-related explanations of German policy-makers which led to contradictory policies. Relying on an extensive review of the related literature and policy documents, together with the personal interviews with policy-makers, academics and women's organisations, this chapter concludes that the relatively conservative outlook of the German government which prioritises the motherhood and caregiver role, and the dominance of the corporate welfare system, has limited developments to improve access to childcare resulting in '*a culture of childlessness*' in Germany (Kreyenfeld & Konietzka, 2017).

Keywords: Childcare; childlessness; de-familialisation; fertility rates; Germany; multiple veto-points

Introduction

Over the last two to three decades, the majority of European welfare states have witnessed tremendous changes both in family and labour market structures resulting in a considerable shift in women's roles. More women entering higher education, the structural transformation of the labour market, the economic necessity for two-earner families and the increasing dominance of service employment have paved the way for an inter-related alteration of (a) the prevalent family model and concomitantly the existing gender roles; and (b) the life-courses of individuals, particularly of women. It is argued that the traditional male breadwinner family model (Esping-Andersen, 2009; Hantrais, 2004; Lewis, 1992) has gradually lost some of its social prevalence with other family models such as the adult-earner family model, or at least a one-and-a-half-earner family model, gaining more prominence. This has resulted in a significant change in the life path of many women. Generally speaking, a typical post-war woman was expected to marry in her early 20s and have children right after the marriage then dedicate the rest of her life to family altruism, acting as a '*domestic servant*' (Esping-Andersen, 2009, p. 27). From the early 1980s, many women have gradually waived dedicating their lives to family altruism. They have come to be less associated predominantly with childbearing or childcare and more with lifelong employment (Esping-Andersen, 2009; McDonald, 2000).

These changes were viewed as improving women's status within society. In pursuing a shift from primarily domestic 'duties' to lifelong employment, they could be freed from the dependency on either their fathers or male breadwinner partners (Lewis, 2009). However, it was also argued that they gave rise to new social risks, including increasing childlessness, a factor which Esping-Andersen (2009) associates with the social policy structure of societies and existing welfare states not being fully ready to off-set this new trajectory. While examining the fertility trend of today's modern world, it is important to note that the decision to remain childless for some women is a positive voluntary choice – a conscious decision; for others, it may be what has been described as a constrained choice. There has been an ongoing debate among feminist scholars in terms of explaining women's behaviour regarding fertility behaviour and employment. Some scholars have argued that women's different choices on fertility and employment depends on their sociological background, whereas others have argued that women's behaviour have always been constrained by laws, regulations and policies. Thus, in some contexts, the decision made by some women is constrained by the socio-political conditions of the day (Hakim, 2000; Lewis, 2009). In other words, certain contexts and socio-economic conditions impact on women's decision-making with respect to having children. There is some evidence (Esping-Andersen, 2009; McDonald, 2002) of a mismatch between the preferred and actual number of children. Statistics reveal that while the expressed desire of a typical adult in terms of number of children varies between 2.1 and 2.3, the actual number of the children they have, differs at between 1.31 and 1.85 (OECD, 2017). This gap between the desired and the real numbers of children may be explained by women's career goals and concerns. It may be that some women want to become mothers but the ambition to build a stable, secure and a lifelong career may result in them making 'choices' to postpone pregnancy or even forgo having children. Comparative analyses have found that the lack of social policies and government support for women's labour market participation increases childlessness. The presence of accessible, high quality, free or at least subsidised childcare provisions are key factors, along with maternity and paternity leave, part-time employment and other financial incentives (Brodmann, Esping-Andersen, & Guell, 2007; Hemerijck, 2013; McDonald, 2002; Stobel-Richter, Beutel, Finck, & Prahler, 2005). Arguably, the fertility behaviour of women has been shaped by whether they can rely on the welfare provisions of their region or not with respect to childcare.

Just like many other developed European welfare states, Germany has also been required to respond to societal changes. Germany's complex historical background and the corporatist conservative welfare state model, which asserts the family as the main welfare provider, means that the effects of this transformation have been felt more acutely than in some other states. After the World War II and the division of Germany, West Germany (FRG) experienced economic recovery under the conservative Adenauer administration (Grebe, 2009 and Roberts, 2016). Here, the traditional male breadwinner and female home-carer model was maintained. In East Germany (GDR) under the socialist-communist ideology, the dual-earner model was dominant accompanied by a system of public childcare provision (Lietzmann, 2014; Ostner, 2010). In both parts of Germany in this period, there was a 'baby boom' – but with distinct differences. While, the FRG provided its citizens with various child benefit allowances[1] and tax deductions[2] in order to encourage them to have children, the GDR encouraged childbearing through comprehensive public childcare places (Ferree, 1993). These differences are explained with reference to political ideologies. The GDR's Marxist ideology saw women's employment and their salvation from private sphere as the biggest part of women's emancipation (Ferree, 1993), whereas the more conservative FRG prioritised women's motherhood roles. A combination of the reunification of Germany[3] and the global trend of moving away from one-earner families towards dual-earner families led to dramatic changes in German women's roles. But according to Esping-Andersen's (2009), the transformation remained incomplete. While German women said a farewell to their sole housewifery roles and welcomed paid employment (Ostner, 2010; Pfau-Effinger & Smidt, 2011), they continued to be responsible for the bulk of domestic tasks. Thus, they came to carry the 'double burden' of paid employment and childbearing and housework. In the absence of appropriate employment-friendly childcare arrangements from the government, they took the decision to postpone the first child or abandon the idea of motherhood.

In the quest for a full understanding of the reasons for falling fertility rates and postponement of the first child, research established a link between childlessness and the advancement of childcare arrangements (Krapf, 2014; Lee & Lee, 2014; McDonald, 2002). However, there is still

[1]Families in Germany were eligible to child allowances if they had children under aged 18 and also children aged 18–27 if the child is still at school or training or registered as unemployed. In 1999, the child allowances were 250 DM (German Mark) per child for the first and second; 300 DM for the third and 350 DM for the fourth and every additional child. This system is pretty generous, as a family with three children would receive 800 DM, which equals to approximately 30% of the time present average net wage (see Ostner, 2010; Trzcinski & Camp, 2014).

[2]The solidarity subsidy and church taxes were lower to families with children in Germany; they also had an easier access to private house and apartment subsidies (see Ostner, 2010; Trzcinski & Camp, 2014).

[3]The fear of East German women about losing their worker identity paved the way for signing the bilateral unification contract 'Einigungvertag', which promised an increased attention on women's employment and exceptional effort on preserving East Germany's family friendly social policies (see Erler, 2009).

a noticeable gap in empirical research on this issue. In that sense, this chapter focuses on the intersection of childlessness and childcare arrangements in Germany, a country with one of the highest childlessness rates, with 1.5 child per woman, in Europe. It explores policy-makers' motivation in shaping care policies and maps out the childcare provision deficits in Germany. With reference to primary research, it examines current childcare policies in Germany and the role and influence of the actors involved in the policy-(re)making process.

The empirical data used in this chapter draw on analysis of findings from semi-structured interviews conducted as part of the author's doctoral dissertation on Europeanisation patterns of work and family life reconciliation policies in Germany and Turkey. Twenty-nine interviews were conducted with (a) representatives of women's machinery and corresponding women organisations as well as lobby groups located in various cities in Germany to understand their contribution to the childcare policy-(re)making process; and (b) political elites – including the former and current Family and Social Policy ministers and the representatives of woman branches of political parties, especially the ruling and oppositional parties. The purpose was to explore their policy-making and/or problem-solving logics and related matters and actions throughout the reform process. All the interviews were conducted between November 2016 and January 2017. The collected data have been analysed via the thematic analysis research method. Ethical approval for the study was provided by Ulster University.

The Intersection of Childcare Arrangements and Childlessness

At a time when many European welfare states are experiencing a sharp decline in fertility, far below the replacement level, it is not surprising that the scholarship on childlessness has exploded. Since Becker (1965), authors have appealed to various theoretical explanations while trying to understand the causes of fertility decline (Krapf, 2014; McDonald, 2000). Although there is some disagreement among theorists, there is consensus on the link between the childcare arrangements and the fertility behaviour of women. Women's decisions about childrearing are mostly based on certain cost-benefit calculations, where the decision to have a child is the result of a positive overall calculation (Luci-Greulich & Thevenon, 2013; McDonald, 2000). It is also argued that these costs and benefits change in line with the conditions of the day. Long into the post-war period, women's childbearing decisions depended on various external factors such as their husband's job or income rather than on childcare provision. In the period from the late 1970s, new considerations came to the fore, such as securing a foothold in the labour market or guaranteeing a sufficient income (Ahn & Mira, 2002; Esping-Andersen, 1999). With the dramatic changes in the life-courses and expectations of many European women, childbearing has argued to become less of a priority than labour market participation. This appears to be the case practically, if not ideally. While many women are still keen on having at least two children, there needs to be appropriate policies to allow them to reconcile their career aspirations with their fertility behaviour (Ahn & Mira, 2002; Esping-Andersen, 1999; Krapf, 2014).

The interrelation between childcare arrangements and childlessness has been evidenced by a range of other studies. In 1994, Richter, Podhisita, Chamratrithirong and Soonthorndhada's study of the fertility behaviour of Thai women found that women with lower fertility rates are those with higher childcare constraints. Esping-Andersen, Gallie, Hemerijk and Myles (2002) in their comparison of 18 countries in terms of their welfare provisions and fertility behaviour found that scarcity of childcare provisions dramatically increases women's likelihood of childlessness. Del Boca (2002) and Ferrarini (2006) also conclude that the presence of comprehensive childcare increases both fertility and labour market employment. In a more recent study, Rovny (2011) revealed that the higher the government spending on childcare arrangements, the higher the fertility rates.

In Germany, the fertility rate fell below the replacement level in 1994 and has stagnated there (Sobotka, Zeman, Lesthaeghe, Frejka, & Neels, 2011). In addition to having one of the lowest fertility rates, it has the highest childlessness rate (23%) (Beaujouan, Sobotka, Brzozowska, & Zeman, 2017) among EU members. On average, the desired number of children for German women is around 1.9–2.0 children (OECD, 2017), 0.5 units higher than the actual numbers. Financial concerns and lack of government support for mothers are the most cited factors contributing to childlessness (Borck, 2014; Hara, 2008; Stobel-Richter et al., 2005). The latest statistics regarding causes of childlessness also highlight the link between childcare provision and childlessness by showing the differences between the East-landers of Germany and the West. Childlessness among east German women born in 1968, who have had access to relatively better childcare services is considerably lower (16%) than among their west German counterparts (25%), who have historically been left with care responsibilities (Beaujouan et al., 2017; Kreyenfeld & Konietzka, 2017).

This evidence suggests a possible relationship between childcare arrangements and women's fertility behaviour, but there has been less analysis of the existing care arrangements with a view to understanding their impact on the childlessness problem.

Theoretical Framework

Building on the premise that childlessness cannot be examined in isolation from childcare arrangements, this section introduces the analytical framework of the discussion. In doing so, it concentrates on two crucial aspects: (a) whether and to what extent German childcare arrangements encourage women's employment and career building; and (b) the roles of the societal actors in terms of shaping those arrangements. The first stems from the feminist critiques of Esping-Andersen's (1990) path-breaking welfare regime typology and differentiates care arrangements on the basis of their women-friendliness. The second classifies the societal actors' norms and values (Pfau-Effinger, 2005; Tsebelis, 2002).

In the wake of new social risks, European welfare states began to make efforts to adjust to fluctuating conditions of post-industrialism, re-structuring childcare services to occupy a major part of that effort. Yet, there are considerable differences between countries with respect to their childcare arrangements. While some states have succeeded in establishing highly subsidised and formalised childcare arrangements, others have continued to rely on families – and more precisely on the female family members (Hantrais, 2004; Lewis, 2009). Differences are not confined to inter-country policies and practice, but are also evident within countries. In order to analyse this heterogeneous nature of childcare arrangements, this chapter uses Esping-Andersen's (1999) concept of de-familialisation. Although Esping-Andersen and notable feminist scholars use the term in a broader comparison of welfare regimes, this chapter applies it solely to childcare arrangements as the central aim is to tease out German childcare arrangements. In a broader sense, familialisation is used to denote producing or reproducing a welfare model, wherein the family is the main welfare provider, whereas de-familialisation refers to seeking to curtail individuals' welfare dependence on kinship (Esping-Andersen, 1999; O'Connor, 1993; Orloff, 1993; Saraceno & Keck, 2010). With respect to childcare arrangements, familialisation means assigning a greater amount of care responsibility to families, whereas de-familialising care policies are designed to transfer care obligations from the private sphere of the family to the public sphere. More precisely, de-familialisation regards childcare as a social citizenship right instead of being a family affair (Esping-Andersen, 1999; Lohmann & Zagel, 2016). If one of the biggest reasons behind childlessness is women's desire for labour market participation, de-familialising policies could be considered as important to reducing low birth-rates.

As shown in Table 1, a wide range of policies can be defined as familialised and de-familialised. Yet, these policies are not polarised opposites of each other, nor are they mutually exclusive. Presence of de-familialising childcare policies does not necessarily mean that familialising ones have been eradicated. In many welfare states, familialising childcare policies have survived alongside the de-familialised ones because policy-making is generally acknowledged as value dependent (Pfau-Effinger, 2005; Tsebelis, 2002). This links to the second aspect of the theoretical framework: *the roles of the societal actors.*

The existence of the aforementioned social risks, childlessness being the foremost one, requires welfare states to change policies or even in some states, due to levels of traditionalism, the whole legislative status quo. This requirement, however, can be limited by the ideological motivations of the existing societal actors, whether governmental or non-governmental (Heritier et al., 2001; Radaelli, 2003). This analysis divides these actors into two major groups, whom Tsebelis (2002) calls *multiple veto-points*. The first group, the so-called *catalysts*, consists of the ones whose presence accelerates the policy-(re)making process and the second group, the *veto players*, consists of the decelerators (Heritier et al., 2001; Radaelli, 2003). In terms of childcare arrangements, the first group, the catalysts, are in favour of more institutionalised childcare. They aim to formalise childcare policy and provision and bring it into the public sphere. The second group, the veto players, hold more traditional views with respect to childcare. To be more precise, veto players are in favour of the idea that women should be the main child carers. Although these two groups hold opposing views they are not mutually exclusive. The primary question is, therefore, what brings about policy change? The answer to this question is not straightforward. The simultaneous presence of these two opposing ideas (Borzel & Risse, 2002; Tsebelis, 2002) plays an important role.

Childcare Policies in Germany

The development of public childcare policies in Germany have historically lagged behind other European welfare states despite demands for

Table 1. Overview of Familialisation/De-familialisation Indicators Regarding Childcare.

	Initiative	Consequence
Familialisation	Childcare benefits Home care allowances	Cash payments to parents (mothers) would provide a disincentive for women to remain in the labour market.
	Fragmented childcare services regulations	Childcare service regulations include the fees and opening hours of those services. Without centralised working hour and price regulation, the opening hours of care centres may not be compatible with parents' working hours; or some of them fees may increase to a point that parents could not afford which discourages women's employment.
De-familialisation	Public and high quality childcare services Universal childcare service enrolment right to children Central regulations on the opening hours	Relieving women from their childcare responsibilities would allow them to engage more fully with the labour market. Entitling every child with a right to a high quality and centrally regulated place is argued to be the most effective way of doing this.
	Legal obligations to private companies to open childcare services	In many welfare states, despite the legal universal right of children for a childcare place, many are not enrolled in a childcare place due to the disproportional supply:demand ratio. Forcing local authorities and private companies, as well as providing some tax incentives to private companies to open a care place, can reduce the gap between supply and demand.

policy reform from the feminist movement, the progressive stance of some Ministers, pressure from the EU, the unification of Germany and growing demographical risks. Two years after unification, Germany made the first legal step towards non-familial state-subsidised childcare (Lewis, 2009), which has been consolidated with three further legal federal laws in 2005, 2008 and 2013 (Schober & Spiess, 2015).

Prior to fall of the Berlin Wall, only the FRG, since then the unified Germany, has often been cited as the perfect exemplar of '*conservative corporatist regime*' (Esping-Andersen, 1990), which holds a strong adherence to the traditional male breadwinner family model, based on the gendered work and care dualism and the principle of subsidiarity which requires an individual to seek help first from the family and to consider the state as the last resort when the family's capacity is exhausted (Esping-Andersen, 1990; Ostner, 2010; Trzcinski & Camp, 2014). A consolidation of these two characteristics played an important role in Germany being laggard in developing non-familial childcare services. However, as discussed above, this gendered work and care dualism resulted in social risks and social inequalities the German government could no longer overlook. In 1992, the Christian Democratic-Liberal government introduced a national law, entitling a right for part-time childcare for every child between the ages three and six (Grebe, 2009). This Act, however, was not implemented. The federal government legislatively required the local governments to supply places, yet remained highly reluctant to increase public expenditure. The increase in annual spending from €8.5 billion to €10 billion was considered highly inadequate (Palier, 2006; Ruling, 2008). While the implementation of this Act was delayed, fertility rates continued to fall, dropping as low as 1.25 in 1995 (OECD, 2017). Linked to the debate about declining fertility rates were discussions about convergence of abortion laws in the former east and west Germanys. While the GDR wanted to preserve existing legislation which was more liberal than in the West, the FRG opposed this, concerned that it might further reduce fertility rates (Meyer, 2005). This political debate about the convergence of abortion law in the end turned in favour of childcare expansion. The unimplemented 1992 Child and Youth Act was actualised as part of the reform of the abortion law 218 (Grebe, 2009; Meyer, 2005; Palier, 2006).

While the passage of this law was the first step towards de-familialising childcare provisions, it contained contradictory elements and impact was limited. As argued earlier, law increasing fertility would most likely be achieved by improving childcare to allow women to enhance their labour force participation. The childcare policy that passed as a part of the abortion law had significant limitations. Firstly, it guaranteed a childcare place only on a part-time basis, portraying the kindergarten as a place where children could go and play for a couple of hours per day rather than provision for full-time working women. Secondly, but equally importantly, the law applied only to children over three – placing another significant constraint on women's career aspirations. Although the law was aimed at preventing further fall in fertility rates, it exhibited high familialisation and very low de-familialisation and fertility rates fell dramatically from 1.45 in 1990 to 1.25 in 1995 (OECD, 2017). Although the rate increased to 1.34 in 2002, it was still low enough to get the newly elected family minister Renate Schmidt's attention.

Renate Schmidt was the first family minister in Germany since the Nazi period to be vocal about falling fertility rates. In 2003, she launched the 'Alliance for the Family', whose slogan was '*Germany needs more children*'. The aim of this alliance was to abolish the care and work dualism through expanding the public childcare provisions (personal interview). In 2004, she passed The Day-care Facility Expansion Act (*Tagesbetreuungsausbaugesetz*, TAG) (Fleckenstein & Lee, 2014; Grebe, 2009; Leitner, 2010; Ostner, 2010). The goal of the TAG, came into force in January 2005, was to increase childcare enrolment rates to 35% by 2013 by adding 750,000 full-time childcare places. The Red-Green coalition, meanwhile, lost its electoral majority in the 2005 elections and Renate Schmidt was no longer family minister. She was succeeded by Ursula von der Leyen, who was also seen as progressive on this issue. She called for more childcare places for children under three years and in 2008, the Law to Support Children in Day-care was passed (Schober & Spiess, 2015). This aimed to increase childcare enrolment rates to 39% from 35% by 2013 and came with guarantees of extra funding (Andronescu & Carnes, 2015; Ruling, 2008). These two pieces of legislation were important steps towards an enhanced childcare policy, yet there was still no statutory right to kindergarten place for children under three years. This particular gap was filled by the introduction of Crèche Plus (*Kitaplus*) in August 2013 (Andronescu & Carnes, 2015), which brought a legal right to a kindergarten place for all children aged one and older. These developments suggest de-familialising efforts through childcare policies and these may be reflected in increasing fertility rates – from 1.34 in 2002 to 1.42 in 2003 and 1.47 in 2014 (OECD, 2017). Although, these developments could be interpreted as significant advances for Germany, progress on reversing fertility decline is still less than in many other European countries.

Since 2001, Germany has also pursued additional initiatives for childcare through tax legislation. Alongside tax reductions, it also provided a separate €1,500 cash transfer for childcare expenses to employed parents (Grebe, 2009). Referring back to the cost-benefit calculations made by women, increase in childcare provision expanded non-familial childcare services while the tax deductions decreased the opportunity cost of those childcare places. As employment is a condition of benefitting from the policy, it also (indirectly) encourages women to be employed. While it can be argued that Germany has made progress in terms of de-familialising its childcare policies, several familialising childcare policies, which could be expected to increase childlessness, are also still on the agenda. Therefore, the process of de-familialising German childcare arrangements seems to be a slippery one, leading some notable scholars to refer to a '*modernized breadwinner model*' (Leitner, 2010; Pfau-Effinger, 2005).

Home care allowances (*Betreuungsgeld*), the €150 monthly payment to parents (mostly to mothers)[4] who care for their children at home until the child turns three (Fleckenstein & Lee, 2014; Krapf, 2014), is an example of the conservative welfare model heritage. Although the government defended this law as '*an essential part of our policy of freedom of choice*', and allocated £319 million to it, it seems to contradict de-familialisation logic. Such allowances induce women to interrupt their careers for three years and push them back into the familial sphere and, as noted earlier, such a long break is no longer desired by many women.

In addition to the conservative corporatist welfare model legacies and its childcare arrangements, the ways in which the TAG and its revised versions were formulated also mattered. TAG assigns all the responsibility regarding childcare place extension and regulation to local authorities (Andronescu & Carnes, 2015), watering down the de-familialisation process and resulting in diversity across lander. Although the federal government increased the amount of government spending allocated to childcare twice (in 2005 and in 2008), the allocated money comprises only one-third of the local authorities' spending on childcare

[4]The law itself is addressing both mothers and fathers. Yet, given the existing division of paid and unpaid work between mothers and fathers in Germany, together with the considerable gender pay gap, women are more likely to interrupt their careers and stay at home to care for the children.

(Andronescu & Carnes, 2015; personal interview with a die Linke deputy, 2016). The other two-thirds come from the lander government, the municipalities and other various non-governmental institutions such as the church and local NGOs (Andronescu & Carnes, 2015; Schober & Spiess, 2015). This multiactored arrangement has two serious outcomes. The first is in relatively poorer lander or relatively more conservative lander, there is more reluctance to invest in non-familial childcare places than in more progressive lander (Andronescu & Carnes, 2015; Meyer, 2005). For example, in Bavaria, associated with a strong adherence to traditional and conservative values, 2011 statistics demonstrate only 23% of all children under age three were enrolled in public day-care and even then, it was mostly in part-time care (Andronescu & Carnes, 2015; BMFSFJ, 2012). Although this could be considered relatively limited provision, and local and national women's organisations were critical of the policy, the Bavarian deputies interpreted the fact that Bavarian woman had the opportunity to work part time as huge progress (personal interview with a CSU deputy and Frauenrat). Similarly, in Rheinland-Pfalz, wherein citizens are argued to be relatively more religious compared to other parts of the country, only 27% of children under three were enrolled in day-care in 2011 (Krapf, 2014). The second outcome of this multiactored arrangement is the opening hours and monthly fees of the childcare places also differ across lander, which at the end assuages the de-familialisation impact. Each local government is responsible for defining their childcare services opening hours and, with places mostly offered on a part-time basis, this presents obstacles to women's employment and thus disincentives their fertility behaviour (personal interview with Frauenrat). In addition, with no centralised childcare fee, the cost of a regular childcare place differs according to the family income, the lander and the age of the child (Krapf, 2014; personal interviews). It has been claimed that parents start looking for a place to enrol their child right after they realise that they are pregnant, especially in crowded lander like Berlin or Nordrhein-Westfalen. Since the demand is much higher than the supply in these kinds of lander, childcare fees are high, resulting in women withdrawing from the labour market and caring for their children at home (personal interview with a deputy from SPD).

Overall, the residuals of the former strong conservative welfare understanding, together with regional variations influence the overall reform picture and dilute the de-familialisation impact of the German childcare policies. The contradictory elements apparent in these policies are related to the ideological motivations of the actors in the policy process as discussed in the following section.

Actors in the Process

A range of actors can be identified as relevant to the childcare policy process. A key grouping advocating policy reform has been women's organisations seeking a better work and family life, and labour market equality for women. Trade unions and employers' associations also acknowledge the need for improved childcare and lobbied for the issue to be on the political agenda. At a political level, the political parties and several commissions within the German Parliament are key players in policy reform. Additionally, due to Germany's federal nature, the local landers also have a stake. Finally, because of the subsidiarity legacy[5] religious organisations too feature in discussions about childcare policy-making. Therefore, as can be seen from Figure 1 below, in Germany the power and the responsibility to make childcare policy are divided between various societal actors. While political parties are the most powerful of these (Meyer, 2005), all are highly tangled in the contemporary German conjuncture to the extent that it is almost impossible to make a sharp distinction between catalysts and veto players.

A consolidation of the literature and my personal interviews indicated that the increasing low birth rate is at the core of all the above-mentioned actors' agenda. Deputies from major parties explicitly expressed their concerns about drastically falling birth-rates and the sense of obligation to intervene. Yet, the ways in which they approach both the cause of the issue and the solution differs immensely. Initially, Eastern women's organisations, and eventually cross-country women's organisations backed by the trade unions and employers' associations, had begun to lobby the German government for more institutionalised childcare services. The trade unions and employers' associations' emphasis was more on increasing women's labour market employment, whereas women's organisations highlighted various factors, such as falling fertility rates and women's attempts to reconcile work and family lives and obstacles to women's employment (Andronescu & Carnes, 2015; Ferree, 1993; Meyer, 2005). Their quest for childcare expansion was strengthened when the unspoken conflict between eastern and western women's organisations ended and western women's organisations

[5]As has been mentioned earlier, the German welfare model has long rested upon the principle of subsidiarity with the state seen as the last resort, especially with regard to familial affairs. Therefore, in Germany non-public providers such as religious organisations and parents' organisations offer childcare services (see Andronescu & Carnes, 2015; Esping-Andersen, 1990, 2009; Ostner, 2010).

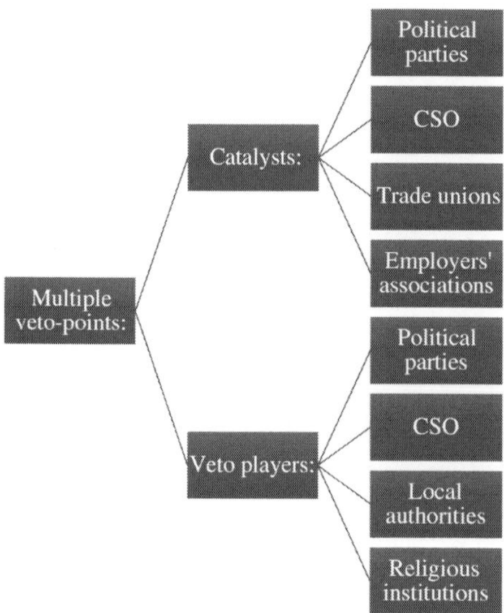

Figure 1. Distribution of the Actors of the Policy (Re)-making Process.

began to focus on women's employment issues as well (Ferree, 1993). The GDR was an anti-democratic country and did not allow any independent political or social movements, including feminist movements. Hence, although the eastern feminists, especially feminist academics, were well aware of the gender inequalities, they could only unite and mobilise after unification (Ferree, 1993). This time, an invisible conflict between eastern and western feminist movements appeared. The western feminist organisations, with less focus on women's employment, distanced themselves from the eastern organisations for a very long time. It was the 2000s, when the west saw women's employment as not only a concern of eastern women's organisations, but a global one (Miette, 2008). Thereupon, a relatively more united German women's organisations successfully got the low birth rate and the need for better childcare provision onto the political agenda. They formed what has been described as the '*velvet triangle*' (Woodward, 2004) referring to the cooperation of women organisations, academics and female friendly parliament members.

The demands of civil society organisations for better childcare provision influenced the SPD's agenda and the party included the issue in its party campaign (Ruling, 2008) with the Family Minister from the SPD,

Renate Schmidt, arguing that expanded childcare provision was the only necessary precaution towards increased childlessness (Erler, 2009; Schmidt, 2011). Yet, there were also some intra-party coalitions which could be considered veto players. An interviewee from SPD Bielefeld fraction argued:

> … [T]he majority of the SPD all around the country are well acknowledged about the misfit between the demand and the supply of the childcare services. We again are well aware of the fact that this situation is either reducing women's labour market participation or the number of children they have. However, we have some relatively older members within the SPD, whose views are more closely aligned with the CDU even though we are their main opposition in German Parliament …. (personal interview, 2016)

Historically, both the CDU and, to an even greater extent the CSU, are highly committed to the male breadwinner and female homemaker family model, which leaves little room for non-familial public childcare arrangements. Additionally, they considered the falling fertility rates and increasing childlessness as a taboo topic and wanted to leave it within the familial sphere rather than treating it as a social problem (Meyer, 2005; Trzcinski & Camp, 2014). While discussing the recent developments with respect to childcare provisions, a senior politician from the CSU stated that:

> … If you love your baby, we expect you take some time off from your work and we support this with our revised leave schemes. In order to support you while you are on the leave, we also pay you… On the other hand, we also know that lots of young couples build a house, they have debts in the bank, they have to pay the money back to the bank so they need money, so we also need to give them the opportunity of work so that, now most of the women leave their children to kindergarten or to kita half day and contribute to family budget ….

For this participant, non-familial childcare place meant only part-time provision, not perceived by women as useful or economically viable. Some change in the position of the CDU is evident with the coming to power of Angela Merkel (Fleckenstein, 2011). As general secretary of the CDU in 2002, when the party lost the elections, Merkel diagnosed that the main reason behind the election defeat was the lack of votes from younger urban women (Fleckenstein, 2011). She argued that 'women-friendly' and more 'gender-equal' policy-making would attract those young women voters (Fleckenstein, 2011). In that sense, the CDU has gradually moved away from their strong commitment to familialising childcare policies. This re-orientation raises the question that if the biggest veto player in de-familialising the childcare provisions had begun to change, then why could Germany not achieve a full-fledged de-familialised childcare policy framework? The answer to this question requires a closer look at the power relations within the CDU and its Bavarian partner CSU.

The CDU/CSU is far from being homogeneous. The majority of the CSU and an intra-party group in CDU are still in favour of the traditional gendered division of labour. While analysing the political parties' attitudes towards leave schemes, Leitner (2010) described this group as '*right-wing fundamentalists*', and these are the strongest veto players in the de-familialisation process. Their historical support for family care has been legitimised in their views of child well-being and in arguments about children's education. For them, the best way of raising a child is caring for them at home until their third birthday and then sending them to kindergarten for a half day until they reach school age. They are not totally against kindergarten. For example, while discussing about the characteristics of an ideal mother, a deputy from CSU mentioned the following:

> ... Children are very important for Germany, they are our future, Germany owns everything to education of its children, it is the only reason how we succeed to stay alive after our difficult times in the past... Therefore, our mothers are so important too, because they are the cooks of the meal, yet you cannot imagine a dish without salt and kindergarten is the salt here, you cannot put much but you should not put less either ....

Alongside these right-wing fundamentalists, there are also a group of deputies within the CDU, described as '*true people in the wrong party*' by women's organisations (personal interview). These people are perceived as highly progressive and modern in terms of childcare provisions and they are concerned about increasing childlessness in Germany. Angela Merkel and the former Family and current Defence Minister

Ursula von der Leyen are the most active ones of those '*moderate Realos*' in Leitner's (2010) words. It is important to note here that these two opposing groups are not just two groups within a party with antagonistic opinions, the tension between them is remarkably high, which results in a weaker and controversial de-familialising process. The 2012 Home Care Allowance Law could be seen as an outcome of this tension. The Law was first proposed by a senior deputy from CSU in 2007. However, although the CDU was highly reluctant to pass it, Merkel had to silence the critical voices in the CDU against the law because the CSU was threatening to leave the coalition unless it came into force (Havertz, 2012; Heineman, 2013). The oppositional parties see this controversy within the CDU/CSU as one of the biggest obstacles to childcare reform. A speaker from the SPD when discussing the slowness and contestability of the reforms stated that:

> … any kind of initiative regarding childcare provision expansion proposed by the SPD have been cut by the CDU in the process of negotiation within the coalition. Sometimes I think I'm being unfair when I say the CDU because it's more their sister party CSU but at the end of the day it is the party's responsibility to find a middle way and speak from the same mouth… And so, I think the enemy is within the government ….

In lander, alongside NGOs and various welfare organisations such as the Red Cross and AWO, the Catholic, Lutheran and Protestant Churches are also responsible for the running of kindergarten and kitas. Due to the federal nature of the German state, there are no countrywide standards[6] with significant potential for policy divergence. Evidence from other studies and empirical work by the author indicate that provisions run by Catholic organisations are primarily for children older than age three and operate part time (Andronescu & Carnes, 2015; Meyer, 2005; Theobald, 2005), and are thus a structural constraint on women's employment. Therefore, while these religious organisations believe in the importance of the family and favour increasing the

[6]Although the SPD and die Linke have proposed to change the constitution and centralise the regulations with respect to childcare, this was rejected by the majority of the CDU (personal interview).

fertility rates, the ways in which they try to achieve this are unlikely to be successful.

Overall, despite the highly tangled views of the actors, it is possible to argue that in the current German conjuncture catalysts who are working towards de-familialising German childcare policy consist of: women's organisations, particularly the ones originating from the GDR; trade unions; employers' associations; and 'femocrats' within political parties. It would also be safe to put the political parties holding a more leftist ideology in this group. Yet, it is important to note that, although all these actors belong to the same category, their expectations and gains from increased public childcare provision are slightly different. The femocrats and the leftist deputies as well as the women's organisations are concerned about the tensions between women's career aspirations and fertility behaviour whereas the trade unions and the employers' associations are more focussed on the need to keep highly educated women in the labour market. However, all are in favour of decreasing childlessness through expanding the public childcare services rather than any other forms of pro-natal family policies – whether be it tax deduction or cash benefits. On the other hand, the extreme rightist deputies; the rightist political parties; the religious organisations; some religious civil society organisations; some conservative women's organisations, mainly the ones established in the FRG times; and some traditional local authorities generate the veto player. That they hold more conservative views does not necessarily mean that they ignore childlessness. On the contrary, they are highly worried about increased childlessness but their way of redressing the situation is more familialising. The fact that the power of childcare policy-making in Germany has various stakeholders, as well as their great tangled nature, might explain why two opposing ideologies regarding childcare simultaneously exist in Germany, and why it has a certain impact on policy.

Conclusion

This chapter aimed to understand why, despite the recent policy developments in Germany, the public provision of childcare services remains a contested policy area and may contribute to childlessness remaining high. For analytical considerations, it clustered childcare provisions under two opposing groups: de-familialisation and familialisation, and regarded their co-existence as product of ideology (Pfau-Effinger, 2005).

Policy actors were placed into two opposing groups: catalysts and the veto players, on the basis of first categorisation.

In Germany, familialist childcare policies have long been the dominant social phenomena. There was a lack of political enthusiasm for defamilialising until the mid-2000s even though German lifestyles had already begun to change. The German government, however, in the long run has acknowledged the need for greater childcare policies, which would enable parents, especially mothers, to combine their career aspirations with fertility aspirations without risking the latter. This acknowledgement has not necessarily been followed by a total transformation in policy. Due to the existence of various veto players favouring familial care, de-familialisation of childcare policy process has been diluted by various familialist initiatives especially driven by the conservative voices within the Parliament.

Acknowledgements

The author would like to thank Prof. Ann Marie Gray and Dr. Markus Ketola for their helpful comments and suggestions.

References

Ahn, N., & Mira, P. (2002). A note on the changing relationship between fertility and female employment rates in developed countries. *Journal of Population Economics*, *15*(4), 667–682.

Andronescu, C., & Carnes, M. (2015). Value coalitions and policy change: The impact of gendered patterns of work, religion and partisanship on childcare policy across German states. *Journal of European Social Policy*, *25*(2), 159–174.

Beaujouan, E., Sobotka, T., Brzozowska, Z., & Zeman, K. (2017). Has childlessness peaked in Europe? *Population & Societies*, *540*, 1–4.

Becker, G. S. (1965). A theory of the allocation of time. *The Economic Journal*, *75*(299), 493.

Bundesministerium für Familie, Senioren, Frauen und Jugend (Hrsg) (BMFSFJ). (2012). Familienreport 2012.

Borck, R. (2014). Adieu Rabenmutter—Culture, fertility, female labour supply, the gender wage gap and childcare. *Journal of Population Economics*, *27*(3), 739–765.

Brodmann, S., Esping-Andersen, G., & Guell, M. (2007). When fertility is bargained: Second births in Denmark and Spain. *European Sociological Review*, *23*(5), 599–613.

Börzel, T., & Risse, T. (2002). When Europe hits home: Europeanization and domestic change. *SSRN Electronic Journal*, doi:10.2139/ssrn.302768.

Del Boca, D. (2002). The effect of child care and part time opportunities on participation and fertility decisions in Italy. *Journal of Population Economics*, *15*(3), 549–573.

Erler, D. (2009). Germany: Taking a Nordic turn? In S. Kamerman & P. Moss (Eds.), *The politics of parental leave policies. Children, parenting, gender and the labour market* (pp. 119–134). Bristol: The Policy Press.

Esping-Andersen, G. (1990). *The three worlds of welfare capitalism*. Cambridge, MA: Polity Press.

Esping-Andersen, G. (1999). *Social foundations of postindustrial economies*. Oxford: Oxford University Press.

Esping-Andersen, G. (2009). *The incomplete revolution: Adapting to women's new roles*. Cambridge, MA: Polity Press.

Esping-Andersen, G., Gallie, D., Hemerijk, A., & Myles, J. (2002). *Why we need a welfare state*. Oxford: Oxford University Press.

Ferrarini, T. (2006). *Families, states and labour markets. Institutions, causes and consequences of family policy in post-war welfare states*. Cheltenham: Edward Elgar Publishing.

Ferree, M. (1993). The rise and fall of 'mommy politics': Feminism and unification in (East) Germany. *Feminist Studies*, *19*(1), 89.

Fleckenstein, T. (2011). The politics of ideas in welfare state transformation: Christian democracy and the reform of family policy in Germany. *Social Politics: International Studies in Gender, State & Society*, *18*(4), 543–571.

Fleckenstein, T., & Lee, S. C. (2014). The politics of post-industrial social policy: Family policy reforms in Britain, Germany, South Korea, and Sweden. *Comparative Political Studies*, *47*(4), 601–630.

Grebe, C. (2009). *Reconciliation policy in Germany 1998–2008: Construing the 'problem' of the incompatibility of paid employment and care work*. Wiesbaden: VS Research.

Hakim, C. (2000). *Work-lifestyle choices in the 21st century: Preference theory*. Oxford: Oxford University Press.

Hantrais, L. (2004). *Family policy matters: Responding to family changes in Europe*. Bristol: The Policy Press.

Hara, T. (2008). Increasing childlessness in Germany and Japan: Toward a childless society? *International Journal of Japanese Sociology*, *17*(1), 42–62.

Havertz, R. (2012). Germany debates plan to pay stay-at-home moms. *US News*, August 17. Retrieved from http://www.cnbc.com/id/48699000

Heineman, E. (2013, March 1). *The debate over Betreuungsgeld*. American Institute for German Studies John Hopkins University. Retrieved from http://www.aicgs.org/publication/the-debate-over-betreuungsgeld/

Hemerijck, A. (2013). *Changing welfare states*. Oxford: Oxford University Press.

Heritier, A., Kerwer, D., Knill, C., Lehmkuhl, D., Teutsch, M., & Douillet, A. C. (2001). *Differential Europe. New opportunities and constraints for national policy-making*. Lanham: Rowan and Littlefield.

Krapf, S. (2014). *Public childcare provision and fertility behaviour: A comparison of Sweden and Germany*. Opladen: Budrich UniPress Ltd.

Kreyenfeld, M., & Konietzka, D. (2017). Childlessness in East and West Germany: Long-term trends and social disparities. In M. Kreyenfeld & D. Konietzka (Eds.), *Childlessness in Europe: Contexts, causes, and consequences* (pp. 97–114). Cham: Springer.

Lee, G., & Lee, S. (2014). Childcare availability, fertility and female labor force participation in Japan. *Journal of the Japanese and International Economies, 32*, 71–85.

Leitner, S. (2010). Germany outpaces Austria in childcare policy: The historical contingencies of 'conservative' childcare policy. *Journal of European Social Policy, 20*(5), 456–467.

Lewis, J. (1992). Gender and the development of welfare regimes. *Journal of European Social Policy, 2*(3), 159–173.

Lewis, J. (2009). *Work-family balance, gender and policy*. Cheltenham: Edward Elgar.

Lietzmann, T. (2014). After recent policy reforms in Germany: Probability and determinants of labour market integration of lone mothers and mothers with a partner who receive welfare benefits. *Social Politics: International Studies in Gender, State & Society, 21*(4), 585–616.

Lohmann, H., & Zagel, H. (2016). Family policy in comparative perspective: The concepts and measurement of familization and defamilization. *Journal of European Social Policy, 26*(1), 48–65.

Luci-Greulich, A., & Thevenon, O. (2013). The impact of family policies on fertility trends in developed countries. *European Journal of Population, 29*(4), 387–416.

McDonald, P. (2000). *The 'toolbox' of public policies to impact on fertility – A global view*. Unpublished manuscript. Australian National University.

McDonald, P. (2002). *Low fertility: Unifying the theory and the demography*. Unpublished manuscript. Australian National University.

Meyer, T. (2005). Political actors and the modernization of care politics in Britain and Germany. In B. Pfau-Effinger & B. Geissler (Eds.), *Care and social integration in European societies* (pp. 281–307). Bristol: Policy Press.

Miethe, I. (2008). From "strange sisters" to "Europe's daughters"? European enlargement as a chance for women's movements in East and West Germany. In S. Roth (Eds.), *Gender politics in the expanding European Union mobilization, inclusion, exclusion* (pp. 118–136). New York: Berghahn Books.

O'Connor, J. S. (1993). Gender, class and citizenship in the comparative analysis of welfare state regimes: Theoretical and methodological issues. *British Journal of Sociology, 44*(3), 501–518.

OECD. (2017). Fertility rates (indicator). Retrieved from https://doi.org/10.1787/8272fb01-en. Accessed on March 4, 2017.

Orloff, A. S. (1993). Gender and the social rights of citizenship: The comparative analysis of gender relations and welfare states. *American Sociological Review, 58*(3), 303–328.

Ostner, I. (2010). Farewell to the family as we know it: Family policy change in Germany. *German Policy Studies, 6*(1), 211–244.

Palier, B. (2006). The politics of reforms in Bismarckian welfare systems. *Revue Française des Affaires Sociales, 5*, 47–72.

Pfau-Effinger, B. (2005). Welfare state policies and the development of care arrangements. *European Societies*, *7*(2), 321–347.

Pfau-Effinger, B., & Smidt, M. (2011). Differences in women's employment patterns and family policies: Eastern and Western Germany. *Community, Work & Family*, *14*(2), 217–232.

Radaelli, C. M. (2003). The Europeanization of public policy. In K. Featherstone & C. M. Radaelli (Eds.), *The politics of Europeanization* (pp. 27–56). Oxford: Oxford University Press.

Richter, K., Podhisita, C., Chamratrithirong, A., & Soonthorndhada, K. (1994). The impact of child care on fertility in Urban Thailand. *Demography*, *31*(4), 651.

Roberts, G. K. (2016). *German politics today*. Manchester: Manchester University Press.

Rovny, A. E. (2011). Welfare state policy determinants of fertility level: A comparative analysis. *Journal of European Social Policy*, *21*(4), 335–347.

Ruling, A. (2008). *Re-framing of childcare in Germany and England*. Working Paper. Retrieved from http://www.agf.org.uk/cms/upload/pdfs/WP/200810_WPcsge_e_re-framing_of_childcare.pdf. Accessed in March and April 2017.

Saraceno, C., & Keck, W. (2010). Can we identify intergenerational policy regimes in Europe? *European Societies*, *12*(5), 675–696.

Schmidt, V. A. (2011). Speaking of change: Why discourse is key to the dynamics of policy transformation. *Critical Policy Studies*, *5*(2), 106–126.

Schober, P. S., & Spiess, C. K. (2015). Local daycare quality and maternal employment: Evidence from East and West Germany. *Journal of Marriage and Family*, *77*(3), 712–729.

Sobotka, T., Zeman, K., Lesthaeghe, R., Frejka, T., & Neels, K. (2011). Postponement and recuperation in cohort fertility. *Comparative Population Studies*, *36*(2–3), 417–452.

Stobel-Richter, Y., Beutel, M. E., Finck, C., & Prahler, E. (2005). The 'wish to have a child', childlessness and infertility in Germany. *Human Reproduction*, *20*(10), 2850–2857.

Theobald, H. (2005). The formalisation of care work and labour market. In B. Pfau-Effinger & B. Geissler (Eds.), *Care and social integration in European societies* (pp. 195–215). Bristol: Policy Press.

Trzcinski, E., & Camp, J. K. (2014). Family policy in Germany. In M. Robilla (Eds.), *Handbook of family policies across the globe* (pp. 137–153). New York, NY: Springer.

Tsebelis, G. (2002). *Veto players: How political institutions work*. Princeton, NJ: Princeton University Press.

Woodward, A. (2004). Building velvet triangles: Gender and informal governance. In T. Christiansen & S. Piattoni (Eds.), *Informal governance in the European Union* (pp. 76–93). Cheltenham: Edward Elgar Publishing.

Postscript: Moving Forward Towards a Feminist Understanding of 'Otherhood'

Natalie Sappleton

Reflection on the Volume

Childlessness, its drivers, manifestations and implications, is a hot topic, and researchers in the Global North and South, in Higher Education, think tanks and policy institutes, and in a broad range of disciplines, are now studying it. Yet, in spite of this interest, published research has been relatively unconcerned with the insight that feminist analysis can supply. To some extent, this is perhaps unsurprising, for feminists hold diverse views about how to achieve gender equality, the types of research questions that should be posed and addressed, how knowledge should be produced and the methodological approach(es) that should be used to produce it (Humm, 2014; Lykke, 2010). The failure of feminists to agree on such points often acts as a deterrent to solidly feminist analysis. In spite of the heterogeneity of approaches, a common thread is that 'feminist scholarship begins by asking questions informed by women's exclusion in the world and from the standpoint of a personal life that has yet to be taken seriously by others' (Taylor, 1998, p. 358). It is in this spirit that we, researchers from disciplines as diverse as philosophy, psychology and public health, have brought together this anthology. As well as highlighting original and novel research into childlessness, this collection should be considered as a general criticism of the dominance and normalisation of the motherhood narrative across the disciplines in which we work, with childless individuals still, in spite of their burgeoning numbers, living lives that are 'yet to be taken seriously by others'. The fundamental ambition of feminist science and scholarship is to challenge exclusion and inequalities, and to empower the marginalised, and each of the essays in this volume make a contribution to those objectives. We hope, therefore, that this volume gives visibility to the transdisciplinary, multimethodological, contextual and politically relevant nature of research on childlessness, united around a feminist methodology.

At the same time, the collection is by no means intended to be an exhaustive reflection of the excellent work that is being carried out in this area, and so we end this volume by considering the gaps that still exist in our knowledge and by setting out a promising research agenda for the future. This anthology has revealed and inspired abundant opportunities for future research which could help to progress knowledge and understanding of childlessness. Specifically, future research directions fall in five dimensions, in line with some of the key ambitions of feminist scientific research.

Five Dimensions for Future Research

Social Locations and Inequalities

The central premise of feminist scholarship is that research efforts should be directed towards understanding and addressing the myriad sources of social inequalities in general, and of gender inequality in particular, with a view to transforming the underlying structures that produce oppression and inequality (Robinson, 2000). Since motherhood is seen as innate to womanhood, it is perhaps unsurprising that studies of childlessness have placed gender inequalities at their heart, by focusing, for example, on the contribution that motherhood and otherhood make to social and economic inequalities. The essays in this volume have demonstrated that in the modern pronatalist society, by occupying the position of 'other', non-mothers experience social stigma, severed social networks and challenges to their essence of womanhood. However, there are several other areas of social inequalities in which the impact of childlessness can be explored, drawing on a feminist lens. The literature on gender and occupations would benefit from research that exposes whether childlessness is a contributing factor in a host of occupational and economic outcomes such as occupational segregation, pay gaps and progression gaps. For instance, there are few feminist studies of the sociological aspects of workplace outcomes that pay attention to the role that parental status and gender play in relation to the meanings that childlessness has for those that experience it, as well as for their colleagues and peers.

Similarly, more research is needed that acknowledges the fluidity of social locations and the way in which this translates into both marginalisation and privilege. For instance, Anna Gotlib (Chapter 3, this volume) points out that 'the process of choosing my choices does not exist in a vacuum'. However, the majority of research on childlessness has failed to fully address the social embeddedness of childlessness by exploring the perspective of those with whom the childfree interact, and who may contribute to the pronatalist ideology. The theoretical offerings of Bourdieusian ideals of social capital have left its legacy upon feminism (O'Neill & Gidengil, 2013). Much existing research on voluntary childlessness attributes to the childless state a solidity and immutability that privileges the sphere of individual agency and overlooks the pre-structured contexts in which actors operate. Feminists have long called for a poststructuralist or pluralist discussion of individual experience which acknowledges the role that actors play in determining the structures of constraint and dependence in which they operate. There is a need for research on childlessness that is conducted in that spirit, which recognises the fluidity of social identities, and acknowledges the interplay of structure and agency.

Unsilencing and Unmasking the Invisible

Across disciplines, feminists are united in their call for topics and issues of interest to be reanalysed and reconceptualised in light of women's everyday experiences of gender oppression (Hesse-Biber, 2011). Through this activity, it is hoped that our 'collective delusions can be undone' (Millman & Kanter, 1975, p. vii). A central objective of empirical feminist scholarship is the valuing, validation and vocalisation of the lived experiences of those that have been marginalised or overlooked in mainstream research.

It is almost an accepted wisdom that childless or childfree women (but not men), experience social stigma as a consequence of being cast as deviant. In introducing her study on stigma management, Park (2002, p. 21), for instance, writes that the childfree 'are faced with the ongoing tasks of accepting [their stigmatized identity] themselves and negotiating it in interactions with others who may view their character and behavior as incomprehensible, strange, or immoral'. Yet, the research focus on stigma, stigma management and coping is predicated on a priori assumption of stigma towards childless women. Research undertaken along these lines adheres to a deductivist-empiricist theory of knowledge, whereby general axioms are assumed to be true in view of their self-evidence, and thus used to support empirical justification. Feminists, however, reject this approach, taking axioms instead to be problematics rather than truisms; research questions rather than hypotheses. This leads us to find, for instance, that some women are privileged as a consequence of their childfree state (Sappleton, Chapter 14, this volume), and that many women do not engage with the concept of coping at all (Mullins, Chapter 6, this volume).

In her critical feminist disquisition on American families, Coontz (2016) is clear that the nostalgic myth of nuclear family that is inscribed and embedded in popular culture and the popular imagination is not congruent with the lived experience of most people. Indeed, we already know that childlessness is a growing trend, both in the Global North and the Global South. Yet, interestingly, studies of childlessness themselves start from the assumption of the conventional family form. There are few studies that take childlessness as the *context* of social lives, rather than an *outcome* that is so unusual as to warrant investigation. We hope that this collection inspires research that gives visibility to childless families as they become normalised in society.

Reflexivity and Participatory Methods

Positivist science proceeds from the assumption that reality independent from the knower, such that an objectivist ontology is demanded. Feminist scholarship contests that basic assumption, calling instead for a reflexive approach to inquiry, in which the researchers' own assumptions, social location and background play a pivotal role in the production and interpretation of knowledge (England, 1994). The emphasis on a reflexive ontology stems largely from the belief that methodologies are shaped by those that deploy them. However, it is also a contention that where the researcher is also an 'insider' at the site of knowledge production, their marginal status sensitises them to the perspective of those being researched, so that the arguments made always take into account one's own personal experiences (Krieger, 1991, Furthermore, feminists view 'listening to the experiences of "the other/s" as legitimate knowledge' (Hesse-Biber, 2011, p. 4). Explicitly reflexive accounts of childlessness, however, are rare, and those employing participatory methods of data gathering rarer still. Chapters presented herein (e.g. Carroll, Chapter 9; Gotlib, Chapter 3) buck that trend, but further work is needed that adopts this methodological approach.

Intersectionality

It has been the tendency of many feminist researchers to generalise women's social situations, either deliberately or unintentionally overlooking differences such as ethnicity and race, cultural and national context and social class. More intracategorical research is needed on the intersections *between* achieved and ascribed characteristics that 'uncover [s] the differences and complexities of experience' of individuals at the intersection of several categories (McCall, 2005, p. 1782). In their study on the decision-making pathways of childless women, for instance, Settle and Brumley (2014, p. 2) remark that

> most research has focused on childfree women who are white, married, college educated, and upper-middle class, with little religious affiliation, and who hold nontraditional gender beliefs .... Few studies explore the experiences of women of color, unmarried women, or lower-income women.

Wood and Newton's (2006) work on female managers, for instance, included a sample of 156 women, of whom only one was of non-Anglo Saxon descent, and heterosexuality was implied.

Yet pronatalist ideologies impact different groups of women in different ways. The notion of the 'ideal mother' applies to white, middle class, heterosexual women, while societies tend to have very different expectations of motherhood for other groups of women. For instance, Mezey's (2013) ethnographic study reports that lesbians are rarely expected to become mothers, and those that do experience prejudice predicated on heteronormative viewpoints. Sexual orientation and sexuality may have implications for parental status as well as for occupational 'choices' and stereotypes yet aside from Wright's (2016) work, this specific intersection has not been addressed in the literature on childlessness, management and occupations. We also know of no studies that have explored the othering choices of disabled women, for instance, although researchers on motherhood have begun to adopt intersectional methods (e.g. Frederick, 2017).

In her call for intersectional approaches, Davis (2013, online) has argued that:

> Feminism involves so much more than gender equality and it involves so much more than gender. Feminism must involve consciousness of capitalism (I mean the feminism that I relate to, and there are multiple feminisms, right). So it has to involve a consciousness of capitalism and

> racism and colonialism and post-colonialities, and ability and more genders than we can even imagine and more sexualities than we ever thought we could name.

It should therefore be expected that childless women experience childlessness differently contingent on their socio-economic class, ethnicity and sexuality, as well as on the context in which these intersectional identities are played out, and we call for more research adopting this approach.

Individualised Experiences and Contextualised Knowledge

As Tanaka and Lowry (Chapter 14, this volume) have demonstrated, lived experiences are constructed both by and within social contexts, as well as spatial, temporal and geopolitical power structures and power relations. Thus it is crucial to understand how 'experience is discursively constructed by dominant ideological structures' (Hesse-Biber, 2011, p. 9). At the same time, we need to value and understand individual's unique experiences. The ascription of gender is something which is shared by all in society, but as Anne Jorunn-Berg has lamented (in Lohan, 2000, p. 896), gender 'sticks more easily to women'. Thus, men are elevated to the position of 'ungendered representatives of humanity'; a status that carries with it the assumption that they are able construct their own identities, while those that sit outside traditional gender binaries are often overlooked completely. The feminist project is about eliminating patriarchal society, which assumes that there is only one (white, middle class, heterosexual) form of patriarchy. Feminists thus call for the deconstruction of hegemonic masculinity – an activity which recognises that there are many *genders*, with each regarded as hegemonic in their own context.

Raising and rearing children can be viewed through the lenses of biological sex, social gender and sexuality; three strands of human life that are 'simultaneously distinct, interrelated, and somewhat fuzzy around the boundaries' (Jordan-Young, 2010, p. 16). The relationship between individual interpretations of one's own physical body, sexuality and the societal norms to which we are exposed are key to understanding individual experiences of gender. Thus, there is a need for research on childlessness that is both *context driven* and *gender-aware*, investigating the experiences of *individuals* embedded in patriarchal societal contexts.

References

Coontz, S. (2016). *The way we never were: American families and the nostalgia trap.* Hachette, UK.

Davis, A. (2013). *Feminism and abolition: Theories and practices for the 21st century.* Speech given at the University of Chicago, May. Retrieved from https://beyond-capitalismnow.wordpress.com/2013/08/08/angela-y-davis-feminism-and-abolition-theories-and-practices-for-the-21st-century. Accessed on 17 February 2018.

England, K. V. (1994). Getting personal: Reflexivity, positionality, and feminist research. *The Professional Geographer*, *46*(1), 80–89.

Frederick, A. (2017). Visibility, respectability, and disengagement: The everyday resistance of mothers with disabilities. *Social Science & Medicine*, *181*, 131–138.

Hesse-Biber, S. N. (Ed.). (2011). *Handbook of feminist research: Theory and praxis.* London: Sage publications.

Humm, M. (2014). *Feminisms: A reader*. London: Routledge.

Jordan-Young, R. (2010). *Brainstorm: The flaws in the science of sex differences.* Cambridge, MA: Harvard University Press.

Krieger, S. (1991). *Social science and the self: Personal essays on an art form.* New Brunswick, NJ: Rutgers University Press.

Lohan, M. (2000). Extending feminist methodologies: Researching masculinities and technologies. In A. Byrne and R. Lentin (Eds.), *(Re) searching women: Feminist research methodologies in the social sciences in Ireland.* Dublin: IPA.

Lykke, N. (2010). *Feminist studies: A guide to intersectional theory, methodology and writing*. New York, NY: Routledge.

McCall, L. (2005). The complexity of intersectionality. *Signs: Journal of Women in Culture and Society*, *30*(3), 1771–1800.

Mezey, N. J. (2013). How lesbians and gay men decide to become parents or remain childfree. In A. E. Goldberg & K. R. Allen (Eds.), *LGBT-parent families: Innovations in research and implications for practice*. New York, NY: Springer.

Millman, M., & Kanter, R. M. (1975). *Another voice: Feminist perspectives on social life and social science*. New York: Anchor Books.

O'Neill, B., & Gidengil, E. (Eds.). (2013). *Gender and social capital.* London: Routledge.

Park, K. (2002). Stigma management among the voluntarily childless. *Sociological Perspectives*, *45*(1), 21–45.

Robinson, J. (2000). Feminism and the spaces of transformation. *Transactions of the Institute of British Geographers*, *25*(3), 285–301.

Settle, B., & Brumley, K. (2014). 'It's the choices you make that get you there': Decision-making pathways of childfree women. *Michigan Family Review*, *18*(1), 1–22.

Taylor, V. (1998). Feminist methodology in social movements research. *Qualitative Sociology*, *21*(4), 357–379.

Wood, G. J., & Newton, J. (2006). Childlessness and women managers: 'Choice', context and discourses. *Gender, Work & Organization*, *13*(4), 338–358.

Wright, T. (2016). *Gender and sexuality in male-dominated occupations.* London: Palgrave Macmillan.

Index